Dying into Grace

✿

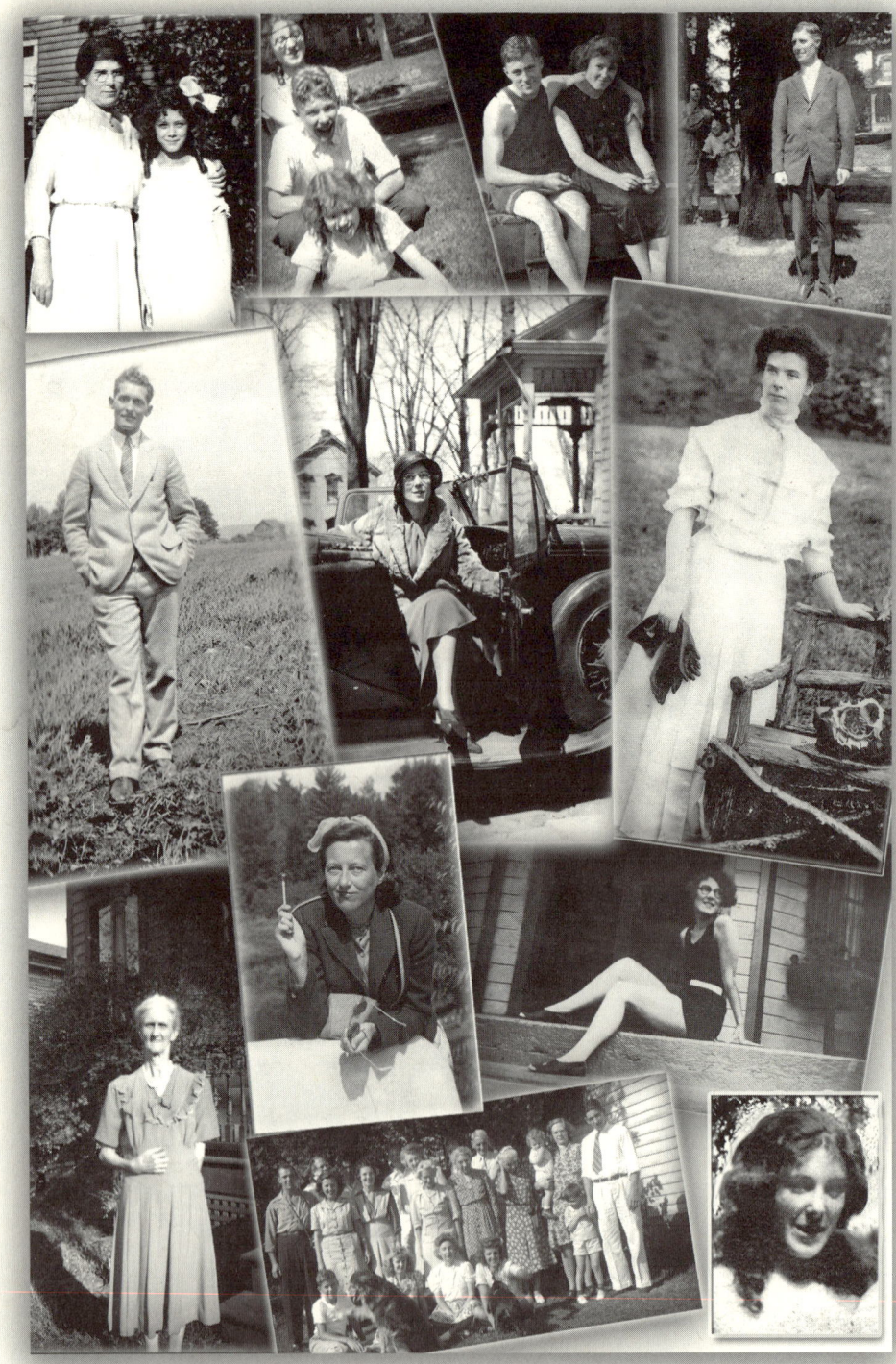

Dying into Grace

Mother and Daughter... a Dance of Healing

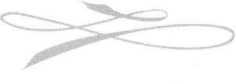

by
Artemis March, PhD

QUANTUM LENS PRESS
CAMBRIDGE, MASSACHUSETTS

Grateful acknowledgment is made to the following for permission
to reprint material copyrighted or controlled by them:
Quotation from the motion picture "The Hours" courtesy of Paramount Pictures Corporation. Quotation from THE PROPHET by Kahlil Gibran, copyright 1923 by Kahlil Gibran and renewed 1951 by Administrators C.T.A. of Kahlil Gibran Estate and Mary G. Gibran. Used by permission of Alfred A. Knopf, a division of Random House, Inc.

Copyright © 2007 by Artemis March, PhD. All rights reserved, including the right of reproduction in whole or in part in any form. With the exception of "fair use" by other authors and reviewers, no part of this publication may be reproduced, stored in a retrieval system, transmitted, or previewed in any form or by any means, electronic, mechanical, photocopying, recording, or otherwise without written permission from the author.

Ordering information: www.dyingintograce.com, or Quantum Lens Press, PO Box 391317, Cambridge, MA 02139. Discounts are available when purchased in bulk for premiums and sales promotions as well as for educational and fundraising use. Special editions, book excerpts, and case studies can also be created to specification.

cover design: Maureen Roche
front cover photo: Mary Wirth
interior design, typesetting, and book production: Arrow Graphics, Inc.
info@arrow1.com
Printed in the United States of America

Library of Congress Control Number: 2007923340
ISBN: 978-0-9793967-9-3

This book is printed on acid-free paper and meets the minimum requirements of the American National Standard for Information Sciences—Permanance of Paper for Printed Library Materials, ANSI Z39.48-1992

This book is intended to help you through a daunting life passage, but it cannot guarantee desired outcomes for the dying person or the caregiving survivor(s). The author and publisher disclaim all responsibility and any liability for how its advice is interpreted or applied. The author and publisher are not engaged in rendering medical, psychological, or other professional services.

To protect people's privacy, many names have been changed—not only of persons, but also of towns, streets, street numbers, and names of buildings. What has not been changed is the story. The events, experiences, interactions, and scenes depicted here happened as described, including our encounters with healthcare facilities and representatives of the healthcare system. This book should not be read as a critique of specific healthcare providers or facilities, but of the paradigms and systems through which healthcare professionals are trained, and of how health care and end-of-life care are organized, delivered, and funded in the United States.

To Olwen,

for gracing herself and me with her final and eternal gifts;

to those who supported us and helped make it possible;

to those who, in their dying, recover the self they lost in life;

and to all those who give the precious gift of midwifing and witnessing the final journey.

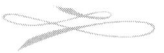

Contents

**Introduction: Why I was Compelled to Write this Book,
and What it Offers You** 1

> *... there is only one person whom one needs for dying.
> To have such a person is a great good fortune. To be that
> person, to have been such a person, is a heavy and blessed
> experience ... Once at least, in each lifetime, we are meant
> to be a blessing to each other.* —Gerda Lerner

Part I. Where are We? 15

> *From out of that primal chaos something true
> can self-organize.* —John Briggs and F. David Peat

Chapter 1. Is this The Call? 17

> *I am always waiting for The Call,
> and always dreading it.* —Artemis, April 28

**Chapter 2. Will Her Body Outlive Her Mind?
Hospitalizations and their Consequences** 29

> *I never thought I would outlive
> anything like this.* —Olwen, May 6

**Chapter 3. Mobilizing to Beat the Odds
and Get Mother Home** 51

> *I want to go back to my apartment
> and live there for a short time.* —Olwen, May 9

**Chapter 4. Detour through Rehab: Buying Time
and/or Losing Ground?** 65

> *I am going to 102!!* —Olwen, May 12

**Chapter 5. Getting Mother Home—
But Can We Keep Her There?** 81

> *We'll know in a week or so.* —Kate, May 20

Part II. Creating Space for the Dance to Unfold ... 93

> *It's come to the point where it's long enough.
> We know it can't get great again.* —Olwen, May 26

Chapter 6. Hospice: Shifting the Paradigm 95

> *You can't do this, dear. It's too much.
> It's too hard.* —Olwen, June 3

Chapter 7. Building Our own Family of Caregivers and Our Private World 111

> We live in a world that is terrified by death and hides its dying. We know the vacuum that forms around the dying. —Marie de Hennezel

Part III. Rhythms of the Dance 125

> Always the years between us, always the years. Always the love. Always the hours. —"Virginia Woolf" in "The Hours"

Chapter 8. Peaks and Valleys:
When a Heart can no longer do its Work 127

> You die in episodes. Dying is an irregular process full of mountains and valleys. It chews away at your life while consuming hers. —a friend, June 15

Chapter 9. How do You Let Go of Your Life? 143

> I don't know what I'm doing, and I don't know if I'll ever finish it ... It's the last thing I am doing, and I can't do it ... I want to let go. I'm trying to let go. —Olwen, June 25

Chapter 10. My Life or Hers?
the Dream versus the Nightmare 163

> You do what you have to do, and I'll do what I have to do. —Olwen, June 26

Chapter 11. Weaving a Path Through the Shadows 183

> I've lived a good life really, but I know I worked at it. I had to do a lot of things, and I was able to do them. —Olwen, October 2001

Chapter 12. Retrieving the Understory 201

> When I go way back, I'm glad sometimes I didn't know— not the answer, but what did it mean? —Olwen, June 13

Chapter 13. The Dance of Grace 215

> Only when you drink from the river of silence shall you indeed sing ... And when the earth shall claim your limbs, then shall you truly dance. —Kahlil Gibran

Part IV. Dancing with the Ancestors 233

> If you know who you are and you know where you've come from, then you'll know what you must do. —Ancient Celtic Proverb

Chapter 14. Unexpected Gifts 235
> *Through mourning we let the dead go
> and take them in.* —Judith Viorst

Chapter 15. The Houses Speak 249
> *To be rooted is perhaps the most important and least
> recognized need of the human soul.* —Simone Weil

Chapter 16. Roots and Completion 265
> *The longing to tell one's story and the process of telling is
> symbolically a gesture of longing to recover the past in such a
> way that one experiences both a sense of reunion and a sense
> of release.* —bell hooks

Part V. Giving Cultural Form and Visibility to the Dance 279
> *Wisdom, then, is born of the overlapping of lives,
> the resonance between stories.* —Mary Catherine Bateson

Chapter 17. The Caregiver's Story 281
> *Family caregivers are the backbone of the long-term care
> system, they are not doing well, and current public policy
> does little to support them.* —Susan Reinhard

**Chapter 18. The Dance of Death:
What do we need to Know and Do?** 299
> *[H]ealing and wholeness are always possible . . . Even as
> people confront death, . . . they can reach out to express love,
> gratitude, and forgiveness. When they do, they consistently
> find that they, and everyone involved, are transformed—
> for the rest of their lives, whether those lives last for
> decades or just days.* —Ira Byock

Chapter 19. Dancing the Dance of Death 313
> *. . . [W]ith the help of another presence that allows despair
> and pain to declare themselves, the dying seize hold of their
> lives, take possession of them, unlock their truth. They dis-
> cover the freedom of being true to themselves. It is as if, at the
> very culmination, everything managed to come free of the
> jumble of inner pains and illusions that prevent us from
> belonging to ourselves.* —François Mitterand

Epigraphs 328
Notes 331
Further Reading 335
Acknowledgments 339
About the Author 345
Reader Commentary 346

Introduction:

Why I Was Compelled to Write This Book and What It Offers You

> *There are all kinds of ties in one's life, all kinds of friendship, loves, complexities, but there is only one person whom one needs for dying. To have such a person is a great good fortune. To be that person, to have been such a person, is a heavy and blessed experience . . . Once at least, in each lifetime, we are meant to be a blessing to each other.*
> —Gerda Lerner

I had no choice but to write this book. What compelled its creation was the most extraordinary, grueling, exhausting, surprising, disruptive, rewarding, and transformative experience of my life: midwifing my mother's death.

The idea that I, who live four hours away, would ever move in and become her primary caregiver was about the last thing I could have imagined in my "normal" life, and no one could have predicted where her/our journey would take us. That journey uprooted my life and threatened my dreams while Olwen struggled with why, in her view, it was taking so long to die, once she—a pragmatic doer who did not know the meaning of procrastination—had decided it was time. Our dance was imprinted with stunning surprises and deep connections, yet it also exacted terrible demands to surrender what each of us held most dear: "How do I let go of my life?"

Ultimately, my mother and I transcended ancient patterns, kept her out of her nursing home nightmare, and healed our wounds and losses, the deepest of which long predated my birth. Shedding her inessentials, Olwen came home to herself, took immense risks, and broke through a lifetime of cautiousness. She was able to complete her relational and spiritual work with me and for herself in a profound and joyous way that was permanently transformative for each of us. Our intimate Dance of Death led to the hard-won and unexpected gift of mutual healing.

Olwen's death and dying were continuous and discontinuous with who she was in life. She looked life and death in the face, never backing away from hard things. A self-starter sustained by durable energy, she had a robust constitution, bones and joints which never broke or ached, and tremendous strength of will. She was the most resilient person I have ever known. Following life-shattering losses, she rebirthed herself three times, weaving a rich life as an independent woman in the prefeminist, prepsychological era. She was sustained by the steel in her backbone, her capacity for friendship, and in-the-bones knowledge that every relationship is part of a larger fabric. Olwen was the quintessential Weaver who understood that when the fabric of connection tears, you mend it, reweaving the fabric as best you can around the holes and absences. A life is as strong as the fabric it weaves, and hers was strong indeed. At ninety-eight, however, she had outlived all her lifelong friends, most of her small family, and most of her networks.

Olwen's willpower, resilience, backbone, and the life she had woven were integral to how she dealt with her last years of subtle decline and her months of dying. Yet, in other respects, her dying was also discontinuous with the path she had been on since before I, her only child, was born to her late in her childbearing years.

Getting on with her life meant closing off the back rooms of her mind and living life in the front room. A friend recalls meeting my mother when Olwen was in her mid-eighties: "I met her once at the Cape and remember her vividly. She was nice—and she was precisely carved out of rock. A definite presence, formidable, not animated. I liked her." It was the closed rooms, the shadows, and the silences that I absorbed in my bones, that shaped so much of my life and our relationship. They were the underside of her survival and triumph over loss.

In those final weeks, however, everything shifted. The rooms that had been closed now opened and the real Olwen shone through more brilliantly than ever. She found again her whole self whom she had locked away before I was born.

I was to discover her letting go were inseparable from my own. While it had seemed her dying was about *her* letting go of *her* life, it was *I* who also had to let go by truly surrendering to the process in order for her life journey to complete itself in a mutually transformative way.

"Transformation" has been overused for trivial purposes, but I must claim it as the only word that properly names the outcome of our journey. Transformation is altogether different from incremental change along a continuous path—a concept modeled after billiard ball trajectories. Transformation is a living process that represents discontinuity with the past, a catapulting into an After which feels altogether different than the Before—so different you can't get yourself back to that old place.

Whereas "change" happens over time, transformation happens in a moment, after which life is never the same going forward, and our relationship to the past is forever altered. We see everything from a larger vantage point and through a new lens. Yet transformative moments are intimately bound to the past, for they do not emerge from fallow ground. Like the order that self-structures from a rich chaos, or the birthing that emerges from months of gestation in the dark, transformation has a mysterious quality, arising as if from "nowhere."

I now look back at all the struggles, complexity, and ambivalence of the Before, and the fundamental fact that Olwen and I never gave up on each other as being the rich ground from which our After sprang. What if we had never gotten there? Having gone through this enduringly transformative process, it is unthinkable that we might have missed it. I discovered that:

> **Dying can be the most powerful and transformative experience in life, not only for the dying, but also for those of us who enter deeply into their process.**
>
> **Yet most of us cheat ourselves and the dying.**
>
> **We *can* do something about that. We aren't in control, but we aren't powerless. We *can* empower ourselves to dance with our beloved dying.**

You will find in our caregiving/dying story a new, relational paradigm—represented as a dance between the dying partner and her caregiving partner—for enhancing the probabilities that the dying process will open to *mutual* growth and healing. ("Healing" means movement toward greater wholeness, through which old wounds and losses become extinct.) While the focal pair in my exposition of the dance is intergenerational, especially mother and daughter, it can be applied to any significant relationship in which one person—or animal companion—is dying.

My dance with Olwen was based on intuition and attunement, grounded through a lifetime's experience of who she was and what was important to her. I had read nothing about "dying well" or its deeper dimensions. As I was finalizing this book, I began to read books by professionals experienced in end-of-life care to help locate our story while clarifying its distinctiveness. Yes, it does happen that dying people become their whole and essential self. Yes, learning and growth do happen near the end of life. Yes, the dying do come to grace. And, most intriguing of all, the amazing things that sometimes happen between the dying and loved ones can be permanently transformative for both.

But, none of these things happen routinely. Indeed, their relative scarcity appears to have been the motivating impetus behind several books. The physical and medical foundations for supporting these emotional-spiritual openings are not even in place: people die badly, whether in pain, alone, abandoned, without witness, without presence, subjected to unwanted treatments and interventions, in alien environments, or at the least, without having made the best use of their precious time with loved ones.

And, these mysterious discontinuities near the end of life are not solo events. They arise in a context of presence and witnessing, and in relationship informed by authentic engagement. This truth is implicit in accounts illustrating what is possible emotionally, relationally, and spiritually at the end of life. The well-timed question, the consistent presence of compassionate witnessing, the ability to listen through symbolic language and engage with what the dying are really saying—all bespeak relational processes that triggered, enabled, or enhanced the more profound dimensions of "dying well."

But, the chroniclers and advocates for realizing full end-of-life potential lack a relational framework for presenting their experiences and observations. Informed by standard personal and transpersonal psychologies, expansion of the dying self is presented as a solo process, even when supported to varying degrees by the living.

The Dance of Death, by contrast, shifts primacy to *movement in and through relationship.* Movement is fostered by the empathic attunement of the caregiving partner who is herself learning and growing while creating a safe, responsive space in which her beloved dying is more likely to open and grow. The Dance of Death is about each dance partner's opening more fully to themselves and each other, and, through their mutually responsive process, helping to heal both the self and the other.

We, as family caregivers—past, present, or future—who will ourselves be dying one day, can stop cheating ourselves and our elders, and enhance the possibilities for jointly experiencing growth, healing, and even transformation by doing three things:

- Reframing and living the dying process as a dance full of growth opportunities for everyone;

- Empowering ourselves to dance as well as possible, even if it is our first time up close and personal with dying;

- Becoming a political force that demands end-of-life environments, care, practices, policies, and programs that support rather than violate the dying and their family caregivers.

These three things are linked: When we understand in our bones what is possible in and through a dying process and that we can make a difference in whether and how those possibilities are realized, we are motivated to build the social-political-medical foundation that enables their realization to become typical rather than exceptional.

Dying into Grace weaves all the dimensions of dying—physical, medical, emotional, relational, spiritual—into a seamless dance, and answers the question, "How do we enhance the possibilities for mutual growth and healing at the end of our parent's life?" The story illuminates our dance, while guiding principles drawn from it make the process more explicit, and show us how to dance.

These principles are not intended to add more layers to the burden of caregiving, or ratchet up the standard so we feel we have never done enough—as has happened with parents who turn themselves into pretzels around their kids. Rather, they are directed to our internally reconfiguring our intention and our priorities—and, when necessary, jolting our mental and emotional default settings—so that the urgent does not crowd out the important. These guiding principles are not about spending *more* time and energy, but paying attention to what we are doing with the time and energy available to us, so that we are doing what truly matters.

As my mother and I were living our story, however, we had no idea how things would turn out. How would the last phases of her life unfold? Over what period of time? Would it be possible not only to get her home again, but also to keep her there? Could I find the right help and would it be enough? Would we run out of money before she ran out of life? Might suddenly escalating care needs use up her money, forcing her out of her lovely apartment and onto Medicaid at some dreadful, fragile moment? Would I use up my small savings intended to launch my "real work" around which my own identity and life are formed? Would I, as I desperately hoped, be with her at the end, or would I have chosen the "wrong time" to go home?

Orienting Caregivers. The on-going trepidation kindled by these unknowns, the emotional roller coaster and totality of exhaustion endemic to caring for our beloved dying, and the necessity of riding multiple learning curves initially inspired me to think about writing a book to provide orientation for those who undertake to live it. As I became consumed by the process of caring for my mother, I was learning on the job in the moment with virtually no guidance. Like most of us thrust into this situation, I had no prior experience for the most important job of my life, and I had read but one book. Trying to get it right the first time with no rehearsals, no retakes, and a level of sleep deprivation that was previously unimaginable led me to realize I was accumulating knowledge and wisdom that was wasted if it never went beyond me.

All around me, friends and acquaintances are going through some stage of this process with one or both parents, or have just been through it, or are holding their breath about what the future will bring. There are millions of us in our forties, fifties, and sixties who are facing the end of our parents' lives, and I daresay, have little preparation, foreknowledge, or grasp of what may lie ahead. Although the unique journey we each undertake with a dying parent is fraught with uncertainty and replete with surprises, there are markers that can keep us better oriented, and learning that can be pulled out of the journeys of those who have gone before us.

I felt a growing urge to share what I was learning in this process with people who may become, or are right now, or have been the primary caregiver for a declining/dying parent or elder. I did not want to write *about* the process after the fact from an expert point of view or cull and arrange material for topical consultation, but to capture the process itself.

What is it like to careen in and out of multiple mind-sets while experiencing a kaleidoscope of emotions telescoping in on each other? How do you cope with all the facets and levels of a mother's dying yet stop on a dime to be emotionally present to profound moments which often come out of "nowhere" and catch you by surprise? I wanted to get hold of the dying/caregiving/healing process I call the Dance of Death from the inside and in real time when you don't know how anything will turn out and are drowning in unbearable uncertainties. I wanted to tell a story that is at once my mother's story, my caregiving story, and the last phases of our journey together, yet simultaneously serves as a teaching/learning vehicle.

Only a narrative told in the first person and the unfolding present tense could weave together these stories and themes, and my expanding intentions. Because more and more of my professional work is directed toward improving the quality, safety, and patient-centeredness of healthcare delivery systems, what I chose to include in my narrative silently speaks from familiarity with the fragmented structure and misaligned incentives of our badly designed healthcare system. Particular encounters with that system are integral to our story and illustrate the devastating human consequences of that system even when that system is not operating at its worst, but "merely" in its routinely mediocre ways.

Validating and Witnessing Caregivers. While my initial intent was to help orient caregivers, it expanded to validating that experience, whether past, present or future. To the extent that this book can bear witness to your experience, it will also have done its job.

If you have already been through the caregiving process, your experience may or may not have received validation from people around you, but certainly it is not recognized by our society. Most of us are lucky to get a day off from work for the funeral. Those who quit their jobs, draw down their savings, and put the rest of their life on hold to undertake this journey may jeopardize their own financial viability, job and/or career, other relationships, and even their own health. For most of us, neither caregiving nor grieving warrant a leave of absence, let alone with pay. No communal structures recognize, honor, and support the full, healthy cycle of grief and reconstruction of identity and meaning. By contrast, indigenous peoples accumulate enormous experience with the dying and the dead, create community structures and rituals that witness, hold, and support the processes of dying, caregiving, and grieving, and integrate the living, the dead, the unborn, and the ancestors into a single socio-cosmic fabric.

Despite social invisibility and lack of cultural valuation, family caregivers themselves instinctively recognize their value. Andrea Sankar, a medical anthropologist and gerontologist, has found that::

> Those family and friends who care for the dying experience their efforts as one of, if not *the,* most important accomplishment of their lives—their "finest hour" . . . People end their care of the dying frequently judging it to have been the "best and worst time" of their lives, and yet they have no one with whom to share it.[1]

Having long valued myself by the originality of my "real work," it was a surprise when I felt as Sankar's interviewees did.

In telling our story, part of my intention is to value and validate all those who take this journey with their beloved dying. Knowing how pushed and pulled caregivers are in daunting territory which healthcare professionals claim as their province, I have also extracted a model of the inherent structure obscured by the chaos of our unique situations ("The Caregiver's Story" in Chapter 17). This model is situated in the present moment from the perspective of the caregiver who is in the thick of things, composing a duet with her dying parent. It is intended as an orienting device for those going through it and validation for those who have completed such a journey. Its purpose is to give visibility, shape, and dignity to caregiving, and make it seem a little less overwhelming because you can see your situation as a whole from the outside, even while you are going through it.

Counteracting Death-Denying Culture. By illuminating what is possible, this book also aims to counteract the consequences of our death-denying culture. It empowers caregivers and their elders by illustrating and explaining ways of navigating and dancing which may help give both partners greater closure and peace of mind than they ever imagined possible. If you can draw from my experiences so as to enhance the dying process in which you are a partner and reduce your potential regrets, this book will have also served its purpose.

Because cultural and medical phobia about death keeps us away from dying, most of us don't accumulate first-hand experience to draw on when we become decision-makers for someone close to us. We have to rely on others to fill us in. Too few of us get honest, reliable information about the dying and the death process even if we ask for it, and most of us don't have independent, informed sources to ask. As a result, we may cheat the dying and ourselves of the potentially most powerful, meaningful, and transformative experience of their or our lives.

I first crashed into this cultural reality in a shattering way a decade ago in the days following the stroke of my mother's friend, Elizabeth. Elizabeth was not just one of Mother's friends. She was the oldest and dearest of these relationships, the two having first connected in high school when Elizabeth admired Olwen's knitting and asked her to teach her how. It was to Elizabeth's family's home that Olwen repaired after each of the three great losses of her life, the losses that forever changed her life.

I was present for the third of these when we moved in with Elizabeth and her family for three years after the divorce back in the days when no one was divorced. During those years of great bitterness between my parents, Elizabeth had the profound emotional intelligence to be able to be my mother's best friend, continue working for my father, and be the only adult who saw me in all this. As I told her many times over many years, I don't know how I would have survived emotionally, or where I would be or how I would be if it had not been for her. At what level she took in the profundity of her gift I do not know, because on the surface she tossed it off, saying gracious things about how difficult it was in those days for each of my parents.

I persisted in telling her, however, because it was the primary way I could acknowledge the essence of who she really was, the largeness and wisdom of her being. I often thought I was the only one who truly saw her, and, since childhood, had gotten angry with each and every member of my family who at one time or another said diminishing things about her. From the day I was born, Elizabeth and I never did not see each other, never argued, never had any "stuff" between us. It was always a soul-to-soul, essence-to-essence relationship that never went off-course. Our ability to see each other even when no one else did was the gift we gave each other.

Although one side of Elizabeth's body was severely affected and her swallowing was impaired, her caretakers maintained she could go on for weeks. They talked about getting her well, got her up and dressed her every day, wheeled her down to the dining table at appointed times, and made a big to-do about the "swallow therapist" who, they made it seem, was going to perform a small miracle. Her big moment was to call for a differently-shaped spoon to facilitate swallowing ice cream and such!

My head was spinning in this surreal environment; I felt like I was bouncing off rubber walls in a fun house. There was nothing to hang my hat on except my own intuition which was being validated by no one at the nursing home. No one seemed to be in charge of Elizabeth's case, and there was no one willing or able to explore my questions from a clear-eyed perspective independent of the party line that will not look death in the face, and insists on pushing the body to be here even if it and the being it houses are ready to move on.

My intuition said: how can our dear little Elizabeth go on like this? If one side of her body is barely working, how can her whole body systems function? How long before everything collapses? Aren't we talking about days or a week here? They would not address my common sense questions about her clinical reality. Weeks, they said, or even longer, is quite possible, and they kept treating her as if she were recovering from a surgery or illness and as if they could get her well or get some improvement.

I had dashed home to see Elizabeth unprepared for a lengthy visit and under the impression that her stroke, although serious, was not necessarily life-threatening. Now I had to make an agonizing decision: should I stay on longer, or leave (as I had originally planned) and come back for Christmas in a couple of weeks (or sooner if her situation were deteriorating) when I would be prepared for a longer visit? Having a realistic timetable was crucial for me.

I did not follow my intuition, however, and reluctantly drove back on a Thursday. I got daily reports from my mother, and on Sunday, she and the caretakers all thought Elizabeth was stronger. (Knowing what I have since learned, I think they were misled by what is called an "awakening" that often precedes death.) But Monday morning the nursing home called my mother to come over, and on Monday afternoon, Elizabeth died.

I, who knew "nothing" about dying, turned out to be right. I wanted to be there and should have been there and could have been there. Because I did not follow my intuition, I failed one of the two people who had always been there for me and mattered most to me in the world.

A core principle emerged for me that I would follow in my Dance of Death with Olwen: be deeply attuned with my beloved dying, always respect and follow my intuition irrespective of what experienced providers or other people say. Intuition was my primary guide, and, scary as the dance was, my intuition did not fail me.

Mutual Growth and Healing. As my journey with Olwen evolved, my reasons for writing this book not only expanded, but also found their center. I wanted to illuminate ways of being with a dying parent that can enhance the potential for mutually satisfying, emotional, relational, and spiritual outcomes. (A "parent" can be one's actual parent, or any elder who played that role and carries that meaning.)

If you haven't yet been through the death of a parent, it is almost impossible to imagine your way into the mercurial kaleidoscope of emotions generated by the ever-shifting situation, the impending loss and its finality while, amidst all the high-stakes uncertainties, constantly having to make all kinds of decisions which can't be undone or redone.

- You may discover you cannot make predictions about your choices or behavior or feelings based on linear extrapolations from the rest of your life experience or from your relationship up to this point, because the death of a parent is not like other losses, and the death of the mother is in a league all its own. You may surprise yourself because the Dance of Death is nonlinear.

- It may elicit behavior and feelings from both of you that is discontinuous with who you thought you were, who you thought she was, and the patterns that have shaped your relationship for a lifetime.

- Being open to the surprises and immediately flowing with them is possibly the most important, most healing, most transformative thing you will ever do.

If the narrative of this book and the themes it highlights can help you to do that, then its central intention will be realized.

Telling Her Story. In the last weeks Olwen's life, I felt a growing urge to "tell her story" and promised her she would not be forgotten. That need became more powerful as I became immersed in creating a collage and writing a eulogy for her memorial service, and found that one mirrored the other. I found myself focusing on her formative years, her resilience, and her capacity for picking up the pieces of her life each time it was shredded. Her "overstory" of triumph over loss was the right part of her Story for that occasion.

The Olwen of her formative and prime years is not our focus here, yet they and her stunning willpower are essential backstory to who she was in those last months, weeks, and days of her life. The central narrative of this book intertwines the story of Olwen and her journey Home with my caregiving story about how I navigated a path through our Dance of Death and how we were each transformed by the process.

Our journey was precipitated by Olwen's hospitalization for pneumonia and a weakening heart. Olwen gave herself and me the gift of clarity: getting home, never ending up in a nursing home, and not "going on and on" while the quality of her life went down and down. Our journey unfolded from my efforts to translate my mother's wishes into reality, while our situations kept evolving and we encountered obstacles we each had to overcome as Olwen moved closer to death.

Working as a team, we emerged triumphant in the early rounds. She mustered her last reservoirs of strength and will, and I negotiated with all the stakeholders to get her home after her hospital and rehab incarcerations. Yet the question loomed: will she be able to *stay* there?

When Olwen started going downhill, the only way to avoid her nightmare of pointless cycling between hospitals and nursing homes was to get her off the endless treatment treadmill, bring in hospice, and shift the paradigm to palliative care. By fully vanquishing the first set of antagonists—the medical paradigm, providers, programs, and pharmaceuticals at cross-purposes with her needs and desires—and bringing in hospice, I unavoidably set up the next round of challenges.

I had to move in as Olwen's primary caregiver four hours from my own home and life. The mere existential fact of two people, each with her own needs, generated tensions between "my life or hers?" This tension between two subjectivities, between caring for the other and caring for oneself, is of course the fundamental tension in any family caregiving relationship. In addition, I had to struggle with our old patterns (always exacerbated by our co-existing in her space), try to stay outside of them, and not map old stuff onto her. Grappling with these internal challenges was much harder than rearranging the landscape to meet her ever-emerging needs.

Ultimately, we were struggling with the deepest and most intractable barrier to Olwen's dying well: her self-negating paradigm. Would it—even after all we had been through together and all we had each tried to do—would it defeat us both in the end? Winning this one was not about working together and being on the same side. It required something profound to surrender in each of us so there were no longer any sides to be on. Through the paradoxical mysteries of love and grace, we finally moved past all that had separated us. The grace through which transformation emerged lay beyond anything either of us had ever imagined.

Mythic Structure. Only when I had completed a draft of this book did I recognize we had unconsciously lived out the structure of ancient myth. Mythic journeys are structured by a series of obstacles (disguised in various garbs and storied as characters in a drama), each more daunting than the one before, each of which the initiate must encounter, grapple with, and overcome, thereby allowing her to gain transformative wisdom for herself and share it with others.

What I now see is that as we "slayed" increasingly interior "dragons," I was going through Initiation, "Death," and Transformation while Olwen was going through her Initiation, Transformation, and Death. And so the prosaic level of what this book is about—midwifing a good Dance and a Good Death—opens to the archetypal Story of the Return of the

Daughter to Priestess the Death of the Mother through which they both find healing and wholeness, and mutually redeem each other.

Olwen's death is the end of her life's journey but not the end of our story. "The Return" begins in Part IV where I, the end of our line, incorporate her loss, reconstruct our family story in the old country, and reconstitute my familial identity and legacy within my transformed self. For me, this process became inseparable from writing this book and making explicit the wisdom I gained on my journey. My journey and this book thereby found their own natural completion. The Daughter has done what needed to be done, and through the doing, has prepared the space within herself to fulfill the legacy of her lineage and bring her life's work into the world.

Part I

Where Are We?

From out of that primal chaos something true can self-organize.
—John Briggs and F. David Peat

One

Is *This* The Call?

> *At some level I am always waiting for
> The Call and always dreading it.*
> —Artemis, April 28

I awake refreshed on Monday, April 28, having slept for a solid ten hours after working twenty-one days straight on a crash project—a project that will pay the bills while I begin moving my life's work into the world during the next several months. Emerging from my cool, dark cave, I discover two new messages.

"Hi, March, this is Sue, it's after midnight." I inhale. Sue has been doing light caregiving for my mother during the past eighteen months, becoming my eyes and ears five hours away. Trained as a nurse but unable to tolerate hospital working conditions, Sue, a poet and grandmother, has found part of her calling in caring for ladies in their nineties. Without her on-the-spot presence, I doubt we would have been able to keep my mother at Village Grove all of these last eighteen months.

In our first conversation and many times thereafter, I had impressed upon Sue that our goal is to keep Olwen at Village Grove, the gracious, independent-living apartments for seniors to which she had moved a few years back, thereby giving my mother the highest quality of life she can have and keeping her out of her nightmare, a nursing home.

Even as a child, I had absorbed her dread of nursing homes. Perhaps it had been shaped by visits to her father near the end of his life. One time she took me along, and only three things registered for my child-self: the smell of urine permeating the place, the fact he was unshaven, and the urge to get away. Her dread and my dread of nursing homes fused at a primordial level decades ago, and any alternative to Village Grove is as unthinkable to me as it is to her.

Sue's message continues, "I was at my son's and got back late this evening. Your mother called me—it was well after eleven. I could hear she was having some difficulty breathing and could tell she was a little frightened." Olwen, the paragon of independence, who never wants to "be a bother" to anyone, had reached out for help. Sue had come over immediately. "I called the medics. They're here right now and giving her oxygen." I can hear them in the background. "She was sitting in her chair when I got here, very alert, but struggling to breathe. We'll be going down to the hospital in a few minutes."

My mouth dry, unable to move, I hold my breath. What will the next message bring? "This is Sue again, it's now about eight o'clock. They took her down to the hospital last night. I stayed with her 'til I had to go home and get the [grand]kids ready for school and then I came back. They took chest x-rays. They are treating her as if she has pneumonia although they are still not sure if she does." Overnight her little cold had flipped into a life-threatening situation.

Standing there listening to my answering machine, my head is spinning. Is this it? Is this The Call? There have been so many health events over the decades, several times when Olwen could have left us, and always she has rallied. Her incredible constitution and tenacious will have surprised those who didn't really know her. We who did came to expect her to pull through and gradually regain her strength. We had learned to expect her to fuss for some weeks or months afterward that her strength was still not 100 percent of what it had been, always impatient to be her old self. At Olwen's memorial service, Sue will describe her own learning curve in this regard:

> When I picture Olwen, I see an elegant lady who dressed meticulously, often in clothes she made herself and had worn for decades. She was ninety-seven when we first met. She had been rehospitalized in the critical care unit, and I went to transport her back to Village Grove. Upon entering the ward, I saw Olwen standing in the doorway of her room, leaning gently on her cane. She was voicing her impatience to be discharged to a bevy of medical personnel too busy to listen.

Olwen marched to a different drummer—or more likely, a Welsh piper. She was absolutely clear about wanting to go home to her apartment where her increasingly simple life was still manageable. I had some reservations about the appropriateness of her going back home. Yet for all her frailty, I was to discover an invincible spirit.

Now she is nearly ninety-nine years old and the oldest member of the Village Grove community. Yet she of the perfectly erect posture still has none of the foot, knee, hip, back, or walking problems that plague so many of her compatriots in their nineties and eighties, and even seventies. An avid walker all her life, Olwen still prefers stairs to elevators and takes a daily walk outside, inspiring some of her younger neighbors to become more active. Until her three hospitalizations eighteen months ago, she often walked to the post office (nearly a mile) and back in good weather.

When outside her apartment, Olwen has taken to carrying the cane that belonged to Grandpa (Elizabeth's grandfather), delighting in its lightness, and feeling utterly confident of its powers to take care of her needs. That includes raising and shaking it at motorists when there is any possibility of their paths colliding. By contrast, one-third of her neighbors at Village Grove are now using walkers, a fact that had prompted Kate, the executive director, to take up the three gorgeous oriental rugs in the great entry hall last Christmas and replace it with wall-to-wall carpeting on which her residents will be less likely to trip.

My mother has, however, become a little less steady on her feet in the last couple of years, particularly on grass, thick rugs, or uneven surfaces. She has also fallen several times in her own carpeted apartment, yet she has never broken a bone or even her glasses. It is not clear just why she has fallen, but as best I can reconstruct from her limited recall, these events were preceded by her getting up from her chair or altering the position of her head. I speculated that the blood wasn't getting to her head because her circulation is getting less robust. Mother has learned, however, to stay put for a few seconds after she gets up, steadying herself before she takes off.

Although Olwen still walks quickly and moves with the agility of a young person, her legs do give her another kind of problem: fluid retention. She has managed her edema for years by elevating them (especially her right leg), wearing support stockings for the better part of the day, and taking Lasix (a diuretic) so that fluid does not build up. Determined to go to church, exercise class, coffee hour, or other morning events, Olwen takes her "water pill" during the night so she is free to come and go by day. From time to time, however, she has been hospitalized when the fluid has built up in her legs, and once about fifteen years ago, in her lungs. Under Sue's watchful eye, Olwen's legs have been quite good during these past eighteen months.

Her tendencies toward falling, fluid buildup, and incipient shortness of breath suggest congestive heart failure (CHF), a diagnosis that her cardiologist, Jack Malone, has not confirmed to me. Given her three leaky heart valves, he acknowledged that heart failure had to be entertained during a lengthy visit three years ago, but opted for a more peripheral explanation of her edema: the valves in her veins are wearing out and give her poor return. I remained skeptical. Her primary care physician, George Noyes, references her atrial fibrillation which has produced many dicey episodes over the past forty years, but become much less frequent since 1979 when Olwen got her first pacemaker. Whatever their source, circulatory problems are also suggested by the fact that she now turns up the heat to suffocating proportions, whereas ten years ago, she wore short sleeves during the winter in a house her younger sister Florence found so cold she did not remove her coat when she came to visit.

So my best guess as I relisten to Sue's messages is that a weakening heart and pneumonia are interacting, each aggravating the other. In the swirl of emotions, questions, and thoughts, only two things are clear. My mother's present situation feels different from all her previous health events, and I cannot possibly leave until I finish the project or I will not get paid and won't be able to keep my own ship afloat.

The Call seems finally to have come. The Call I have for years half-expected, always holding my breath, the one that will change my life forever though I know not how. Never knowing when The Call might come, or whether Kate would tell me Olwen had had a stroke or that she had passed away in her sleep is a tension I have carried in my body for a very long time. My tension level has ratcheted up over the last few years. At some level, I am always waiting for The Call, and always dreading it.

Intuition tells me that this might well be the beginning of the end of Olwen's long journey and I want to be with her now, not next week. I want to make my own direct assessment of the situation calibrated to my intimate knowledge of her and her medical history, and be on the spot to identify what needs attention and action. Although she has always tried to handle her health events without "bothering" me, I have found out about and come for most of them and she has always responded well to my presence. With the loss of six close friends and family members a decade ago, there is no one—except for Sue—with whom I now share this responsibility.

Had I not been with Mother in 1995 throughout the second pacemaker surgery and its aftermath, she might not have survived because no one was paying attention to the serious complications that arose mid-evening on the day of surgery and demanded immediate attention. I dragged the nurse into her room to bring her suddenly skyrocketing blood pressure under control, and literally ran to the phone to call the Malones, who were Olwen's neighbors. I figured, correctly, that if Malone weren't home, his wife would always be able to locate him and get him there pronto, whereas the charge nurse had demonstrated over the past several hours her inability to cope with both paperwork and an influx of post-operative patients. Malone was there in minutes and spent an hour with her, completely redressing the bleeding incision while her blood pressure ratcheted down.

Now I want to leave immediately to be her guardian, nurse, and advocate, as well as do hands-on Reiki, but I cannot. (Reiki is a gentle healing practice in which the body wisdom of the recipient "decides" how to use subtle energies for its relaxation and well-being.[1]) Olwen enjoys Reiki, and it is one of the few ways I can get her to relax. Frustration with the client (who is not behaving in a timely way) mixes with panic and dread: Can I get there soon enough? Might she die in the meantime? Might something irreparable happen? To be trapped here by the need for my own economic survival when my mother might be dying feels like a war inside my body.

How to bridge the wrenching gap between finishing the project and going home as soon as possible? I cannot extend the client's drop-dead date because I am preparing the proprietary discussion materials for the annual, off-site conference where their top one hundred executives will gather in two weeks. I must squeeze more days out of an already impossibly short schedule.

Mid-morning on the twenty-eighth, I am beset by fear, panic, and anxiety. After calling the hospital and leaving messages for Sue, I shunt aside my emotional turmoil to go into overdrive on the seven documents I am preparing.

My anxiety skyrockets again this afternoon during and after a conversation with Kate who raises the question of where Olwen will go after the hospital—if indeed she comes out of the hospital. Kate always goes to the hospital to see "her people," often being their first visitor and a surrogate for family who weren't there yet or couldn't come at all or don't exist. More than once, she has been with Olwen in the emergency room.

Kate has never seen Olwen so weak. Even before this latest event, Olwen's staying on at Village Grove was becoming a bit borderline, Kate discloses. We both know that Olwen, although still amazing, lost ground after her three hospitalizations in the fall of 2001, and so we both know her recovery from this round might not be sufficient to keep her at Village Grove, even with more help.

Kate has finally verbalized the unthinkable elephant in the room in our every conversation and encounter. It is the very last thing I want to hear at any time, but especially at this moment. Kate seems to sense that and quickly takes it off the table, saying we will talk about everything after I get there and we see how Olwen is doing.

I go back to work, and late in the afternoon get reaffirmation from the point man that they will abide by their commitments: no substantive changes after Friday. I impress upon him I am operating in the dark vis-à-vis executive input, feedback, and sign-off with only four days left on their clock and mine. He lassoes the vice-president who owns the project. The VP finds my approach to the key framing document absolutely dead-on and loves what I have done. Yet he still wants to superimpose a structure that assumes a level of maturation in this conceptual territory that simply does not exist. Tension creeps up my shoulders and neck into a headache.

Between Olwen's dicey condition, Kate's uncertainty about Olwen's ever returning to her apartment, the client's contradictions and disappearing acts, and my having to be here when I want to be there, I am ready to explode. I put on Beethoven's Fifth Symphony, turn up the volume, and, borrowing a page from a therapist friend, yell at the top of my lungs while smashing a telephone book against the molding in one of my doorways. I've never done this before. It works. Interestingly, by completely letting it rip, I do not get a hoarse voice and my headache improves. After exercising and a shower, I finally reach Sue in person and fill in the backstory.

The evening shift won't give me an update because my name isn't on their paperwork, and HIPPA privacy rules have just gone into effect. They want written permission from my mother that her medical information can be shared with me. Pointing out the obvious, I finally get them to accept a fax of her power of attorney. This all takes an hour during which my headache grows ever worse. The evening nurses still don't know whether my mother has pneumonia but they are acting as if she does. She is weak, her condition is serious, and she is on six liters of oxygen—the maximum they run.

So ends Monday, April 28. I do not sleep nearly as well as I did the night before.

Tuesday morning I talk to Noyes after rounds. He says, "She is confused, but she's breathing okay. She has fluid in her lungs which is due to congestive heart failure and probably pneumonia. We are using oxygen—she's still on six liters—diuretics, and antibiotics. We'll know more in three or four days." Three or four days—just when I most need to be there, I absolutely cannot leave. And, he has acknowledged congestive heart failure.

Immersing myself in the client's contradictions and the missing or non-fitting pieces, I synthesize a new whole. It appears in the guise of the VP's structure, yet I bend his structure so as to maintain much of the deeper integrity of the piece. I perform smaller miracles with the other six pieces, get sign-off from all key players, and send everything to the client Saturday afternoon, four days ahead of my original, impossible deadline.

Interspersed with finishing the project, I am calibrating reports from my local sources. I am hearing from some of my mother's late-life friends that she looks poorly. Elizabeth's cousin Mary offers a more encouraging report Tuesday afternoon. Olwen was sitting in her chair and looked "pretty good." Her intravenous (IV) line was running, but she was not on oxygen when Mary arrived. "She knew me right away, and remembered that I had taken a recent trip. But from there, she talked in a dream-like way about things like going to do the laundry, and seemed pretty disoriented." Since Elizabeth's death, we three have grown closer, and Mary and I have become the primary keepers of Elizabeth's story, artifacts, and anniversary dates—birthday, stroke, and death within three weeks of each other.

Thursday, Sue is most struck that Olwen "doesn't seem to have any drive." Sue also observes that "she is not focused. She was more present on Monday than yesterday. She seems disconnected from her situation, from where she is, and from her body. She seems to have no sense of why she is here." Sue is picking up disorientation from the hospitalization itself and/or a potentially core shift. Olwen's relentless drive, although it has often driven the rest of us to distraction, is at the very center of her being and has always kept her going.

I speak with the social worker in charge of discharge planning on my mother's floor. We had talked quite a bit during her last round of hospitalizations. She describes Olwen as very weak, still on six liters of oxygen, confused at times, and struggling with the combined effects of CHF and pneumonia. The social worker will be calling in the occupational therapist and physical therapist when Olwen gets stronger, and we will be figuring out what is next. She speculates Olwen will be too weak and perhaps too confused to go home. Olwen is more likely to go to subacute rehabilitation (rehab) to get stronger and potentially clear out some of the confusion. Medicare pays for rehabilitation but only if you are discharged there directly from the hospital, and only so long as you are making progress. Plateau or go downhill, and *you* start paying the bills.

Friday morning, I call Noyes after rounds. "She still has fluid in her lungs and definitely has pneumonia. She is getting better, but she is weak. She can't take a lot of therapy." This is the first time I ever remember him describing her as weak. It is a subtle clue that he, too, is seeing this round as being different from earlier rounds. She is still on five or six liters of oxygen, and he is pushing diuretics. He will be away all next week, and after rounds on Sunday, he will transfer her care to his associate.

Damnation! An incident from the summer of 1999 immediately flashes to mind. Mother was having alarming symptoms on a Sunday evening that neither of us recognized as a urinary tract infection, and we were trying to get some help. We had no luck reaching any of her doctors. Noyes' associate, who was on call, finally called back—the same associate in whose hands Noyes is now about to entrust my mother's care. He didn't have a clue about what might be the source of her symptoms—this, despite the fact that they are quite a distinctive subset, serious enough for tracking by the Centers for Disease Control, sometimes fatal—and, I will learn long after the fact, sometimes present as disorientation or delirium. What's more, he apparently didn't care. His tone came across as bored, irritated, unconcerned, and impatient to get off the phone. In the moment, Mother agreed he was rude and uncaring, but could not grasp my point that Noyes' choice of such a person as his associate reflected badly on Noyes himself and raised a spectre about her future—and that future had now come.

Following a long bike ride on Saturday afternoon, I pick up the house a bit, pack, gather all the papers and numbers I need to take for her, scan a month of my own mail, pull out the bills, and put them and my own banking stuff in my briefcase. I do long-distance Reiki healing with my mother Saturday night and Sunday morning, sleep better than I have in a week, and leave late Sunday morning, going straight to the hospital with my flowers.

Her bed is by the window. I see a different Olwen than I have ever seen. She is lying there very still, eyes half open in a kind of sleep that isn't sleep, from which people are not easily roused when you speak to them, or take their hand, or even lean in close and talk to them. It is a state of consciousness that comes to the very ill and dying. It is some while before she gives any indication of recognizing I am there. She barely speaks. It is hard for her to talk and she enunciates poorly—also dramatic changes. After a while, the more forceful actions of an aide bring her to a semi-sitting position.

Her recognition of me is not the "oh, I'm so glad to see you" kind, and her way of talking is not conventional give-and-take. Very intimate and confiding, she speaks as if I am already inside her mind so there is no need to explain all the "it's" and "they's" and "this's" and "that's" which have no reference. Context is assumed. More precisely, I *am* the context and translator of her images and thoughts. We are a single entity. It is as if no one but us exists. The world is us and we are the world.

She keeps doing something with her mouth. I look at her tongue which is red and furrowed rather than pink and smooth. Her mouth must be sore and painful. No wonder she isn't eating much or talking much! I call in the nurse who has no idea what to make of it. Unbelievable! Figuring out the source of this problem and doing something about it will be my first order of business tomorrow.

Given their inattention to her mouth, I suspect no one from the hospital has helped her to brush her teeth either, so I improvise a method for doing so in bed. I am concerned she will swallow the swizzle water, but after swishing it around for a long time, she does spit it out. Even the simplest things we in our prime take for granted now become mini-projects in which we hold our breath because something can always go wrong.

I drive to Village Grove and bring my stuff upstairs to her apartment. Then I go up to the roofdeck to be alone with the stars on a beautiful clear night.

Just a year ago at this time, my mother and I spent a couple of hours in this very spot, watching the sunset turn to dusk, and the stars and moon appear. Now the tears come, and with them, panic. The panic that yes, Olwen, the survivor of her generation of family, friends, and admirers, Olwen the invincible, really is going to die, and I am going to have to clear out this apartment before long. Pain and anger and grief all pour out into my tears. Not now! Not when I am on the verge of bringing my real work into the world and have just bought myself the time to do it! Not before she gets to see at least the beginning of how all her support and hopes for me turn out! My race against time to publish the book before she dies has, I have no doubt, been forever lost.

Yet I am vaguely aware my dread will be manageable compared to what it would have been fifteen or twenty years ago. Back then, I was sure I would totally crack up if she suddenly up and died, leaving things so unfinished and unworked through between us. My dread was proportional to a three-way truth: the depth of our connection, the difficulties in our relationship, and my intuition that if only we had enough time, we would have The Conversation that would magically bridge whatever had separated us, heal old wounds, and usher in a new level of connection, understanding, and peace. My intuition was grounded in the fact that underneath everything, we have always been connected by a bottomless love, our acutely shared history, and the searing bond of an only child with her only real parent—the kind that will do anything and everything for you.

I realize now that our relationship began to change when I stopped brushing aside her worries about me, and stopped protecting myself from what I experienced as her criticism. So, for example, instead of glossing over the difficulties in my life which had kept her safely out of it, I began sharing them with her.

The downside of letting her into my life was that I carried the double load of her anxiety as well as my own. She had a special knack for asking exactly the questions I least wanted to hear because they stirred up the very pools I was trying to keep out of, the deep pools where her fears and mine merged. When I finished a project, she would ask, "How are you going to get more work?" Not, "How wonderful you've bought yourself some time to concentrate on your real work."

The upside of letting her into my life was that it opened up new levels of sharing, of connecting, of being on the same side. It also initiated conversations about our early history.

Having these conversations was risky for both of us. I struggled to keep her out of the right or wrong, all-or-nothing paradigm through which she framed everything. If the overly-responsible Olwen felt she had not done everything "right," she collapsed into a space in which she felt she must have done it all wrong. "No, no, no, you didn't do anything 'wrong'!" I would exclaim. "These are *my* problems to deal with. You did the best you could. You thought you had to do it all yourself."

Because she was able to accept responsibility for behavior that had had less than ideal consequences for me, I found myself growing out of the adolescent, blaming mode my generation had grabbed hold of, into forgiving her and taking responsibility for myself. Because we have each been able to see and apologize for ways we wounded one other, we have become closer and more real to each other. Despite the fact that our minds and lives are rooted in different worlds, we have found ways to reach across these barriers, have good times, moments in The Conversation, and moments of great intimacy and connection. As I have become more able to see my earlier modes of behavior, I have become awed by Olwen's capacity to overlook them and endlessly forgive my trespasses and long adolescence, teaching me something of the profound mystery of mother love.

Downstairs, I throw out milk and food that is spoiling and pull out one of the leaves of her cherry dining table for working space. I put the felt pad on top of it; I'm not about to damage a pristine table that my mother has kept free of scratches and blemishes for decades. I begin making lists and plans, and prepare my favorite comfort food: Reggiano parmesan cheese melted on a particular multi-grain bread with spinach leaves, red peppers, pesto or fresh basil, and a glass of sauvignon blanc, often eaten in the late evening while talking to Sue about the day past and the day coming. So ends May 4, the first day of being with my mother in what I already sense are her days of dying.

Two

Will Her Body Outlive Her Mind? Hospitalizations and Their Consequences

I never thought I would outlive anything like this.
—Olwen, May 6

Who *would* know what to make of Olwen's mouth? A while back I had discovered a hospice nearby. I call at eight o'clock. The first question from Jane, an intake professional, is a bull's-eye. "Is she getting intravenous meds for the pneumonia?" "Yes." "Then it's likely to be thrush." "Oh, yuk. What do they use for that?" "Nystatin." "How long does it take to clear up?" "You start seeing results quickly, but it takes a week or more."

Why didn't Noyes foresee the side-effects of antibiotics (especially given her age and compromised condition), and prescribe or leave standing orders for nystatin? I immediately call the nurses' station to check out our hypothesis and, if confirmed, get nystatin started. It is early afternoon before the prescription comes over, and I have to prevail upon Mother's nurse to give her the first dose sooner rather than later.

Outwardly, I am clear, firm, and insistent. Inwardly, I am outraged I have to be the one to see there is a problem, do the detective work, get staff and doctors aware of it, and get a remedy. Seven days she had been here with no one else noticing how miserable her mouth is! No one is paying close enough attention. What else are they missing?

Anger at their inattention is tempered only partially by my recognition that much of the problem lies in a fragmented healthcare system oriented to insurers and providers rather than to patients and families, a system whose interventions and "care" are delivered through work processes strangling in non-value-adding activity—"waste" in the efficient world of Toyota.[1]

Because each handoff is an opportunity for error and a point of potential breakdown in communication, I never assume the content of any conversation I have with a hospital staff member gets communicated beyond themselves. I can talk to only a fraction of those caring for my mother, but alert each of them to her concerns and preferences.

I suggest using lotion on her dry skin and feet which are cracking from dry hospital air, making use of the boombox and tapes I have brought, recognizing she feels trapped in her chair by its locked-in tray, not positioning the tray too tightly to her body, not handling her roughly, not grabbing her around the left side where her pacemaker leads are always sensitive because of her dwindling muscle mass—something I had seen a hefty aide do, causing a shock of unnecessary pain—getting to her as quickly as possible when she needs to pee, and not trying to remove her glasses or to put them on her.

Although my mother has always been continent, her bladder is aging. When it sends a signal that she needs to go, it has become difficult to wait. If staff are slow to respond, they might draw the wrong conclusion, setting off a self-fulfilling cycle of enforced incontinence in which they do not recognize themselves as the culprit. Such a prospect makes me shudder for her.

Two caregivers tell me she refuses to let them touch her eyeglasses. I get the sense they think she is being a bit irrational. I simply ask Olwen why she doesn't want anyone to touch her glasses. "I'm afraid they will get broken." Why didn't *they* ask her?

I devise an approach *with* her: let her take off her own glasses, offer her the case, work together to put them in the case, and show her where they will be safely stored (in the top drawer). Reverse the procedure in the morning. I tell this to every caregiver who comes in while I am there, and put up a sign to this effect. How many will read it?

I tell my mother I am making changes that will help her mouth feel better in a few days, but it is hard to tell if she understands her mouth will improve, or indeed, that there is a future unlike the moment in which she is now caught. Although she is more able to talk and more energized this morning, her face is fairly expressionless, she is barely active on her own behalf, and she is not engaging with the world around her. The get-well cards dropped off by the mailperson sit on her tray unopened. Occasionally she turns the envelopes around in her hands, but with no indication that she knows what they are, or even cares.

Her interaction with these cards—or the lack thereof—is symptomatic of the most dramatic change I see in her: not grabbing hold of life in this world or connecting with anything around her. The external world seems to have evaporated. She looks straight ahead (in truth, she is not "looking" at all), not choosing to move her head or shift her gaze on her own.

After an hour or so, I pick up the cards and put them in front of her. I ask if she wants to see her cards, but she shows no interest. After a while I open them and ask her to read them to me. She is able to read them, but I do not sense she takes in the meaning of the words, or connects them with the sender and the sender's intent. I do not think the trail of words makes an image or warm feeling that friends and well-wishers are thinking of her and praying for her.

I spend many hours Monday and Tuesday just attending Mother, listening intently whenever she speaks. I unplug the bed alarm and sit close, leaning in toward her to catch what she says. I say little. I am simply a containing, attentive presence giving her my full attention, but exerting no pressure. Mostly I wait. When she says things that are novel, important, or insightful, I jot them down.

The official line is that she is "confused," but I am not finding that a helpful or satisfactory descriptor. More precisely, she doesn't answer directly or immediately the questions of the ever-shifting cast of strangers floating in and out of her space. She is not following our conventions of thought which are invisible to us until someone violates them. Then we judge them by these conventions and classify them as "confused."

Nor is she giving clear referents for her "it's" and "this's" nor signalling when, *from our point of view*, she changes topics. Although my mother has never been strong on supplying context or connective tissue, now there is none at all. Things have no chronology; they flow through the now of the endless present. The assumptive rules we have learned for separating and connecting what we are talking about are not in evidence. She is operating at a deeper, more holistic level where our conventional rules of thinking are no longer relevant.

Rather than abiding by the artificial linear order those rules impose, she is speaking in holograms and fractals: each phrase is an expression of the whole, and many of her phrases have multiple layers of meaning. Her quiet intensity and prolonged focus convey her felt urgency to finally communicate her experience of this dreadful and shattering week now that there is someone who is really listening, and can hear and hold it all. She needs a daughter who can meet her where she is, sit quietly by the hour, fill in missing contexts, and sustain an expectation that despite her "confusion," she has meaningful things to say.

Olwen is not in the least self-conscious. She is completely absorbed with pulling up and into words her anguish and bewilderment. She is intensely serious as she finds her way slowly through the strange world where her inner and outer landscapes and she and I all flow into the same primordial currents. From their undivided flow, Olwen begins to bring order from chaos just as our ancestors did: through the power of the word.

"This is a really big house ... a lot of rooms ... it's a big family." She repeatedly comes back to the theme of a wedding or a party. The "party" is apparently right here with all the people that are "not *our* family" floating around in the "big house." Most of all, she expresses over a period of days her longing to finish up:

> I have to finish something ... I don't know where it's at ... I don't know how we got here ... It's gone so far ... I didn't want to be in it in the beginning ... We've got to get out of here ... Let's finish it up ... I never was so upset in my life ... Please finish this out so we can get out of here ... We have to stop all this stuff to come out of this somehow ... We've got to finish it ... I never thought I would outlive anything like this ... I want to get out of their party ... They're not *our* family ... This is a big wedding ... Let's not ruin this ... I'm out of things (pointing to her head).

It is not only Sue and I who have recognized that something has shifted at a tectonic level, but also Olwen herself. Her insight into her situation and her yearning not to be trapped longer than necessary in an intolerable, not-me situation gives me a North Star by which to guide my work as her guardian, advocate, and translator, and begin to clear a path through the medical labyrinth which now entraps her.

※

Olwen's soulful utterances do not come out of the blue. For years now since all of her close friends, siblings, and niece have died, she has asked repeatedly, "Why am *I* still here?" and, "Why am I *still* here?" Sometimes she elaborates. "I don't know why I am still around, I'm so old. All my friends have died." She has informed us repeatedly that, "I don't want to be hanging around forever," and that, "sometimes you can live too long." But often she follows the first part of her litany with, "but I think I'll stick around a little while longer to see what happens." Or, "I'd like just a little more time to finish some things."

Her ambivalence sometimes took the form of, "If something happened to me, I don't know if I would want to call 9-1-1. Maybe I just wouldn't call them." I said to her, "Honey, you can't answer that now, and you can't answer it in the abstract. If a time comes, you'll know then what you want to do. You will have an impulse in that moment, *and that impulse is what you act on.*"

To give her more options, I persuaded her to have her apartment hooked up with a Lifeline Emergency System. Pushing the button on its necklace summons the paramedics directly, thereby keeping the phone line open. She fussed about the ten dollars a month, but agreed to it.

An emergency moment did come in the fall of 2001 when, home alone a week after having had tests in the hospital, she began hemorrhaging profusely. She called Noyes who immediately dispatched his nurse. Next, Olwen called me. I was interviewing a physician vice-president about quality and safety in hospitals, but intuition told me to interrupt the call and check the click on my call-waiting. She was wildly upset (rare for her), said there was blood everywhere (which told me she was moving around), and what should she do? I tried to get her to lie down in her recliner chair next to the phone. My first impulse was to call her local 9-1-1 or hospital to dispatch an ambulance. Then I remembered the thing around her neck and told her to push it. The village fire department medics were there in three or four minutes, hot on the heels of Noyes' nurse who echoed Olwen that there was blood everywhere.

I called Sharon, my first and favorite playmate in early childhood who is very fond of my mother and lives nearby, to go over and please report back. She was able to talk to Mother on the gurney before the ambulance took off, and found her lucid and relatively calm now that help had arrived. Olwen received two units of blood in the emergency room (ER) where Kate and Noyes soon turned up. Olwen told Kate how much she loved her apartment (lobbying for herself to stay at Village Grove even when she was in the ER!) and that she wanted a little more time.

Thus in that frightening moment eighteen months ago, Olwen answered her own question. The push-pull between "I don't want to be here forever" and "I don't want to die right now in this way" was tipped in favor of the latter.

Now, in this moment, it seems the toll taken by the last eighteen increasingly difficult months and her present situation is tipping the scale in the other direction. Has the scale tipped permanently? Or might it tilt back?

A North Star is essential for basic orientation, but I need more. What is producing the changes I am observing? Is her disengagement, her new mode of communicating, and her desire to finish up temporary or permanent? Are they an indication that she is finally starting to let go of this life? Am I witnessing the first stage of her dying? Or, can she rally—does she or will she even *want* to rally?—from this grueling ordeal as she has done so many times before?

※

Trying to assess where she is on her journey is complicated by her being in the hospital since hospitalization itself can be so disorienting and debilitating for the elderly, especially by the time they are in their nineties.

When we are in our prime and living safely quarantined from the ground-level realities of aging and dying, it does not occur to us that someone might become disoriented just by being in the hospital, let alone that their post-hospital functioning may never return to pre-hospital levels. Imagine being alone in a strange "big house" with myriad strangers floating in and out, none of them *our* family, none of whom know us, none of whom we recognize, yet they are picking and poking and positioning our bodies and controlling our movement. In this nether world, day and night blur, bed alarms go off for reasons that make no sense and that we cannot control, words are said but float away as quickly as they came. There is nothing familiar rooted in its familiar place to remind us who we are and where we are or structure our day. Our visual-spatial field of orientation has disappeared. We cannot remember yesterday or this morning, and tomorrow has no shape. Time has collapsed into an endless present whose beginning we cannot remember and whose end we fear we will never come. It is hardly surprising if in this unstimulating blur of confusion we are disoriented and/or present an affectless, listless, unresponsive hospital personality, and/or behave in ways that assert our suddenly remembered selves over and against this nightmarish environment.

Further complicating my assessment of what is going with Olwen is the near-term impact of drugs. Common sense tells me what I will later confirm with a hospice clinician: drugs have a more powerful effect on old, thin, poorly functioning bodies than on the young, healthy subjects used in clinical trials. The therapeutic dose for a ninety-eight-year-old is likely to be lower than for a thirty-five-year-old, and the cumulative effect far greater.

This morning, my second full day of being with her, I discover that thrush is only part of the nightmare generated by the antibiotic ("Q") in her IV bag. According to some staff, Q produces some of the worst drug-induced consequences, mental and physical, of anything in their dispensary. It is also a new, high-end, blockbuster antibiotic. Why, I ask, give such a heavy-duty, new drug to an old woman? Why not something less heroic, more tried and true, with a longer track record?[2]

As if these reasons were not enough to vote no on Q for Olwen, Noyes had prescribed it for her eighteen months ago, and just one pill had made her so nauseated that we had to stop it. Yet he has represcribed it in a far more potent liquid form flowing continuously into her fragile body.

No one had consulted with me about medications she has had problems with, and her well-kept list on that account is long indeed. She has had close calls at least twice from the medication choice and dosages, and has had many bad reactions to drugs, several of which were subsequently taken off the market. In our drug-oriented, medical system whose orientation is to cure symptoms no matter what short-term or permanent consequences may ensue, "side-effects" of drugs are often trivialized and treated as seemingly inevitable—particularly if the patient is very old. Those "side-effects" are monumental for a disoriented, elderly patient, and can sabotage their future independence.

The Q situation comes to light when I get to the hospital Tuesday morning. As I walk down the hall from the elevator, I can see Olwen sitting in a chair by the nurses' station. Staff members converge toward me, "Oh, we're so relieved you're here!" They had brought her out there because they were having such a time with her. She had ripped out her IV line, climbed over the bed rails and out of bed, thrown a tray of food, rejected condescending "now, dear" talk, refused her meds, refused to let anyone touch her glasses, and was said to be brusque and rude in speech. Secretly, I am thinking, "Way to go, Olwen!" Obviously, she is getting stronger! And asserting her subjectivity over and against their patronizing erasure of her adulthood.

It is only an hour later that Olwen confides during her long interior monologue punctuated by intermittent expressions of a few choice words, "I never was so upset in my life." Of course!! Hospitalization and the antibiotic were driving all kinds of alien thoughts and behaviors which must have been terrifying for her. *Olwen* climbing over bedrails!!?? *Olwen* throwing food!!?? Mustn't she have been wondering if she were losing her mind? And trapped in this nightmarish place where nobody knows her? Where she has no control over her situation?

By ripping out her IV line, Olwen has actually said no to Q in a direct, physical way. I complement her actions by stopping the drug at the source when Noyes' associate finally returns my call. He sounds as bored, impatient, and disinterested as he was four years ago, and equally eager to get off the phone. When I later get hold of her medical record, I see they did not stop Q yesterday as I asked, but did discontinue it today, the reason given as "confusion." Thus even her medical record acknowledges a causal or contributory link between Q and confusion.

Olwen's record also notes the existence of oral *candidiasis* (commonly called "thrush"), but makes no mention that it was discovered by her daughter, the same daughter who connected the dots about its cause, and demanded it be stopped and nystatin begun. One would never know from reading this medical record that the hospital staff were not paying attention, not observing closely enough. One would never know her physician made a questionable choice of antibiotic and made no provision for its eminently predictable consequences, thereby inflicting unnecessary physical, emotional, and mental stress and discomfort upon a frail elder. One would never know that the reason changes were made in her medications was not that a doctor came up with a better idea, but that the patient's daughter forced them to pay attention. *Olwen's medical record erases her experience and the role of healthcare professionals in unnecessarily making her dreadful situation more nightmarish.*

Unlike those who simply mark Olwen's chart "disoriented" with respect to place and time (though not to persons), one aide takes the "side-effects" of antibiotics seriously, and she separates their effects from the person who is suffering from them. Regina is a fabulous young woman with the potential to become anything she wants. Tall, strong, smart, unafraid of anything physical or emotionally real, she speaks directly and to the point. Of Olwen's behavior this morning, she says, "I said to myself, 'that's not the lady I met on Saturday. That's not *her* mind, that's not *her* behavior. That's the Q talking.'"

Whereas some of the other caregivers seem intimidated or don't know what to do with Olwen, Regina is not afraid to be real with her. She has actually read my notes about the boombox and audio tapes, and, in an effort to soothe my mother, played the Native American music she enjoys so much, but to no avail. The Q has built up in Olwen's ancient body for many days, and, in combination with her increasing strength, some of its consequences are peaking today.

Between her hospitalization and the antibiotic, it is difficult to assess where my mother is on her journey, and how she might be in her familiar home environment and also gets these chemicals out of her system. I suspect she has inflected toward dying and that her disengagement is integral to this shift but that it is also compounded by illness, hospitalization, and medication. Disengagement is a normal and necessary part of the movement towards death. To expect engagement or push reengagement on someone in that phase is to impose the medical/cultural party line on the dying just to make things easier for ourselves.

I simply listen, attend, and observe, allowing her mind to flow as it wishes. I bring things into her visual/tactile field and allow her to engage or not. I draw attention to things, offering possibilities, but not pushing. I create a space for her to expand or contract, to speak or not. The medical record reads, "Daughter's presence calms patient." An accurate observation, accompanied by no interest in exploring why and how she calms the patient. Is her ability to calm her mother due not just to who she is but also how she attends and listens to her?

Where Olwen is and why she is where she is are critical pointers to the two underlying questions with which I am grappling and to which I cannot know the answer: How long will she live? Will she be able to go home and stay there?

The answers are intertwined. The longer she lives, the harder it will be sustain her at home. Given the long-term consequences of each of the last two rounds of hospitalization on her functioning, I anticipate that the present and far more serious round will have more devastating effects and may well sink the ship as far as Village Grove is concerned. It is difficult to see Olwen coming out of this and still being able to continue living independently, even with help from Sue. With summer coming, Sue's grandchildren will be at home during the day, and she will have less time available. At a minimum, I will have to find more help, but will that be enough? As I watch Olwen get stronger before my eyes and her drive beginning to intermittently reassert itself, the knot in my stomach is churning: Will Olwen be able to get back to Village Grove *and stay there?*

Delirium is a marker of poor hospital care for older people: it is associated with serious complications; it often goes unrecognized by physicians and nurses; and its occurrence is integrally linked with processes of hospital care, such as overuse of medications and iatrogenic events. Unfortunately, delirium is common and can lead to increased mortality, morbidity, and loss of independence.

—Sharon K. Inouye, MD, MPH

I first glimpsed the delirium and disorientation of hospitalization and its potentially permanent effects in March 1998, but did not know then what it was, and no one clued me in. My mother had been hospitalized for a couple of weeks, which I thought was a long time just for bronchitis.

When I finally got hold of her hospital records after she had died, I found she was also diagnosed during that episode as having gastroenteritis, dehydration, pneumonia, and congestive heart failure, yet CHF—the possibility of which I inquired about—was never acknowledged to me (or, as far as I know, to her) until her April 2003 hospitalization.

In contrast to prior hospitalizations, in 1998 she did not want a phone, a television, or even her little radio that she took everywhere, and I could not prevail upon her to do otherwise. Nor did she want me to come up. I thought I could be of most use when she first came home, so I went up toward the end of her hospital stay.

I was shocked when I walked into her hospital room. She had no animation in her face or her body. Her demeanor was summarized by one word: grim. I thought, "Oh, my God! Is this what it's going to be like from now on? I don't know if I can handle this."

In the months that followed, she slowly regained much of her physical strength but it became evident that something had changed. This was not obvious to others when she was out and about in company because she was quite animated and seemed like her old self. But inside her apartment and away from being "on" socially, her baseline demeanor was subtly altered. Diminished expression in a face that had always been somewhat inscrutable made it harder than ever to know how she was feeling, responding, and whether she was understanding what I was saying.

When I had walked into the hospital and seen her condition, I had wondered if something had happened to her. Might she have had a minor stroke or TIAs? Malone and Noyes each maintained nothing indicated that. Neither mentioned the possibility of delirium. In fact, *no healthcare provider or caregiver ever mentioned delirium to me at any point during Olwen's life.*

There is a world of difference between marking off boxes on medical charts ("disoriented to place") whose real-world referents are passed off as inevitable ("What can you expect at her age?") and disembedding symptoms by recognizing them as a potentially preventable, hospital-induced syndrome. In the latter instance, the hospital takes responsibility and acts to forestall or reduce their occurrence rather than blaming the elder or chalking it up to old age.

I first learned of the concept of "delirium" nearly a year after Olwen died when a client mentioned the work of Dr. Sharon Inouye, a pioneer and leading authority on the subject. In retrospect, I realize Olwen's expressive and cognitive changes during and after this 1998 hospitalization may have been ushered in just by the long hospital experience itself. Drugs and surgery are major triggers for delirium, but so is simply being thrust into the unfamiliar, disorienting environment of a hospital.

Unlike the slow encroachment of the dementias, delirium comes on in hours or days and occurs frequently in hospitalized elders—especially in their eighties and nineties. Delirium represents a sudden drop in cognition and attention. Recent memory is often affected, and the patient may become disoriented to time, place, and/or person. Speech may be slurred and not follow our rules of organization. These changes in functioning fluctuate over the course of the day as can the elder's affect: from agitated and hyperactive to withdrawn and lethargic (or "hypoactive").[3] Delirium may be an expression of infection or underlying disease.[4]

Textbook distinctions between delirium (acute confusional state) and dementia (chronic confusional state) are tidy enough, but the real world is messier. Preexisting dementia greatly increases risk of delirium during hospitalization, and delirium can trigger or accelerate incipient dementia, but we still understand little about their interactions. Doctors and nurses often fail to recognize it, "in part because of its fluctuating nature, its overlap with dementia, lack of formal cognitive assessment, underappreciation of its clinical consequences, and failure to consider the diagnosis important."[5] Further, because hospital staff often don't know the patient, they may assume the acute confusion *is* chronic confusion, and treat the patient as if they were chronically demented.[6]

Olwen's grimness and rejection of communication devices in 1998 may have expressed the withdrawn, hypoactive form that delirium can take, a form missed by 30 to 70 percent of nurses and physicians.[7] Inouye has developed interventions that help prevent delirium, but it resists being reversed. Delirium may clear up or lessen for some people in the hospital if the situation is recognized and their drugs are adjusted, or, more likely after they return to their familiar environment, but frail elders often do not regain their prehospital level of functioning. Many do not recover sufficiently to live independently.

Whatever the source(s) of the changes in Olwen, I began to see her nineties as divided into the "before" and "after" of this 1998 hospitalization. Although she had had many health events over the years, she had recovered from all of them and her mind had been clear until this hospitalization a few months before her ninety-fourth birthday. The spring of '98 marked a watershed—the first major inflection point in the gentle trajectory of her aging—after which I began to feel uneasy about her long-term future and its implications for mine.

※

This downward inflection from a fully independent life to incipient decline was accentuated by Olwen's decision made during that hospitalization to stay ahead of her curve by not renewing her driver's license and giving her car to her nephew Michael. The ensuing contraction of her range of movement, the lessening of her independence, and her having to depend on others for rides reduced her quality of life. As she became more housebound with less to do, mild depression, intermittent anxiety, and diminished affect colored her life and our relationship. When I wasn't problem-solving, I spent more of my time with her trying to buoy her up, validate her feelings and life experiences, and get her out and about.

Not that she spent all day alone in her apartment. She walked daily, attended exercise class, went to coffee hours and most events offered at Village Grove, and played cards with her neighbors twice a week. She enjoyed the library, living room, large enclosed porch, the solarium where they watched movies and had parties from time to time, and the views from the roofdeck onto which it opened. She discovered that on July Fourth, you could see fireworks in three directions from the roofdeck, and over the years, others began to join her.

Olwen continued to manage her daily life in her home surroundings very well, and dressed so elegantly that she continually received compliments on her appearance. She had made some of her clothes herself and had worn them for decades. She was very pleased they continued to fit and that people often asked if they were new. She kept tabs on her financial and administrative affairs, took care of Medicare and health insurance paperwork, did her own taxes with the help of an AARP volunteer, managed her chronic conditions and her medications, and continued to make new friends and neighbors. She made her own medical appointments, and walked to many of them. She also walked to the bank, drug store, opticians, and other stores in the village.

Olwen still had a respectable support network and people lining up to take her to church, appointments, social events, and sometimes to lunch. She went to all Welsh community events, relishing the contact and polyphonic hymn singing. "Oh, how the Welsh can sing!" she would burst with pride. She regularly attended the church she had joined in the 1920s, and stayed for the coffee hour downstairs, sitting with a group of folks who became very fond of her. She was able to visit her lot at the cemetery because the couple who took her to church most often went to the cemetery after church, after which they sometimes took her to dinner.

Nonetheless, bits of memory loss, repeating herself more often, reviewing and shuffling old papers, and increasing anxiety about what to do with legal, financial, and administrative documents and mail suggested we had started down the slope of age-related, cognitive declines. Knowing how strong her constitution and willpower were, I thought we should plan for the long haul. To compensate for these incipient losses as well as the loss of her car, I thought she would be needing more structure, support, and stimulation.

I began to look for help and resources, but what I found didn't match her emerging needs. Self-care (bathing and dressing) was the first thing everyone offered, but I knew Olwen would be on her deathbed before she even had such needs, let alone accepted help. There was an adult day care program nearby, but I knew it would hold no appeal for Olwen. Meals-on-Wheels was redundant because the major daily event at Village Grove was the dinner hour. I checked out the senior citizens' center, but it was dominated by youngsters in their seventies and early eighties who exercised vigorously, played bridge, and could still hear each other.

We explored a bill-payer program later on, but Olwen wasn't ready to give that up, and the safeguards made it cumbersome. Besides which, it wasn't keeping the checkbook or paying the bills that was becoming problematic, but her coping more broadly with financial and legal matters. As Olwen had worked in accounting for many years, actually enjoyed going over her finances, and prided herself on her frugality and money management, I knew she would be loathe to relinquish control in this area, that it would be one of the last skills to go, that she could continue doing it herself for some time, and that it was important for her to do it herself as long as possible.

This gap between activities, programs, and centers for fully able and alert seniors and services for people who had decreasing ability to self-structure or self-care was frustrating. I surmised that Kate and her staff were noticing the same gap. Village Grove began developing more weekly activities and special events to structure the days of those who chose to participate. But what Olwen needed didn't fit into an activity, a program description, or a job description.

It was more let-your-hair-down companionship that she needed, and more ways to get outside walking distance and do outside things. I fantasized a personal health resource who could check on her regularly and be available by phone at odd hours to answer questions about troubling symptoms of (what could turn out to be) a cataract or a urinary tract infection or a Baker's cyst. As time went on, she needed someone to help her deal with mail that confused or upset her.

The gestalt formed by her needs was hard to define because it blended skills and a relationship in which trust and friendship had emerged. Helping mother with her mail, for example, would open the door to private information for which confidentiality and trust were essential.

The forays I made in these directions did not produce a fit between what she needed and what the agencies could offer. Although she liked the social workers and agency heads who came to visit her, the people they sent to be with her were not a good fit. Since, in addition, Mother could not see the need for any of these things, and was not especially receptive to my suggestions, my efforts during the 1998-2001 period did not bear much fruit.

I filled the bill as best I could through frequent visits and phone calls. A pattern emerged in my visits. I would arrive with treats or gifts and input from the outside world and the hope for meaningful moments together. We would do our high-priority appointments, go to the cemetery, go out to dinner, take rides, and visit with someone who was still alive. All of these things kept her anxiety at bay, but it could become all-enveloping when we were inside the apartment. Her going round and round with the current object of her anxiety and her unraveling whatever we had seemed to settle drove me up the wall. Nothing could ever get done. Nothing could ever move forward.

Sometimes I exploded, but increasingly, I imploded. During one visit, a blood vessel broke in my eye. Shortly after another, I developed shingles. Each time, I arrived feeling like myself and looking forward to our time together. Before long, I would feel defeated, ineffective, and at least a few hundred years old. Somewhere near the dawn of a sleepless night I would awaken with the beginning of a plan which I would start to flesh out in my mind and later on paper. The plan targeted the reality-based, present-tense factor(s) in her current expressions of anxiety or what I perceived to underlie them. I would spend time exploring the idea with her, explaining it, and writing down short summaries so she could review it whenever she chose to. When I got home and called to let her know of my safe arrival, I also reiterated whatever it was we had been talking about and settled. Often, however, she had already started unraveling it or had moved onto something else.

⚜

Conversations with social service agencies did lead me to an excellent book, however: *The 36-Hour Day,* written for families of people with age-related memory loss and dementias. Dementias are clusters of symptoms than can have multiple causes; although Alzheimer's is the biggest and most deadly cause, it is but one. Nutritional deficiencies, dehydration, and vascular insufficiencies can contribute to memory loss, and I suspected all of these were operating in Mother's case. It is sometimes possible to slow down or even reverse memory/cognitive losses when they are of more benign origins. Given Olwen's remarkable constitution and willpower and their implications for her longevity, I thought anything that might retard decline was a good investment.

It meant we should get an assessment by a multi-disciplinary team of geriatric specialists, but we would have to go out of town to find such a group. Mother flatly refused my proposal in the summer of 1999 to see any other doctors even on a specialized or supplemental basis or for an assessment. "Noyes is my doctor," she declared. Our views about Noyes and about doctors were at complete loggerheads. She did not separate professional relationships from personal relationships, and would defend him by saying, "a lot of people like him very much." I would say, "Some people think he is behind the times. A confident doctor welcomes questions from family members and works *with* them, but he gets uneasy and apprehensive when I go with you to see him and ask questions. His uneasiness speaks volumes to me."

I argued for my view that, "Doctors are not gods. *You* are the center of things, not him." This concept of patient-centered healthcare relationships did not compute for her because in her world, people looked up to doctors as authorities. I tried another angle, "Remember how you found good medical help for Florence? Well, now I want to help you find good help for you. I want you to let me." No go. I reminded her how miserable, uncaring, ill-informed, and impatient we both thought Noyes' associate was. I pointed out that no matter how long you have been with a physician, the time you need them most is precisely when they will not be available, and then you will have to make do with their associates. Many rounds, many angles, all to no avail.

I finally had to give up. I remember ending our discussion/argument by standing up and wagging my finger, presciently pronouncing, "If you won't see anyone but Noyes, you will pay the consequences for this down the line."

Over the next couple of years, Mother expressed growing frustration with her memory and not being as "quick" as she had been. She had to go over and over her checkbook. I and others reminded her it was amazing she was still doing her checkbook at all. Still, we were both worried about the possible trajectory portended by her memory problems and cognitive mixups. She catastrophized Alzheimer's. I didn't think that was her problem, but I worried about the gray area into which we were headed. Somewhere down the road covered in murky mist, Kate and/or Noyes might decide she could no longer stay at Village Grove. I again brought up the idea of doing a geriatric assessment now that a team of specialists was spending a couple of days a week in town. This time she agreed to go.

I wrote up three pages of observations contextualized as being extensions of life-long patterns or new developments. The primary symptoms were short-term memory loss and problems with processing connections and sequences between things (which depends in part on being able to remember the pieces long enough to put them together). She could recall concrete things of emotional importance (for example, that I was coming to visit or had a new cat, or *another* new cat, or that I had had a problem with the air-conditioning in my car and was it working now?), but was having increasing trouble understanding abstract matters and papers, such as form letters from Social Security, or the name of a medical condition she had (such as a urinary tract infection), or the fact that she had had a similar problem before.

The team included a neurologist, a nutritionist, and a social worker. Their modern, open, collegial style was a delicious contrast with the archaic, patriarchal, autocratic mode of medicine that seemed to infuse local medical practice.

They spent several hours with us, singly and together, at the end of August 2001. They were delighted by her elegance, dignity, and wry humor, and found her the most charming and lucid person to have passed their way in some time. They found no signs of the deadly plaques of Alzheimer's, nothing beyond modest, age-related memory loss.

With their recommendations reinforcing what I had suggested for some time, I encouraged her to take her supplements and drink more water, touting its virtues and the dangers of dehydration while constantly sipping water myself. All to no effect. Nor did I succeed in improving her nutrition. I brought non-GMO, soy protein powder to mix in things. Although she thought it tasted fine, she never added it to anything on her own. She always had celery to chew on and ate salads when I made them, but never bought ingredients to make a salad for herself. She liked the real soups I made, but for herself, poured boiling water over a commercial soup powder or opened a can of soup.

I didn't wear myself out with these efforts, however. After all, this is a woman who has never broken a bone, has perfect posture, walks like someone in her prime, has all her teeth, and had made it through all kinds of health events to age ninety-seven.

A few weeks after our gerontology visit, Mother came down for a visit. She was keen to see my place again, and be reminded of how I had integrated many of her treasures and pictures of the good times into my home. It was a testament to her classic taste that things which had worked so well in her home worked equally well in mine.

I had an elegant dinner party for her, inviting two of my oldest friends whom she had known for decades. We used her crystal and silver and one of her lace tablecloths. I opened a Sancerre which turned out to be spectacular, and added another dimension of memorability to the occasion. Three other friends came by on other days. Olwen's social skills were still excellent, and she charmed all of them. Those who hadn't met her before were bowled over by her grace and dignity, and my old friends wished their much younger mothers were doing half as well. It was a good moment.

Barely two weeks later, a second and larger inflection point got underway when Mother was hospitalized three times in six weeks: first for tests to which I was opposed (and which she had, on her own, decided against), then for their hemorrhaging complications, and finally, for edema in her legs. Although she knew why she was going to the hospital each time, once there, she was fuzzy about it and couldn't name where she was. She was always clear, however, that she wasn't at home, was surrounded by an ever-shifting cast of strangers, and wanted to go home. As she got stronger, she demanded to go home and had little patience for why they might want to keep her there another day or two. On one of those occasions, she got completely dressed in the middle of the night, put on her beret, got out her coat and cane, sat in the chair, and insisted they let her out. In the weeks and months that followed, she could barely remember having been in the hospital, and the reasons she had been there disappeared.

The permanent toll taken by these hospitalizations—at least two and probably three of which were completely unnecessary—and the disorientation they caused was a reduction in her ability to organize her thoughts or make connections. The problems she was having were continuous with what had been going on for a couple of years, but the gaps in thought were more frequent and sometimes took on the quality of tires spinning in the snow—going over and over the same thing, but going nowhere. Increasingly, she said many of the same things in many of our conversations. Nothing new seemed to be happening. Her litany, I speculated, kept the cornerposts of her slowly disappearing world in place, reducing her anxiety.

Fortunately, I had found Sue through a high-school friend during the first of these three hospitalizations. Sue had cared for my friend's mother during the last two years of her life. The most important things my friend told me were that Sue was completely trustworthy in every way, and that her mother and Sue had really come to care very much about, indeed love, each other. It was a total blessing that Sue had some availability, and that she and Olwen clicked from the start, soon becoming fast friends.

This last drop in Olwen's memory and cognitive processing made Sue's help an absolute necessity. One of her most defined activities was medication management. For years, Olwen had managed her own meds, putting them out each morning into a tiny crystal dish. Although there had been changes in her meds and their frequency over the years, she always made those shifts in her mind, knew her meds by heart and what they were for. Now, however, she was not always clear about which day it was and, more troubling, wasn't looking for clues to tell her because she thought she knew. Concurrently, Noyes was tweaking frequencies and dosages more often. He had also taken away baby aspirin and put her on the potent blood thinner Coumadin whose effects have to be monitored closely with frequent blood tests.

Sue introduced a pillbox, and either Sue or I filled it. She talked to my mother most mornings, checked on whether today's pills were gone, and what was on her mind. She came over a couple of times during the week and at some point over the weekend. Observing that Olwen did better when she was not in her apartment all day, Sue took her for rides and errands as well as to appointments. She tried to enhance Olwen's nutritional intake by preparing or bringing lunches, or taking her out for lunch. With her nursing background, she monitored Olwen's numerous minor but irritating medical problems as well as the edema in her legs. She helped Mother with mail and getting rid of papers whose existence bothered her. "There is so much paper around here!" Olwen would lament. By anyone else's standards, her apartment was impeccably neat and the amount of paper was modest.

These particulars were important and essential, but they paled beside the friendship Sue and Olwen formed. Olwen was able, for the first time since the flood of losses had taken away her life-long friends, to let down her hair with someone besides me. Before long, Sue was familiar with the major players in Olwen's life, the gist of their stories, and most important of all, the arc of Olwen's story. Olwen could replay parts of her story with an interested witness who was willing and able to supply the emotional context and meaning for story fragments and validate her life experience. Sue provided a mode and level of friendship and safety that contrasted significantly with the point-to-point exchanges which dotted Olwen's social space and during which she was always "on." She gave Olwen a sense of security, of being less alone, of knowing there was a reliable, caring, and trustworthy friend nearby who could and would come if needed.

Equally wonderful for me, I now had someone else who was observing the private Olwen and with whom I could calibrate observations and express my frustrations. Now I was working with someone else to identify changes, themes, needs, and problems, and find solutions or ways to improve or counteract the situation.

✂

As the months had ticked by, small, but to Sue and myself (and we feared, the Village Grove staff), perceptible changes kept me continually and increasingly on edge about being able to keep Olwen at Village Grove. I had had a somewhat reassuring face-to-face conversation with Kate during the fall of 2001. When I mentioned the recent mental assessment by the team, she laughed and said, "I could have told you she doesn't have Alzheimer's." I replied, "It was helpful to have that validated by a team of experts." I asked about criteria for people to remain at Village Grove. "Safety." Safety for whom? What does that mean? "Safety for oneself and to the community."

A few days after I left following her first 2001 hospitalization (too soon? if I knew then what I know now, I would have stayed longer despite my deadline pressures), Olwen put the kettle on at 5:30 in the morning, and then forgot about it as she started going over papers in her bedroom. The fire department came, but there was no real damage except to the kettle. I, like many people, have destroyed at least one teakettle in the same way, but when we are in the prime of our lives, we don't usually run the risk of being asked to move.

With safety on the table, I told Kate that I had bought Olwen an electric tea kettle that automatically shuts off after it has boiled a couple of minutes or as soon as you pick it up. I offered to disable the oven, and if necessary, the stove. Olwen didn't use it for anything but boiling water and had adjusted quickly to the new kettle. She knew her toaster oven's operation in her bones; it didn't start without the timer, and when the timer went off, so did the heat. We decided to take the dial off the oven.

Noyes came into the conversation at some point. To be accepted into Village Grove, one has to be certified as able by one's physician and recertified annually. He was noticing changes in Olwen, too, and raised the idea with Kate of assisted living. Kate reported she had chuckled and said, "Olwen is still one of my best people."

How ironic. Olwen trusted Noyes who was apparently ready to do her in, and, like all the residents in a complex like Village Grove, a bit afraid of Kate who ultimately called the shots as to whether someone could stay or not.

Because Olwen had for thirty-five years been on the non-profit board that built Village Grove and hired Kate as its second executive director, she and Kate had a relationship which predated Olwen's residency. They had immediately gravitated to each other because each has style, dress impeccably, is her own person, and speaks her mind. I suspected all this might mean Kate would go a good way into the gray zone with Olwen and would be extremely reluctant to ask her to leave, but I knew she would do it if she felt she had to.

✺

During the last year or so, I have condensed my fears into the question, "What if her body outlives her mind?" Now we are at the cusp of a third major inflection point. How much will her body recover? How much will her mind recover?

It is beginning to look as if bodily failure may keep pace with mental failure or even get ahead of it. Yet Noyes keeps "saving" her body. Every time he saves her by putting her in the hospital, the hospital experience robs more of her mind and brings her a step closer to her nightmare, a nursing home.

I don't know what the aftermath of this round is going to be. Will she be clear enough to stay at Village Grove? Will she live so long and need so much support that we will run out of money before she runs out of life? What if he keeps "saving" her? How many rounds can she take?

Three

Mobilizing to Beat the Odds and Get Mother Home

> *I want to go back to my apartment and live there for a short time.*
>
> —Olwen, May 9

Olwen's assertion of her will and her strength in climbing over bed rails demonstrate she is indeed going to graduate from the hospital. Where to? Kate doesn't think Olwen is ready to come back to Village Grove. Our only viable option right now is subacute rehabilitation. The hospital social worker concurs. "Rehab" will buy us some time. Medicare will cover it, thereby stretching our dollars for whatever lies ahead.

The premise of rehab is that one goes there to get strong enough to go home, but many frail elderly never leave. Rehab often becomes the gateway to nursing home placement, decline, and death. Will we be able to beat the odds?

Complicating our planning is the fact that we don't know what day Olwen will be released. When Noyes' associate calls back, I describe antibiotic consequences, insist Q be discontinued, let him know she cannot return to her apartment at this time, and that he needs to sign off so she can go there directly from the hospital. He is noncommittal and seems to resent and resist the idea of even conferring with the family, let alone sharing power.

Midafternoon, I check out rehab facilities. Small rooms are even smaller because the bathroom carves out a big chunk of space, yet even singles have windows that open. Although there is a "rehab wing," fluctuating numbers of rehab patients and variable room availability mean that, in practice, people from rehab and skilled nursing may intermingle on some corridors and around some nursing stations, as well as share a dining room.

That sets off an alarm in my gut. Elizabeth spent her last three years in another adult home and ate in a common dining room where some residents pounded the table and banged their tableware, while others, including some at her table, were too listless to hold their heads up or talk. Is it any wonder she began deteriorating as soon as she went there? Who could eat in such a setting? Who would not be depressed? Who would not think death a blessing?

I reiterate my request for a single room with the social services coordinator and find out more about how rehab works. Medicare pays 100 percent for up to 20 days, and 80 percent for up to 100 days. No guarantees, however, because one must need services—skilled nursing, physical therapy (PT), occupational therapy (OT), and/or speech therapy—yet also be making progress. A patient has to be assessed within a 14-20 day window; the team reviews all the information on the patient. I am welcome to come in person or by conference call.

Staff appear competent, seem to care about the patients, and are proud of their facility. They know patients by name. The place does not smell bad, and the windows open. Yet I feel suffocated by its very nature, and panicky anticipating Olwen's being cooped up here. Our gut responses of repulsion and attraction to people and place and things are usually one and the same. Once outside, I can breathe again. I weep for Olwen that it has come to this.

&

I need to know more about congestive heart failure, how it plays out, and how it can be managed. I drive to the hospice office. Jane, the woman who clued me into the thrush yesterday morning, sits down with me. Although it is near the end of her official day, she is generous with her time, exudes no indication of needing to rush off or do something else, and answers my questions with a clarity that is missing in the Noyes/hospital fuzz. She draws me pictures of what happens in CHF and pneumonia, and explains her drawing.

"The failing heart cannot handle the fluid. The lower chambers of the heart, the ventricles, pump out the blood that has come back into the upper chambers, the atria. When the left ventricle can't keep up because it is getting weaker or the valves are getting leaky, you get fluid overload. It can cause swelling (edema) in the legs and ankles. Some of it may 'back up' into the cavity between the linings of the heart and of the lungs. That makes it hard to expand the lungs and take a deep breath."

"What I worry about is an end-game scenario in which she won't be able to breathe or is struggling for breath. I don't want her drowning in her own juices or gasping for breath. Can that be prevented? Can it be managed?"

"Yes, it can. We can control it with the 'CHF protocol.' We keep them on their diuretic so the fluid doesn't build up, and we use oxygen to help them breathe. At first the oxygen might be on only at night, or if the weather is humid or hot. We use Ativan to reduce anxiety—including anxiety about not being able to breathe. For pain or breathlessness we use Roxanol which is a form of morphine sulphate. It is a vasodilator so it dilates the major vessels in the bronchials. That takes some of the load off of the heart and helps people to breathe. Most people do not experience pain in the terminal phases of CHF."

"What are some of the end-game scenarios with congestive heart failure?"

"There are several. She could sleep away. She could go into a coma. She could have a stroke or cardiac event. She could be going along and suddenly become short of breath. She could just fade away."

Jane has met Olwen once—eight months ago when her weight had dropped from 120 to 96 pounds in less than three months, and Noyes thought nothing of it. I asked hospice for a consultation. Despite the weight loss, Jane and a colleague found Olwen far too vibrant, immaculate, active, and socially adept to be seriously concerned for the near term.

Now I briefly recap Olwen, her health background, her current crisis. I quote several of today's statements including, "I never thought I would outlive anything like this." We discuss end-of-life dignity and the right to refuse further treatment. Jane explains that Medicare pays for hospice after one's skilled nursing benefit is exhausted. One can also choose to go with hospice before that benefit is exhausted, but one cannot get coverage for both hospice and skilled nursing at the same time. One must choose.

The hospice choice carries heavy responsibility for the family. During Jane's visit last year I learned that hospice can provide only two hours per day of care and requires a full-time caregiver or set of caregivers before they can become involved and oversee medical management of the case. I would have to move in with my mother.

I remember rolling my eyes and dropping my jaw at the very idea, and looking at Jane as if she were out of her mind. Now, here I am eight months later, exploring what then seemed out of the question.

※

A funeral home partner comes to the apartment to go over our contract. Olwen and Elizabeth decided in the 1980s to be cremated and to prepay their funerals, and they each took out a certificate of deposit (CD) with the funeral home. Will the CD's current value cover the funeral and memorial service expenses? Would the CD be counted in the "spend-down" limit if we have to apply for Medicaid? Can it be protected so that it goes for her burial and her memorial service?

We go over each item, and I get rid of a couple to compensate for rising costs on others. I must identify line items for her memorial service, because, as he explains, "Medicaid can only take the difference between the value of the CD and what is not budgeted in the contract." Her CD will cover the cost increases and memorial service expenses. If we have to apply for Medicaid, then, he explains, "we will need to convert the CD into an irrevocable trust."

※

At the hospital. Olwen continues to make observations about the party, the big house, and wanting to finish up. I sit close, leaning in to hear, and continue to make notes. She rarely turns her head to look at me, nor does she look at anything with her unfocused gaze. Yet we are fused together in an intimate universe in which she confides the images and ideas crystallizing from the flow of her inner landscape.

Tuesday evening Barbara stops by to see Olwen. Barbara is the niece of Olwen's niece who died some years ago. Barbara tells Olwen she called her a few days ago to see if she would like to go to the Gymanfa

Ganu *(guh-mahn'-vah gah'-nee)*—a festival where people sing Welsh hymns and sacred music in four-part harmony—being held at the Welsh church.[1] The church, Gymanfa Ganu, and Welsh singing all register for Olwen. She brightens and acts almost like her prehospital self.

Watching Barbara with Olwen, I speculate about how interdependent Olwen's responses and demeanor are with the person in her space. Barbara sits directly in front of her and looks right at her so they are on the same eye level. She tells Olwen she looks well. She speaks firmly, clearly, and not too quickly about matters of interest to Olwen. Olwen's "socially appropriate" responses make it clear she is tracking what Barbara says and connecting the present moment to her real self and her past.

By contrast, a friend who came earlier stood up, shifted her weight from one foot to the other, looked around nervously, didn't know what to say, and started talking to me, shutting Olwen out of the interaction. I cut her off a few times and said, "Let's talk with Olwen," but she didn't take the hint or didn't know how. She seemed oblivious to the fact that none of this was lost on Olwen. Watching Olwen's face and body language, I sensed that what was being communicated to her was, "there's something not right about me. I guess she thinks I'm beyond the pale." Olwen looked hurt and bewildered, igniting my protective ferocity.

This person-dependent contrast in how Olwen responds, acts, and speaks inflects what I will later read in her medical record. Day after day, nurse after nurse checks off boxes that indicate she is "oriented to person" but not "oriented to place."

When an elderly person is disoriented by place and situation, it seems obvious to me they become even more dependent on and vulnerable to how we reflect them back to themselves. If our eye contact, our tone, our body language, our way of being connects with who they really are, they brighten, become more themselves, and respond more "appropriately." If, on the other hand, we cannot get past their current circumstance and shuffle around awkwardly, they pick that up, too. They are less likely to talk and more likely to act "confused."

As the days and weeks go by, I will muse upon how important it is that friends and family recognize that it is they themselves who are creating the context through which their person is responding, and conduct themselves accordingly. It is critical that nurses, residents, and attending physicians—those with the power to define the situation by checking off boxes and creating medical records—understand how they co-produce what they have learned to see as independent of themselves.

Our culture and the mechanistic training of clinicians predispose them, however, to believe that what they observe is an "objective" fact about the patient when, in fact, they are witnessing "quantum events" in which *they themselves are co-creators.* (There are no objects and no objective events in the "quantum world," only interacting "subjects" co-creating a momentary reality through their interactions.) A fragile, elderly, ill patient responds to the contexts generated by the body language, expectations, and behavior of clinicians, caregivers, family, and friends. She is as much their creation as her own.

Likewise, those residing in a standard nursing home are co-created by its physical, structural, and cultural environment, as well as by the staff and other residents. I was appalled by how Elizabeth's isolating, depressing, annihilating situation erased the magical and wise being who had been the beacon of my childhood. Only when long-term care is radically redesigned on quantum principles of co-creation can elder care become life-enhancing.[2]

Wednesday, I begin sorting Olwen's clothes. Sue has warned me that in nursing homes, they tend to scoop up everyone's clothes daily and throw them into big vats that can ruin good clothes, and certainly anything woolen. So we must mark everything, and I have to look at everything I set out as potentially expendable. Olwen's clothes don't require frequent washing because they are always clean and have no spots. Sue will put up big signs saying, "family will do laundry," and she and I will take care of her laundry ourselves.

It is strange and difficult to go through Olwen's clothes, make selections, and begin to pack. I know her clothes fairly well, but have never intruded upon the privacy of how she puts herself together. I find this process of selection one I resist emotionally and cannot complete this morning. I am caught between, on the one hand, wanting her to have familiar things that she likes and that may help to orient her, and on the other, not wanting her things to be stolen or damaged. I start making inventory lists for myself and Sue, and head to the hospital.

Olwen is still talking about the party this morning. The OT and PT people come in to evaluate her; she is improving but needs to get stronger so they support the rehab plan. The hospital social worker comes in with an intake evaluator from rehab. Kate arrives. The mood is upbeat because all of our presences are connected to Olwen's improving sufficiently to graduate to rehab. Olwen picks up the mood, enjoys the attention, affirmation, and sociability. She is smiling! I joke that Olwen has been talking about a party, and now here it is!

After a bit, Kate and I walk down the hall to find a place to sit and talk. She offers to be of help in any way at all. She says she has an "open mind" about Olwen's returning to Village Grove after rehab. I take a full breath for the first time since this began ten days ago. After we discuss a number of issues, I ask Kate if she would come with me to meet with Noyes when he gets back. I explain why. "Sure, I'll come with you." I sketch out my agenda.

The following Monday, May 12, Kate and I go over to Noyes' office around five o'clock. It's after hours, only Noyes is there, and the three of us sit down in his waiting area. Tension is palpable.

I talk about my being the primary decision-maker in Olwen's stead, listening for what she wants and translating that into action on her behalf. I have phoned and written him about my role several times over the last few years, but he still doesn't include me in the loop, let alone consult with me before the fact. He just acts on his own.

He mildly demurs, making reference to Sue's being there on office visits with Olwen or phoning over to his office about this or that. He doesn't really grasp the difference between what Sue is doing as liaison and reporter and my being the family decision-maker for Olwen. I repeat my point that all major decisions and actions require dialogue with me and my consent *before the fact*. Kate expands the context by talking about participation of the family in choices about care, but his words, expressions, and tone suggest he does not really understand what we mean, and therefore cannot see the vast difference between it and what he has been doing.

I move on to the need for a plan of care that relates to Olwen as a whole person, and not just her physical symptoms. Her quality of life and the dignity of her entire being must trump his treating symptoms in ways that have the effect of reducing her quality of life and artificially prolonging it. Olwen has told us all she does not want to go and on, and we all know the hospitalizations eighteen months ago have taken a toll. I remind him I had written him at the time that I was opposed to her doing those tests and she had come to the same decision on her own. Then I found out he had put her in the hospital for these tests, following which there were very serious physical complications which required another hospitalization. The hospital-induced disorientation has never fully dissipated and is threatening her future.

"Each time she is in the hospital, it reduces her ability to function as well as she did before. Each time you treat a set of symptoms and rescue her body, you are driving her closer to her nightmare of ending up in a nursing home. All she wants is to get back to Village Grove. The longer this cycle of hospitalizations goes on, the less likely it is that she is going to be able to get back there *and stay there* until she dies. We don't know yet if she can come back from this round, but I cannot imagine her being able to come back from another one. Being able to stay in her own apartment until she dies is what she wants more than anything in the world."

He does not respond to the totality of what I have said but quibbles with my choice of words. "I don't think I was 'rescuing' her, just treating her. When someone has pneumonia, you give them antibiotics."

"Well," I said, "whether and how much to 'treat' is exactly the gray area in which we are headed. Maybe you *don't* use antibiotics. I am concerned about what happens when there is another event, another round. I am trying to understand the difference between 'treatment' and 'palliative care' or 'comfort care.'"

This is a distinction that he seems not to have thought much about, or maybe he doesn't want to talk about, or is not comfortable talking about. Treatment is treatment in his lexicon. Although Kate elaborates on the palliative care theme, it doesn't seem to go very far.

I ask if he is familiar with the "CHF protocol." He is not. In his view, it means taking the standard approach to edema, not a comfort care protocol for managing the end stages of CHF in a dignified way.

I come away feeling the meeting was pretty unproductive. Kate thinks he heard more of what I was saying than I do. I am glad she was there.

Back at the hospital on Wednesday May 7 after our "party" around Olwen's bed and my conversation with Kate, I still hadn't decided whether to go back to the city that night and keep the appointments I had made for myself in the post-project world I had once imagined for myself. Daylight-savings time and longer days make getting a late start more viable.

I finally decide to leave and come back in four days on Mother's Day. Either Olwen will have just moved or be moving the next day. I get things more together for rehab and leave notes for Sue in several places. Kate has given permission for Sue to have keys to Olwen's apartment and the front door, and I make arrangements for the pickup. When I leave on Wednesday, I don't know which of us will be taking Olwen's stuff over to rehab.

Thursday morning begins with a call from the social worker. Olwen will be discharged tomorrow. Damn! I arrange for Sue to bring things in early so that Olwen's room will be more personalized for her arrival and Sue can stay with Olwen for a while in the strange place.

A long e-mail from Mary Thursday evening affirms Olwen's growing strength. Mary writes that Olwen, who has hardly eaten at all these last two weeks, polished off a full dinner while reporting that, "the lunch was lovely" today. Mary observes a stronger, more alert and more cogent Olwen—now off the antibiotic by a good forty-eight hours:

> She looks almost like her old self. She kept asking questions about whether the doctor had authorized her discharge, if the nurses knew, who made the arrangements, who will be with her, where she's going, what she needs to do, what she should avoid doing so as not to jeopardize it, why she couldn't go home tonight, how fast the night would pass. She was too jittery to understand and remember most of the answers, so would keep asking the same questions. I tried repeatedly to prepare her for the fact that she wasn't going home to her own apartment yet, but was going to the rehab center for a while to build up her strength. Sometimes she seemed to understand and said, "Why do I have to go THERE? I'm feeling fine right now." Most times she would say, "So I'm going to 102 tomorrow."

With great insight, Mary notes that, "Olwen has the ingrained habit of feeling in charge of everything, so how could anything possibly go smoothly when she doesn't even know exactly what's supposed to happen?" Yes, I think, and that's why I implode during my visits and that's why I got shingles. Even when I am doing things for her that she can no longer do for herself, she still wants to know everything (which she then can't remember) and inserts herself back into the middle of the process, unraveling it, delaying it, going over and over it so it feels like nothing gets done or stays done.

∞

Olwen is discharged to rehab on Friday, May 9. Mary and Sue work out the logistics. We have been reminding her that Hugh is here, too. Hugh is a unique link to Olwen's mother and her own childhood because their mothers, both from Wales, were friends and neighbors until my grandmother died when Olwen was still in high school. His family's business is a funeral home, and Hugh's father buried Olwen's mother. Thus my mother's choice of funeral home for herself has been set since her childhood.

Hugh moved to Village Grove soon after my mother did, living on her corridor. He sometimes gave her rides, and they used to make their ear/hearing appointments back-to-back several times a year so that they could go together and have lunch.

Olwen is keen to see Hugh, and manages to see him this afternoon and again around supper when they talk awhile. She immediately concludes, however, that "Hugh is not doing well." In the days to come, she does not show much interest in visiting him again, and she cannot say why.

In the rooms of her being where her emotions are housed, it must be painful for her to see Hugh in this condition. Like her neighbors, she had held to the view that he would be coming back to Village Grove. That is the code they use when one of them is at the hospital or in rehab: "Will s/he be coming back?" or, "S/he won't be coming back." But during my April visit, I had asked Kate if Hugh would be coming back and the expression on her face said it all. When Olwen would state that, "Hugh is coming back, you know," I would say, "Honey, I'm afraid Hugh is not coming back." She uncharacteristically resisted taking in this news, but I know it settled in somewhere, and now she knows it from her own direct experience.

In the coming days, Sue tells me Hugh is talking less and that whenever they see each other, they wave and acknowledge each other, an image that tugs at my heart. Somewhere inside Olwen's remarkable being, she is both distancing from and dealing with the impending loss of Hugh in her own way while mobilizing her resources to get her own self back to Village Grove.

The afternoon of her admission, I talk to her day nurse and check her medications. I try to get her hearing-enhanced phone connected so she won't feel so isolated. They can't do anything until Monday. Damn! I get reports from Sue and Mary. So far things have gone well, more smoothly than we would have thought. Too smoothly, I think. I can't believe it.

My intuition is correct. At 7:30, the phone rings. Olwen is on the hall phone near the nurses' station. We talk for over a half hour. Her voice is strong with a lot of energy behind it. She is far more focused than she was in the hospital. I am elated by these improvements.

". . . So what will we do?"

"You are there to get stronger and see if your mind clears up some more so that maybe, we hope, you can go back go your apartment."

"Where is my apartment?"

"You know where it is because you've just been telling me. It's at 102 Main Street. Nothing has changed. Everything is still there."

"Where are you staying?"

"When I'm here in town, I stay in your apartment."

"Who else is in my apartment?"

"Nobody, just me." In the days to come, she will ask repeatedly, "Where is my apartment? Is it still there? Where are my things? Who else is there?" I try to address the underlying fears: that Kate has given her apartment away, and that it and her things no longer exist.

Whomever and whatever Olwen cannot see or handle physically seems to have less and less reality for her, and she doesn't go looking for things as much as she used to. I have come to suspect that one of the things that happens to an aging mind/brain is that the very existence of whatever is not immediately, physically present seems to erode. Loss of "object-permanence" may be the counterpart of learning it as a child.

Her laser focus on her apartment continues, "I want to go back to my apartment and live there for a short time." Another incisive statement about what she wants, and her recognition that time is getting shorter.

"Well, that's exactly what we're trying to help you to do."

"I can't go back there now?"

"You can't go there right now. That's what I have been telling you. That's what Sue and Mary have been telling you. I know it is very hard."

"I am believing your words."

"Well, good."

"Then what do I do? Because I am *not* staying here."

"Honey, I am very sorry you can't go back to your apartment right now, I wish you could. But now there are a lot of people involved in deciding where you can be. I don't have the power to take you where you want to go. I couldn't even get them to keep you at the hospital until Monday. Noyes' substitute dumped you in here today."

"What should I do about Doctor Noyes?"

"He is not back until Monday. I will call and tell him that he and I and Kate need to sit down and talk, okay? He does not include me in things. He thinks he's in charge of you. I think YOU are in charge of you, and I'm trying to be your advocate. Do you understand that?"

"Yes."

"Okay. I am trying to get the best situation for you, so that is why he and I need to talk. His way of practicing medicine is not the way the best people are doing things now. Now it's more of a partnership and a conversation among the patient, their family, and the medical people."

"I will do just what you say but how the hell am I going to do it?" Olwen never swears, so this question is startling.

"I don't know. You have incredible will power."

"I'm feeling fine now. I'm up and everything."

"I can hear that! I can hear how feisty you are! That's a good sign. You've come a long way in the last five days! There are people there with skills to help you get stronger and take care of you."

"I don't need anybody to take care of me. I'll stay on here and you tell me what to do, but my God, I should be able to say how I feel myself!" She never says "my God" either.

"Well, of course you should! I hope you are as outspoken when you see Noyes as you are being with me."

"Well, let's take care of it."

"We're trying. I'll be back there in a couple of days to make it work as well as we can for you, okay? The people who are supposed to work with you won't be around on Saturday or Sunday, and this is Friday night, so it is going to be boring for the next couple of days."

". . . giving me pills, and I don't know just . . ." Her voice trails off.

"I have told the nurses there that whenever you have been in the hospital, you have *always* challenged the pills. And I told them that I have always supported you in doing that." Olwen, as usual, has been decades ahead of the curve by personally interrogating the correctness and safety of her medications. "Right now, it is confusing because you have some new pills in addition to the ones you have taken for years."

"I'm leaving it to you. Otherwise, I would shoot myself."

"Well, you don't have a gun, so that's a good thing! Right now you are saying that you would like to have a little more time in this life, and you want that time in your apartment. Let that be our goal. That *is* your goal. The only way we can get back to your apartment is for you to show improvement with what you are able to do. So that's what you need to do in order to achieve your goal to get back to your apartment."

"All right then. What do you want me to do right now?"

"I guess try to relax, get sleep, and bear with it. I will be there in a couple of days. We'll get your phone hooked up so you can talk to me and Sue and other people from your room and not feel so cut off. Sue is coming over tomorrow and Mary will be over later in the day."

"I don't know how to do it, but I'll do the best I can."

"That would be the best thing to do even though it's hard. And you have done a lot of hard things in your life, and you've done them very well. This is another hard thing that you have to do. And you have made amazing progress in the last two or three days. You are starting to eat, you are starting to walk again, you're being really feisty. You've come a long way!"

"I don't know what to do. I thought if I was back at 102 Main Street everything would be fine." In retrospect, she may have been right while all the experts may have been wrong. "I'd like to be over there. What do you want me to do?"

"I'd like you to go along with the program as best you can. You won't always like the food, so just eat what appeals to you. You won't like every person, but most of them will be trying to help you."

"Okay, but I would like to see my house—102. I can't see it?"

"Well, we'll see about your seeing it. I think we have to get permission to go out."

"I would love to be at 102!"

"Of course you would!"

"And I can't go there, huh?"

"Not right now, but that's what I am trying to make it possible for you to do."

"Okay."

"Okay?"

"You'll get me over there, you mean?"

"I am trying to do that. I can't make it happen right now."

"What do you want me to do? What have I done that isn't right?"

"You haven't done anything wrong! It's just that you've been sick and have become less able to take care of yourself fully, and people want to make sure you are safe. That you are not going to put yourself at risk. So they have put you in a protected environment. Try and bear with this, give it a little time, give them a chance to work with you."

"I'll try and do it. What'll I do now?"

"Well, pretty soon you might want to go to sleep."

"It's now going on eight o'clock. I'll go to bed. I'm so tired."

"All right then, you go."

"Okay."

"Okay. I love you."

"Well, I thought you did."

"Well, I do!"

"Ay-yuh."

I talk with her nurse, summarizing our conversation, and ask if there had been a crescendo leading up to this phone call. She replies, "No, she's been very good until after dinner. She talked to Hugh for a while. When I said, 'Are you ready for bed?' she said, 'Oh, no, I'm not staying *here* tonight.'" Her nurse and I talk a bit longer and then she interrupts, "Oh, there she goes up the hall. She is walking, *pulling her wheelchair behind her!*"

"That's Olwen! That's the old Olwen! She's making another comeback!"

Four

Detour through Rehab: Buying Time and/or Losing Ground?

I am going to 102!!
—Olwen, May 12

When Mary visits on Saturday, Olwen is dressed in a teal blue outfit, sitting in her wheelchair, Grandpa's cane across her lap. She has wheeled herself right up to the edge of her room, with her feet in the main hallway. Mary asks if she is going somewhere, and Olwen says she doesn't know.

They enjoy the flowers and sunshine. Mary e-mails, "she noticed everything and asked good questions. When she gets tired and anxious, she tends to get mixed up; but when relaxed, she's very good." When the nurse comes to collect her for dinner, Olwen asked Mary not to leave. The nurse assured her she wouldn't be alone, there are many people here. "But I don't know them!"

On Mother's Day, I bring lilacs—our favorites—and an ultra-fine, white cotton top with a sweet neckline and gathered sleeves. She sniffs the lilacs when I bring them close, and seems to enjoy the feeling of the exquisite cotton.

I point out our route when I take her to the front lobby and outside, and encourage her to try it on her own. I assure her they will know who she is and where she belongs even if she doesn't know who they are or where she is. I can tell she is afraid she will get lost in this sea of strangers. This is the woman who for so many years drove by herself to all her daughter's apartments, even in Manhattan.

A ferocious thunder and lightning storm erupts and circles around us for hours. Lightning has always made her agitated, but now she pays no attention. I begin marking clothes, play tapes, and we hang out. When she is tired, I put her in a new pink nightgown, play one of the restful Native American tapes she likes with sounds of the forest, do some Reiki, and stay with her until she falls asleep. I talk with the nurses on my way out, and to Sue after I get in.

❧

When I return Monday morning, Olwen is sitting exactly where Mary found her on Saturday: in her wheelchair at the edge of her room with her feet in the hallway. As soon as she sees me, she announces, "I am going to 102!" Her voice is angry, defiant, purposeful, as is her body language.

She restates her intention several times, yet she is afraid to venture past the border of her room, and has evidently been waiting for me to take her there. She didn't just happen to reach the edge of her room as I arrived. She has no doubt been sitting like this at the edge of her little hallway for some time, agitatedly moving back and forth a few inches. I squeeze by to put down stuff I've brought for her, and we talk.

She is ferocious, energetic, determined, and single-minded about getting back to 102—NOW! Clearly her energy is stronger and can be self-directed and focused. I am very pleased.

Today there is no comprehension of why we have to wait, or that I don't control the decision-making. She is angry I haven't taken her home. It takes a good hour for her to come down from this anger-ferocity place and take in the idea that I am not in charge here, that we have to work with a lot of players and rules, and that they won't let her go home right now.

I have brought her bedroom chair so she and a visitor will each have a place to sit. She has only the wheelchair to sit in and the bed is alarmed. I begin working to get another chair from their inventory, the bed unalarmed, and her hearing-enhanced phone connected so it works with their phone system. The phone and alarm each turn out to be major projects that take a lot of back and forth with staff and a couple of days to resolve.

Until then, every time any of us touch the bed or Olwen moves in the bed, it screams. The bed alarm is completely counter-productive. It does not act as a deterrent to Olwen's getting up when she wants to go to the bathroom, so it does not protect her against falls. But it does deter her from lying down as often as she might—and she suddenly tires during the day—and it does deter visitors from staying for very long as they have no place to sit.

When I bring her home-made ice cream, she polishes it off. The food they bring she hardly touches, and I ask for the nutritionist to stop by.

The nutritionist is low-key, attentive, respectful, not at all rushed. Olwen is comfortable with her, tunes into the conversation, proactively participates, and answers the question being asked. What does she like for breakfast? "Shredded wheat and banana with low-fat milk." We rule out big, heavy meals and large portions. When the kitchen starts sending her favorite breakfast, fruit, a half-sandwich for lunch and dinner, and puts juice and Ensure in smaller glasses, she will start eating better and finishing her beverages.

Next I take up the issue of where she eats. I tell the nutritionist they've been taking her to the nursing station area. Those who hang out there all day or are taken to eat here are in pretty bad shape. Heads droop, hair is unkempt, few can participate in a conversation, and they wear hospital attire or sloppy-looking clothes.

The ostensible reason for bringing my mother down to the nurses' station to eat is to "see how she is eating." Presumably, one has to eat decently to "graduate" to the dining room.

"Well," I said, "*there's* a self-fulfilling prophecy! Bring someone like Olwen down to this depressing place, and why would she eat anything? If she won't eat while sitting under their noses, they conclude that *she* has a problem rather that the setting itself being a problem, and so won't let her out of there to sit with the grown-ups."

The nutritionist agrees the nurses' station is depressing, and Mother should not be taken down there to eat. She will tell the nurses to take Olwen to the dining room. I caution, however, that until this awful, antibiotic-induced diarrhea is over, it would be best if she could just stay in her room to eat because the bathroom is close by and she knows where it is. Agreed. I then work these same issues from the nursing end, and they also agree on all points.

Olwen brightened during our upbeat conversation with the nutritionist. I use it to reinforce the idea that even though she doesn't know the people here, they are trying hard to help her. "Soon you will start getting food that is more like at home. You won't have to sit in that depressing area down the hall to eat. Pretty soon, you will go to the dining room."

It's hard to say how much of this is making sense to her. Do my words float by her and away because she has no place to stash them?

Later in the afternoon, Olwen has three rounds of the most appalling diarrhea. The staff are slow to come each time or at all, the fan doesn't work in the bathroom, and I shove the window as far open as I can. What if I hadn't been here to help?

I try to reassure Olwen the diarrhea is only temporary, it will go away, it is due to antibiotics—the medicines she was taking only for a short time. She no longer understands what an antibiotic is, however, and I cannot find a way to make a separation in her mind between her regular meds and temporary ones. I am deeply frustrated by my inability to convey that this dreadful aspect of her current situation is going to improve fairly soon.

Mother is tired and starts to get herself ready for bed soon after supper. I help her, play music, and do soothing things like Reiki and putting lotion on her hands and feet which are so dry from the hospital. There is a lovely, quiet, intimate flow between us, more physical than verbal. She is receptive, quiet, taking in what is offered. Olwen is so rarely easy, always fussing, interrupting the moment, pushing back, but tonight she is simply in the moment, in the flow, and everything feels easy.

※

On Tuesday, May 13, Fran, who is head of social services, is back from vacation. She is also Olwen's social worker and visits her first thing. When I meet with Fran a couple hours later, it is obvious she likes Olwen and is impressed by her in many ways, beginning with her appearance, her dignity, and her independence. She seems particularly struck by Olwen's understanding that her daughter has a separate life, apparently a rarity among the residents. Olwen is quite lucid and interactive with her, clearly states her needs to be out of here, get back to 102, and not go on and on.

I am pleased but not surprised. Fran exudes warmth, caring, positive expectations, and, despite all she has to do, is not in a rush. She conveys that being with you in this moment is the only place she wants to be. We have a meaningful conversation about the Olwen that is and the Olwen that was, her situation, and her ability to look death in the face.

We turn to practical matters. "No feeding tubes." "We don't use them." "Dining room, not the nurses' station." "Absolutely." "No restraints." "We don't use restraints." "Let's get the alarm off her bed." "Yes." "Will she be able to take rides or have outings?" "As soon as she is assessed by physical therapy and they approve it."

Only after the fact did it register that Olwen had not yet been seen by PT, yet she had already been there four days.

"Do you have any idea how long Olwen will be here?"

"We'll know better when we have our case conference on the twenty-second. She is still weak and gets tired suddenly, but she is getting stronger. She can already get dressed by herself and do most of her self-care. She is confused about some things and clear about other things."

We explore post-rehab options. Given Olwen's current upward trajectory, Fran's sense and mine is that we need to think in terms of several months and perhaps even as long as a year. Fran strongly favors her returning to Village Grove if it is possible. "She has already been uprooted into two unfamiliar situations in the last few weeks. I would rather not see her put into yet another." I am relieved and encouraged.

A second option is adult care where you are relatively independent and must be able to pay for a year. A third option is an intermediate level of care which usually runs about 50% more than adult care. You can come in as private pay or on Medicaid.

Yet when I visit a couple of facilities and levels of care, I can barely distinguish them from each other or from rehab, and Olwen has already voted with her feet on that. Level-of-care distinctions evaporate when it comes to the physical environment, institutional lighting, institutional furniture, plastic floors, the mood, and the feeling of being trapped. Despite the cheeriness of staff and some tenants, the all-pervading ambience is that life is over.

When I get back to Village Grove, I am bowled over by how lively are its tenants even at a median age of eighty-seven and even on their walkers, and how upbeat and gracious is its atmosphere. I greatly miss the three beautiful Oriental rugs in the foyer, yet antique tables, wall sconces, Italian lamps, and the grandfather clock do wonders for the new, high-quality, wall-to-wall carpeting. Cherry dining tables, matching high-back chairs, real tablecloths, lamps on the sideboard, and wall sconces suggest a fine restaurant. Attractively upholstered sofas and living-room chairs, a grand piano that Olwen's ninety-eight-year-old friend and tablemate plays for holiday gatherings, and an exquisite, leather-paneled table in the library all create a warm, welcoming, elegant yet homey feeling.

While the spectre of death and dying is never more than a table or neighbor away, there is still sparkle in these old gals (and the few guys). Despite their age and being survivors of vast losses of friends, spouses, and, in many cases, of children, residents are still very involved in living day by day. Village Grove never feels like a place where people are just waiting to die.

The decision I make about where Olwen goes next entails weighing many risks and placing my bets. How long will she live? How will her dying process play out? Will there be major events, a series of little ones, or just a gradual ebbing away? How much will her needs escalate, at what points, and for how long will she need to be sustained at each level of care?

These uncertainties chew at my insides. When I am fresh in the mornings, I diagram possible scenarios, and in the evenings, I run the numbers.

We might just be able to squeeze under the wire for admittance to adult care right now. It would not leave anything for private help, however, and we are going to need Sue to prop up her sagging quality of life. Her needs are going to escalate, and we will need more help than Sue can offer, especially during and after future health events.

Even from a purely financial perspective, Village Grove, at one-third of adult care's costs, is the best choice *as long as* Olwen's needs don't escalate beyond eight hours a day, and *as long as* her life is measured in eight months or less. Big if's. If her situation escalates toward 24-hour care, we could handle that outflow for only a few months. Obviously, I would have to become much more involved and take on a lot of the care to slow down the hemorrhage of funds.

The image of having to suddenly vacate Village Grove and be applying for Medicaid in the midst of a seriously deteriorating or dying scenario (and handling the apartment liquidation on top of everything else) is too dreadful to contemplate. Equally dreadful is the image of having to sell my condo because my savings have been wiped out. The risks attached to the financial calculus and the spectres of future scenarios keep me awake long into the nights.

In considering options, my innards are gnawed not only by financial risks and visceral responses to adult care, but also by questions about how the people in charge or on duty would respond to another health event or acute episode, and the residential implications of a downward spiral that a series of events or gradual deterioration could generate. Would Olwen be allowed to deteriorate and die at Village Grove? Would Kate let her bring in the level of help she may need? Or would she have to be moved out at some point? What happens if she goes back to Village Grove next week and, as vets and doctors like to say, "gets into trouble" again? Would she again be dispatched in an ambulance to the hospital, and be sent off to rehab again?

It is hard to imagine her ever getting back to Village Grove after yet another round of hospitalization. The possibility of rounds of see-sawing between hospital and rehab is nightmarish.

Even if we become better able to define the gray area where treatment is scaled back and passes into comfort care, and even with advance directives and standing orders, some nurse or aide could still summon an ambulance and set the heroic machinery in process again. A friend who launched and ran an ambulance service with her husband has alerted me to the possibilities of such mistakes being made, and to the requirements that caregiving staff continue to do their utmost to "save" patients. "They would probably call for an ambulance and get her to the hospital. Only if she is a hospice patient can you be reasonably certain that they won't call an ambulance if the fluids build up and she starts to have trouble breathing."

We could better define the situation and move to comfort care by bringing in hospice to manage her case *if* they think she has six months or less to live. For hospice to take on medical management of her case, she would need a full-time caregiver and there is only one candidate: myself. Yet only if hospice is in charge can we be reasonably assured that should an emergency or new event arise, "comfort care" rather than "treatment" would be the operative guideline.

On Wednesday, May 14, Noyes shows up for weekly rounds. He hasn't seen Olwen in ten days and is impressed with her progress. Her edema is so good he cuts back the Lasix—so important for her quality of life. Her lungs are nearly clear. Her heart is behaving—no fibrillation—and her vitals are good. He prescribes Flagyl for the diarrhea, treating it as a trivial, expectable occurrence.

Why then didn't he leave standing orders for this expectable side-effect? In the absence of his standing orders, why wasn't Flagyl prescribed by his associate?

Noyes actually looks at me and smiles, and says she can go home—probably next week. His manner is still paternalistic and pseudo-jocular, however, and he refuses to engage seriously or respectfully with her statements about not wanting to hang around much longer and wanting to be done with it. "You're not at the head of the line yet, Olwen. You'll just have to wait your turn before you see St. Peter."

This is a replay of what happens during their office visits. Neither Sue nor I have ever observed him engaging seriously with her thoughts and preferences about death and dying. Nothing has changed despite the gravity of her last round of health events. Not to mention the years of non-reciprocal, first-naming that pervades his and most medical practice.

Olwen does not say much during his visit. She is not her feisty self but becomes quiet and expressionless. She does not respond expressively or verbally to anything he says or does. She does not even really look at him or make eye contact. She stares down vacantly at the lunch tray.

I am again reminded of how interdependent her responses are with the person creating the context. Olwen was lively and assertive with the nutritionist yesterday, answered her questions, and actually seemed to enjoy the conversation. She was alert, interested, fairly lucid, and held up her end of the conversation with Fran yesterday. I watched two nurses who snatched/created quiet time for a sustained period with her, and the interaction was not bad. Even though each of these four people was a stranger, Olwen did pretty well with them.

What did all of these professionals have in common? They were respectful of her as a person. They were present to the moment and conveyed no sense of being rushed or that they really needed to be somewhere else. They communicated an expectation that she was a mentally capable partner, and listened to what she said and let *her* concerns lead the conversation.

By contrast, Noyes exudes paternalistic, condescending authority, and that the important issue here is *his* precious time. It's all about him. It is evident that at a deep level, Olwen knows the difference and responds accordingly.

Thinking back on it now, I am even more struck by how person-dependent her demeanor was. Not that her synapses weren't failing or drug-impaired, but the other person's behavior, tone, style, and body language formed the context generating what officially passed as "her" behavior, *and this person-dependent context is absent from the official calculus.*

After Noyes leaves, I sit down opposite her, look right at her and say, "Dr. Noyes has given us three pieces of really good news. I want to make sure you understand them." She still has no expression on her face. She continues to stares off into space or down at her uneaten food. It's as if I have said nothing.

I ask her to listen because we have good news, but she keeps blocking her ability to hear the most wonderful news she could possibly get. Wherever she disappeared to while Noyes was here, she is still gone. She is not making eye contact, but commenting about the food or that she should have what I am saying down on paper.

After a while, she half-gets what it means to take less of the water pill, so I move on to the diarrhea. I tell her yet again that it is temporary, and now she will have a new pill which will help it go away sooner.

"How will I know it?"

"You won't have the problem. It will go away."

"But I have to take the pill."

"Yes, you take the new pill to help it go away."

"Uh-huh."

"Okay? So Noyes is saying what the nurses have been saying and I have been saying: this is a temporary problem."

"They're going to tell me that?"

"He just did. It will go away."

Then I focus on the really big news. "The third great thing is he thinks you can go home next week! That should have you jumping for joy. He said it with a smile on his face. He thinks you are going to be able to go home!! ... Do you understand that? ... You look totally forlorn."

"Yes, but ..."

"There is no happiness in your face."

"It's because I can't remember all these things. I can't remember four or five things."

"I'm telling you the best news you can hear. And you don't look happy."

"I'm wishing they were down on paper."

We continue in this vein for quite a while. I am starting to lose patience for the first time since all this began because she is/we are actually achieving her/our goal, and it isn't even registering!

Perhaps I should have just let her drift a while and recover from Noyes's visit before I started trying to reinforce the good news. Perhaps I should have started with the news about going home because by the time I got to that news, there were too many things to remember and I had lost her along the trail somewhere. Perhaps I should have started writing things down, very simply—one, two, three—right then and there. Why didn't I?

I had been observing the difficulty she was having in connecting written words with what they represent, and so I didn't think it would do a lot of good. I knew it was likely to lead to hours of going over and over each thing on the paper, and I had a four-hour drive ahead of me. I was in her face and pushing when I should have just backed off for a while. All the tension I had been carrying wanted to share a celebratory moment of release with her: We've done it! We're going to get you home! You are going to 102! Instead, she was caught up in her own world, blocking out what she most wanted to hear.

This contradiction flashed through my mind as a paradigm for so much in her life, its familiarity making me at once sad, frustrated, despairing, and irritated. The difficulty she has taking affirming stuff all the way in blocks not just big things, but extends into the capillaries of her life.

Take blueberries. Olwen has adored blueberries in any form all her life. Being Welsh, she also loves good scones. I would bring her wild blueberries, blueberry scones, the best of blueberry jams, blueberry ice cream. Of the scones which she liked very much, she did not say, "oh, good," but, "oh, they're so big." "Well," I would say in exasperation, "then cut them! Cut some of them in half and put them in the freezer."

Even such a simple "transaction" as this could not be completed easily and directly. Instead, we bumped into detours which denied her the pleasure of simply receiving, and me the pleasure of seeing her pleasure. Multiply the blueberry events by thousands of other such exchanges. It is so wearying and so sad.

I keep pushing, nonetheless, probably because while I am still here in person, I can try saying it different ways, observe her responses, and use body language to make my point. As I get more frustrated, I am probably making her more anxious, and then she doesn't process things as well as when she is relaxed. The more I try, the worse it gets. I'm doing this all wrong.

Fortunately, Sue arrives and listens. Olwen asks what she thinks. Sue is judicious, using different words to explain the same thing. Olwen still registers no joy, no response. I leave the room to give Sue a chance to triangulate things out of the rut I have dug.

I may head home this afternoon, which is no doubt contributing to my anxiety that Olwen "get it." Should I stay longer? The goals of this visit seem to have been achieved. I have met and talked with several of the key players in rehab, made important improvements to her situation here, gotten all the players on board for the next step, and unless something unforeseen happens, that next step is going to be the achievement of her/our immediate goal: Village Grove. We have changed the food she gets, she is starting to eat, her dining venue will improve, the bed is no longer alarmed, the phone is working, and she is beginning to learn how to use the phone.

What is the best use of my time? How do I balance what I do here this next week with what I can do for myself at home and what I will need to do for her in the unknown future? If this rehab tenure and getting her home and getting her reacclimated for a few days were going to be the end of it, then I should stay longer now.

I don't think we are at the end of anything, however, but at the beginning. There are going to be many trips, probably more health events and rounds, and I have to pace myself even though I don't know what I am pacing myself for. I don't know when or why or over what period of time those trips will be happening. Certainly my car must be in top condition and seeing my mechanic is at the top of my list for when I get back.

Most of the drive home is rainy, as my other drives have also been. I enjoy watching the ever-shifting patterns of clouds that range from white to black and every shade of gray, and the way the fog hangs in the valleys, hiding one hill from another.

Suddenly a rainbow appears, and I am driving toward it for the better part of an hour. The rain lets up, but the entire sky is still blanketed with clouds—except, finally, one tiny opening of blue appears straight ahead. Out of nowhere, a full moon appears in this blue aperture. Amazingly, the clouds leave this precise opening for an extremely long time, making the moon visible, framed by clouds, with the arc of the rainbow embracing the entire pictorama.

I take all this as a sign. "Trust the process. Everything will unfold as it should. Out of this darkness will come new birth, something transformative. I must, we must, trust the process."

Acutely aware this may be the last time for a long, indeterminate time in which I can concentrate and do any sustained work to move my work and life forward, I plunge back into my book proposal on May fifteenth, initiate a number of marketing threads, and take the car in.

I am also spending hours on the phone each day, placing over ninety long-distance calls to or about Olwen from May 15 to May 22. I am trying to keep her oriented, motivated, and feeling less alone in an alien place, and get her discharged to Village Grove as soon as possible. I am encouraging her friends, former neighbors, and church members to call or visit her.

Physical therapy is no longer covering her. Seeing how well she was walking, PT took away her wheelchair, and encouraged her to walk. This seemed precipitous to me because she gets tired very suddenly. What if, instead, she took her wheelchair with her, wheeling it along as she had that first evening, and could sit down when she needed to rest?

Rather than kicking her out of PT, why can't they gear their support to her real needs: to get out of her room on her own? They could do that by walking her routes with her three or four times a day, which would help build her strength and endurance and install a new habit so that she is more likely to attempt these outings on her own. Don't they understand how that mobility would make her feel less trapped, more empowered, more herself, more oriented? Or is it simply not possible to meet patients' real needs in a protocol-driven, Medicare-reimbursed world? If your needs don't fit the system's categories, forget it.

When occupational therapy gives her tests on the fifteenth, she is offended by their simplicity ("they had me doing all these funny little things and I did them all fast"). Sue says, "she wants to distance herself so much. She was mortified that they think she could not do these things. She is really angry at the people in OT." Olwen tells me on Monday, the nineteenth that, "I'm through with that and everything is fine."

Because Olwen is now being cut from OT coverage and will soon be cut from skilled nursing because she has been doing most of her own self-care right along, Fran calls me on May 20, ahead of the scheduled conference date. Her team believes Olwen does not belong in rehab any longer and is ready for the next level. We agree Noyes needs to cut the orders tomorrow when he is here on rounds so she is not stuck here over Memorial Day Weekend with me footing the bill.

Only later when I get Mother's rehab records do I fully realize how few services she got, and how her reality contrasted with the picture everyone had painted. She sat there for six days bored out of her mind because assessments, I later surmise, have to be ordered by one's physician before services are rendered, and Noyes was not there for rounds until the fourteenth. As far as I can tell, she got no real support from PT, and used OT services for only three days.

No wonder Olwen was angry and frustrated. She saw more clearly than any of us what was going on and what her situation was.

> *"I want to be done instead of string along, string along, string along! Why? Because they get more money!!"*
> —Olwen, May 18

Olwen's anger and frustration peak on Sunday the eighteenth. Thus energized, she makes a number of sharp, incisive, penetrating comments about her situation and she is crystal clear about her wishes to get out of rehab and off the merry-go-round.

"This room I am in is a very tiny room. I can hardly move . . . Why are they trying to keep me here? I am in good enough shape to be out of here . . . I went and took a nice long walk. I went to the beginning of this place. I do things like this just to keep myself going. I don't need to keep myself going; I'm all paid up, it's all taken care of a long time ago."

She is acting on her recognized need to keep herself going while in rehab by getting out of her room, and immediately juxtaposes that with the recognition that in a larger sense, she does not need to keep herself going because she has prepaid her funeral expenses, headstone, and her perpetual care at the cemetery. I have little difficulty tracking her changes in context or in supplying missing contexts, but a stranger might think she is contradicting herself.

Because I can provide the unstated changes in context, I find the ways her mind is working on multiple levels to be rather fascinating. She keeps choosing phrases which have layers of the "same" meaning, or whose words themselves form the connections among her thoughts.

She continues, "Most of the people around me just ride along all day long." Her imagery is vivid and dead-on. Knowing Olwen as I do, I have been certain from the outset that she has been constantly comparing herself with the people around her, and that she is recoiling from the idea that anyone could think that *she* belongs in the same place as *them*. I know it's hopeless to paint a distinction between people in rehab and those needing skilled nursing on an on-going basis, and to contrast those technical niceties with the *de facto* reality that they intermingle. She is sensibly marshalling her survival instincts by distancing. "Yes," I affirm, "you are in much better shape than most of the people around you."

"Of course I am! . . . Well, I can't go along living like this. I do not want to be here *period!* . . . I want to be done instead of string along, string along, string along. Why? Because they get more money!!"

Wow! This "confused" woman has seen through all the gauzy layers and right to the heart of the matter. I howl with laughter and compliment her.

After I recover, I say, "That's exactly what I am trying to prevent happening further. Your doctor has been rescuing your body when it says it wants to go. That just strings out the process, and it's very hard on you, and it's what you have told me all my life you don't want. We have to stop him from continuing to do that but make sure you are at all times comfortable. That's what I am trying to do. Does that make any sense to you?"

"Comfortable!!?? Comfortable is not lying here thinking that I don't want to be here! I am ready to go, and I want to go, period! I have had it over and over, and I'm tired of it."

"I am trying to make your wishes happen in the real world."

"I'm sure you are."

"You shouldn't be fixed anymore, you should be allowed to go. I am trying to get everyone on board with this, but it is difficult."

"Well, I'm sorry, but I'd rather have that be taking your time and just getting it over with. It's long enough, and the weather is good now, and it would be a good time. I just don't want to go on and on and on and on. A couple of days ago I walked a long ways, and I was so tired, and I got back and I thought, 'gee, my bones are doing pretty well, but I don't want them to break and be in the hospital again,' because I don't want it. I want out, not for you, but for myself!"

"Yes."

"I've lived long enough, and I don't want to keep on going. I don't want to be in this horrible, weasy little room I'm in here."

Where she pulled up "weasy" from I don't know but I again roar with laugher at her immaculate choice of words. "That's a great description! A perfect choice of words!"

"I just—I am ready to go, dear."

"I know you are, dear, I know you are, you're right. And I am trying to make it possible for nature to take its course rather than intervening to hold you back. In the meantime, I really hope you will find a way to get out of your weasy little room today and take another walk."

What Olwen achieved during her incarceration in rehab, she did on her own. She mustered her willpower and last reservoirs of strength to escape from her weasy little room. She did this *despite* OT and PT, not because of them or even with their help.

In fact, I should not have been repeating to Olwen the bill of goods I had been sold. In fact, Olwen's direct experience of the irrelevance of these services to her situation was the one truc thing in all this. For someone who was "confused," she revealed laser-like perception about their irrelevance and the reason why she was being "strung along" in rehab: because there *is* money to be made here. *Of course* she was dismissive toward OT and PT. Whatever the reasons she articulated, she understood at a deep gut level that they were not doing anything for her, and she did not really need what they offered.

Which is not to say she didn't need something they might have provided. She did, but she didn't get what she needed.

What she needed was a patient-centered approach and what she got was driven by protocols shaped by regulatory agencies and financing mechanisms.

What she needed were multiple, short sessions daily from Day One, and what she got was left alone in her weasy, little room.

What she needed was help with disorientation and the mental side-effects of drugs and being in one alien environment after another, and what she got on this account appears to approach zero.

What she needed was targeted interventions for her whole self.

As her situation continued to unfold, it became more and more evident to me that she had not gained anything in rehab; in some ways, she actually lost ground. All the more amazing she got out of there. Too few frail elders ever make it home.

Five

Getting Mother Home— but Can We Keep Her There?

We'll know in a week or so.

—Kate, May 20

Fran is encouraged Olwen can follow verbal directions, but has some concerns about her "confusion." Even so, she still favors her returning to Village Grove and that will be her recommendation to Kate and to Noyes.

I discuss options with Kate. She agrees to Olwen's coming home but anticipates she will need more help. "Let's try her at home and see how it goes. We'll know in a week or so." Her last statement catches my ear. I wonder: How could we possibly know anything so soon? Kate knows much more about these things than I do, however, so I note her statement and store her words in an empty memory slot.

Even though Kate, Noyes, Fran, and others are gearing toward Olwen's return to Village Grove, I am privately uneasy. It is still too soon to tell (especially in this alien setting) what she is going to be able to handle, but I am noticing changes that do not bode well for independent living even with increasing levels of support.

Although she knows in her bones what to do (to make or receive a phone call, for example), she cannot describe her actions. She cannot always connect written and sometimes even verbal instructions to an action that implements them. Only her immediate physical situation is real. Absent realities do not sustain themselves. Her sense of sequencing and how much time has elapsed is diminishing. The present moment is her overwhelming reality. She is not really *in* the moment, wherein one brings one's entire, self-aware being into connection with one's situation or other people, but she *is* the moment.

What underlies these difficulties is hard to disentangle. How much is hospital-and-drug-induced delirium and disorientation? Might it lessen in her home environment as the chemicals erode? Have these nearly four weeks in two institutions accelerated incipient dementia? Have her systems and organs begun to fail to a degree that toxins are building up, fogging her brain?

On Thursday, May 22, I head off for the third trip this month, this time to bring Mother home to Village Grove. After spending time with her at rehab and double-checking with the nurses that everything is set for tomorrow, I bring home her bedroom chair and some of her clothes. Sue meets us at rehab Friday morning, and off we go for our triumphant return to 102.

After we get into her apartment, Olwen looks around a bit, and heads directly to the places where she keeps her pocketbook and little stashes of cash. Satisfied with what she finds, she settles into her recliner chair in the living room and says to me in a calm voice with only the slightest hint of puzzlement, "I thought it would be a yellow house."

I am completely dumbfounded. She is finally here at 102, but doesn't fully recognize it. She does acknowledge, "it looks similar to our place," and does seem to know exactly where things are and where they should be. She also observes, "this looks very nice."

I am wracking my brain to think of any yellow houses that might represent "home." I think of two, one belonging to Elizabeth's family where Olwen lived after her mother died, and one in Florida belonging to her friend Ginny and her husband who insisted she winter with them, which she did for twenty-five years until Ginny died nineteen years ago. Neither house rings a bell for her. Of Ginny she says, "long time since I've seen her."

I observe, "You seem to know where things are here." She immediately says, "yes." "Have you been here before?" After a long pause, "Yes, I think so. When we drove up, I thought it wasn't just what I was looking for."

I am glad Sue is here because I need to collapse somewhere by myself for a while. All the tension and anticipation of the past three weeks that was supposed to reach a moment of shared triumph and satisfaction has just flipped off in another unexpected direction.

We've done it. We've gotten her out of the weasy little room she despises. We've gotten her home, the first big step on her journey Home. We've done it together, as a team, with her stubbornness and willpower marshalling her deepest reservoir of resources and my orchestrating the sets of players and rules who now have so much control over her fate. Yet she cannot herself fully savor the fruits of our work, and we cannot fully share this moment in the ways that I would have hoped and had expected.

I weep for all she has lost and is losing, and what it portends for her future and mine as well. If she lives for many months or even a year, how can we possibly keep her at Village Grove for the duration? Not only did rehab not do anything for her, but, it is now beginning to appear, she actually lost ground while there.

Later, when I can think about such things, I realize her drumbeat about getting to 102 was concentrated during the transition period and her first week in rehab. Sue, Kate, and I had been uncertain about her making a visit to her apartment (what if she refused to leave? what if her distress got worse?), but now I think a visit might have anchored its eroding reality. Once again, Olwen was right.

I go downstairs. Kate is in her office and welcomes me. I uncork.

With no problem, Olwen finds her way to Kate's new office. Though she has lost weight and muscle, her energy, agility, and alertness are almost like her prehospital self. We focus on what she might like for food. She wants small portions of any dinners. Sherbet, fruit, and cottage cheese have appeal. She can have dinner sent up to her room or come downstairs. She opts to stay upstairs tonight.

Mother continues to behave inside her apartment as if it is *her* apartment because she knows where everything is. She is obviously pleased to be sitting in her recliner chair again, her command post as I called it when we set it up six years ago with essential things within sight and reach on either side of her. We return her picture of her mother to its rightful place on the marble-top coffee table.

After a rest, she is keen to go up to the cemetery. I take the usual route to Florence's grave, then Elizabeth's, and then to our place. On Saturday, we repeat the process. We don't get out of the car because it is raining. Later it becomes evident Olwen isn't satisfied, and doesn't really feel she has even been there.

I finally figure out the problem. My route is now too circuitous and somehow, our place hasn't registered. We need to drive directly to our lot. I do that on Sunday.

The sharp approach to our lot from the road is now too steep for her, so we stand in the road with the sun shining directly on her headstone and her mother's. Olwen stands there looking right at them, reading aloud what is written, taking in the entire scene. For the first time since this all started, she is fully engaged. Her body language is strong, erect, sure of herself. "This is where I'll be, right next to Mama."

This time it is right, it is perfect, and, I recognize in that moment, this is it. Something has connected, permanently locking in place for her. What she needed from coming up to the cemetery is now done and she is deeply content. Her anxiety and uncertainty have evaporated and her full self is present to this moment.

I know that we do not really have to come up here again. We will, but our subsequent trips will in a way be superfluous because she will have gone past this moment. Every time I have been to the cemetery since, I remember this moment with her, this image of her standing in the road looking so bravely and with such satisfaction and sense of completion at her eternal resting place.

※

Over the next few days, I drift into the slow place of life here and am a quiet presence to Olwen's reacclimating to her life and her space. Every day I take her for drives. I am trying to help her reorient, but mostly I want to get her outside. She does pretty well with the streets and where things are in relation to each other. "My house was up that hill ... the school is way down the other end of this road ..." The hills and trees are all shades of spring green, and she always loves going up and down the hills.

Saturday we go for a drive to visit with the niece of my favorite teacher who died ten days ago. We sit as always in the huge cozy kitchen overlooking the gardens and steep hill, all acutely aware of her absence, none of us sitting in her spot.

Olwen remembers on her own that the niece is from the West Coast. I find this amazing as she has met her only once, last Christmas, when they had a long, animated conversation. Being in company like this in a familiar setting and being the center of admiring attention is clearly affirming for Olwen.

I am disappointed I could not come up "between trips" for the memorial service, but the niece tells me about a dinner on June 5 at which her aunt is to receive a lifetime achievement award—an award about which she knew and was thrilled, and which will hereafter bear her name. I note the date in my book. Who knows?

By Sunday the twenty-fifth, Olwen is looking forward to going down to dinner. I let her friend and tablemate Helen know. Helen has really missed Olwen at dinner, and had told her so in a note on special stationary with the red Welsh dragon on it. I walk Mother down early, and Helen comes down early, and the two old Welsh friends catch up with each other.

―――✂―――

Noyes has reduced dosages, so I am cutting old digoxin and Lasix pills in half. Mother takes digoxin only on alternate days now, and her Coumadin alternates between four milligrams and two milligrams; one is pink and one is blue. Even with only four-to-six pills total, the alternating rhythms require more concentration to set up the pillbox than before, a fact I point out to Sue. As our fixed point of reference, I mark the wall calendar as to which are digoxin days and which are four-milligram-Coumadin days.

Last week I found a digital atomic clock which tells the month, date, day, and temperature as well as the time. If Mother could match up the day on it with the day on the pillbox, maybe she could quasi-manage her pills?

Although she can read and understand all the separate information offered by the clock, I now doubt she can or will use it to always check what day it is, let alone match it to the right day on the pillbox. She is much more interested in the control buttons on the back, buttons she does not understand but with which she insists on playing.

The pillbox itself is presenting problems. Not every day has the same number of pills. This is new, and she is bothered by it. "How can it be right?" she keeps asking. The different colors of the Coumadin also bother her. Yet on her own, she is still opening one box, today's, and taking her pills in the morning. She may not finish taking all of them, however. Someone will need to check that she has taken all of her pills for the day and coax her until she does.

Sue does this when she is here. This coming week she can see Olwen every day, either in the morning or in the evening and can spend much of the day and evening on Friday.

A companion agency owner graciously meets with us over Memorial Day Weekend. Olwen warms to her and they have a good chat. I decide to start the companion on Tuesday with a couple of hours daily in the late morning or early afternoon. With a potential life span of 6-12 months with who-knows-what escalation in care needs, I need to manage the money very carefully.

Monday May 26 is a particularly lazy and pleasant day for us, and that ease continues despite the fact that Olwen feels a pain in her chest. Later she says, "I almost didn't tell you, then I thought I had to tell you." "Well, I think it's good that you did." After a while she recognizes it is a familiar pain around her left rib cage. I call Noyes anyway. When he calls back, we decide it is the recurring problem of tenderness and pain she gets from the pacemaker leads as there is less and less muscle mass to support it and them.

In the meantime, I get her to rest on the couch where I do Reiki and we flow through a profound conversation—assisted, I now see, by my frequently repeating the words she had just spoken. I ask her if she wants to go to the hospital and she is firm, "No! I don't want to go to the hospital. I think it's come to the point where it's long enough. We know it can't get great again."

"No, it can't get great again, we know that."

"I've paid for everything so it's all taken care of. I want the end of it to come. I want to get along with it."

"A faster ending is easier than a long, lingering, declining ending."

"Yes!" She is emphatic in her agreement. Connections between her readiness to get on with dying, her peace of mind from having taken care of her funeral expenses, and yesterday's completion of her emotional and spiritual work in relation to the cemetery are all evident. "This isn't the first time it's done this" (referring to the pain), "but it was hurtful, and at the time I thought, 'Oh, I've gotten that all taken care of.' This time we went to the grounds and right to where they were and stopped right there."

"Yes, we did this time."

"Uhm-hmm."

"We took a direct route this time."

"Uhm-hmm."

"And you liked that."

"Yes."

"So that's what we'll do from now on, just go there directly."

"Uhm-hmm. And I think, this is it. This is long enough. I am not going to try to pull out of this like I have some of the others." It is only months later when I am transcribing this tape that I realize she did not say, "I am not going to pull out of this like I have some of the others," but, "I am not going to *try to* pull out of this."

She continues, "It's better that I'm gone. Of course it is. Causing you lots of problems to begin with. That's enough. You can't go on like this forever. And I don't want to. I don't want to. It can't be great again. So you know now just how I feel about it. And it's all paid for."

"Yes, it's all paid for."

"And the stone. I saw the stone."

"Yes, you saw the stone."

"We went right to the place yesterday."

"We went right to the place yesterday."

"And that's good."

"That's very good."

"So."

"You took care of all that a long time ago."

"Probably it's much more expensive now than it was."

"To be sure."

"But it doesn't change? It's still paid for?"

"You bought the CD, and it's invested and builds up interest, and the interest stays in the account. This kind of account gets a much better rate of interest than we are getting in general these days."

"So it's growing bigger." She's drawn out the logical conclusion! Still following the implications when it comes to money. Accounting and practicality are in her bone marrow.

"So it's growing and it has stayed ahead of their increases in costs. Because their costs have gone up quite a bit. I went over this with the guy from the funeral home a couple of weeks ago, and there's plenty of money for everything."

"How much money is there?"

"You bought the CD for $2800 about fifteen years ago. Now there is over $5000 in the account."

"I'm glad to hear it."

"That will cover all the funeral expenses and there will be enough for your memorial service."

"Well, I'm glad I was smart enough to do this."

"I am, too."

"I'm a smart girl."

"You're a smart girl, definitely!"

Once again I am torn about whether to leave this evening or tomorrow. Her lucidity, logic, and ability to make connections or draw inferences is stronger than in any of her recent conversations. I am encouraged by this, and hope that it portends her making some improvement in her home environment. Eventually I head back when it is going on six o'clock.

※

Sue comes over Tuesday morning after Olwen tells her she has been up all night and can't find her glasses. Sue is startled to find Olwen is not dressed and her bed is not made—a first on both accounts. Sue and the companion find her confused, and both observe her being able to cover her confusion when downstairs or outside with other tenants.

Wednesday morning, Kate calls to express concern for the first time about Olwen's walking, and wants someone to walk her down to dinner and back up from dinner. I ask the companion to come back at three o'clock and take Olwen down to dinner at five, and Sue can get there in time to bring her upstairs. Olwen and Sue call me Wednesday evening after dinner. Olwen tells me she doesn't like the companion and that, "I don't want her around," so that's that. I call the agency owner to try someone else.

During this same call, Olwen tells me that she is "not in good shape" and that she is "feeling very weak. I'm not myself." Sue confirms Kate's observations that Olwen is having a little trouble with her walking.

Sue can cover Thursday dinner and Friday dinner and evening. I will try to work out a longer-term solution and return Saturday, earlier than planned. During these few days at home, I am getting a cell phone and my hair cut, seeing my chiropractor, and putting the air-conditioner into my study, but my top priorities are car repairs and converting Hi8mm tapes to VHS format.

Olwen has expressed repeated interest in a birthday party, and always wants to know about the cats and if things are still the same at my house. "How are my rugs doing?" With a friend's camcorder, I had made a slow tour around my house highlighting family pictures, ancestral objects, and Olwen's things. I had also taped the party and captured the spectacular acrobatics and kitten play of the first of my new cats. These videos are ways of assuring her that I am "settled" and will be okay because I have extraordinary friends and have created a home that is warm and alive and integrates the ancestors into the fabric of my life. It gives her a preview of how she will be remembered and honored in death.

Thursday, Sue reports Olwen continues to complain of nausea from the medications and sometimes resists taking them. In the house, Olwen holds onto the edge of the dining room table and the backs of chairs as she makes her way from her command post to the bathroom or bedroom. Photo albums have become too heavy for her to manage in her lap. She is lethargic, but she made her bed this morning.

When Sue arrives early on Saturday, Olwen is not dressed and her bowl of shredded wheat is soggy. Olwen is intermittently nauseated and alternating between being hot and cold. She has no fever, but is fanning herself so Sue turns up the big Vornado fan which pulls air through the entire apartment. Olwen is anxious, confused, and wants answers right away to any question, a pattern that alternates with falling asleep. She is weaker, and for the first time, having a bit of trouble getting out of her chair. Her lower abdomen is tender to touch, but the problem is not constipation. Sue calls Noyes, fills him in, and asks what he thinks of Compazine to suppress the nausea. He concurs and stops the digoxin for a few days.

On the drive up, I talk to Sue several times and to Olwen when she is awake. She is eating and drinking in small amounts. The Compazine seems to be helping her to feel more comfortable. Sue says that Olwen is worrying about what to wear and speaks of getting her clothes out to "be ready." We note the meaning of her statement. After my arrival, we compare notes for a few minutes and Sue goes home.

This agitation does not feel like an extension of Mother's life-long patterns of worrying or the anxiety that surfaced in recent years as she had less and less to do and no car. It feels like it is being driven by a body that is failing and thereby clouding her mind. She does or says the same thing over and over. Many of the actions seem to have no purpose.

By eight o'clock, she is telling me how tired she is, and I put her to bed. For the next hour, she keeps repeating how tired she is, and that, "I gotta go to sleep," but she keeps getting up and doing things that keep her awake. "How will I go to sleep?" she asks more than once.

My suggestions are useless. I resort to bribery, promising her, "If you go to sleep now and get some rest, you'll be more able to enjoy our special movies tomorrow, okay?

"I'll try. I hope I can do it, dear."

"Don't make it something you *have* to do. I brought them as a way to *reduce* your anxiety. You say you can't remember how my apartment looks. I wanted to be able to show you so you could see it for yourself, okay? I thought that would be one little thing that would be more settled for you, yeah? Do you understand what I am saying?"

"My throat is getting dry again."

She is also hot, and takes covers off and puts them back on again in the same minute. I have brought my small fan for the bedroom which helps circulate the air. A third Compazine does quiet her, and she is finally able to go to sleep.

Sunday, I awaken at six to find Olwen in her chair in the living room. She is hungry. I make her cereal and banana and bring her a small glass of chocolate Ensure. I don't know if she finished them because I fell asleep again, and she had washed the dishes before I woke up!

When she is in an alert phase, I take her upstairs to the solarium to see some of the tapes which she watches with fascination. For this adventure, I have enlisted the old wheelchair that someone left in the tenants' storage area long ago. I make a game of it, running behind her down the hall so we can go fast. She likes that.

On the way out, she reaches for her keys in a tiny leather box on the top shelf of the bookcase we use for kitchen storage, pushes the elevator buttons, and later returns the keys to their special place—bits of important independence I will caution every caregiver to abide by and support. I had anticipatorily set up such a place a couple of years ago, hoping she would establish a key habit that would stick. She did and it does.

Sunday night and Monday morning I work on leads for used wheelchairs and walkers, becoming aware of their many features and variations. Would she even have the upper body strength to use a walker? I suspect not. Olwen has in just days gone from walking virtually unaided (Grandpa's cane is more a prop than a necessity) to needing a wheelchair for outings.

I set up a time on Monday to replace her recliner chair which has been wearing out for a long time, but she has refused to buy another. One of Sue's clients has recently given her a virtually new lift chair, and she wants to loan it to Olwen. No more heavy lever to pull to get the footrest up or down. It has an electronic control with one button. Push it one way and it pushes you up from a sitting to nearly standing position—something that Olwen is just starting to need this weekend—while automatically retracting the leg rest. Push it the other way, and it takes you from standing to sitting while still in contact with the chair so you don't fear it won't be there to support you—something she is going to need.

I have arranged with a high-school friend's brother to come over midday to help us make the swap. We ooh and aah over the new chair and let Olwen try it out and begin to learn the new control. She only has about an hour to play with her new chair and enjoy its plush rose-colored fabric and firm seat before we are due to see Noyes at 2:45.

It is finally a beautiful, sunny day so I wheel her down the street to his office. She likes me to run so she can go fast.

He listens to her heart and hears fluid building up again. He puts her on oxygen there and then. He wants to talk outside. I tell her I will be right back.

We stand in the supply pantry. She needs to be on oxygen, she may be retaining urine, and he wants to put her in the hospital immediately. As always, he exudes impatience. He expects immediate compliance.

My mind is trying to grapple with what he has said and all its implications, and my whole being is shouting to myself, "No!! No more hospitals!! She doesn't want that!" What about alternatives to hospital? He offers none. Can I manage her at home with support? "It would be too hard. You can't possibly do that." Besides, he adds, "Kate doesn't want to run a nursing home over there." How long does he think she would be in the hospital? A few days. I am spinning. He is impatient. What can I pull out of this for her? "No ambulance. I will drive her." He agrees, somewhat reluctantly.

I go back into his office where she is sitting quietly in the wheelchair hooked up to some oxygen. She looks so dear, so trusting, so sweet. I tell her that she needs oxygen and some help with fluids building up, and that although neither of us want any more hospitals, we don't seem to have a choice this afternoon. I tell her how sorry I am that I can't keep her out of the hospital today, but that at least she won't have to go in an ambulance. I will get the car and drive her down. I will be back in a few minutes.

It is hard to leave her there, but I tear out of his office walking-running toward Village Grove. The sidewalk seems like it is spinning right up and will crash into my head. My mind is exploding and imploding. I am supposed to be going to get my car, but I am grasping for hospital alternatives. Kate's words come crashing back through the din, "We'll know in a week or so."

It is evident Mother is not going to make it on her own. Her body has begun a downward spiral and cannot be sustained without oxygen and other props. She is not, as she herself said so clearly to me a week ago, going to pull out of this one—or try to. The time line has just shortened. We don't have a year or anything close to it. She is beginning to die.

Part II

Creating Space for the Dance to Unfold

It's come to the point where it's long enough.
We know it can't get great again.
—Olwen, May 26

Six

Hospice: Shifting the Paradigm

> *You can't do this, dear.*
> *It's too much. It's too hard.*
> —Olwen, June 3

I stride right past my car in the Village Grove lot and into the building to look for Kate. She is just coming out of a meeting and is having quick moments with people who want to see her. I catch her eye and exaggerate the motion of my mouth so she can read my lips: "I need to see you—*now!*" Within two minutes we are seated in her office.

I pull two questions out of this crisis. Can we find any alternative to hospital this afternoon? Can I bring in hospice to support her dying at home?

Yes, I can bring her home to die. The aging of tenants has led to serious conversations among Board members about its philosophy and policies. Kate herself is an advocate for the Aging in Place philosophy the Board has adopted. That does not mean everyone gets to die at home or that no one is ever asked to leave. It does mean residents can bring in support that may turn out to last a period of years and potentially expand to 24-hour care. An event or precipitous decline may, however, finally (or sometimes suddenly) lead to a transfer, either to a hospital or a nursing home.

Kate cannot find a way to avoid hospital. Noyes' office tells us to use the ER entrance, go to admitting, after which Olwen will go directly to the third floor. When we arrive, there is a snafu due, apparently, to the way Noyes communicated the orders. We must go back downstairs and be admitted through the ER, and they can't guarantee this room, or

/ 95

indeed any room, even though it is available at this moment and the staff are ready for and expecting her. What!!?

The ER people have no rooms so they put her on a gurney in a curtained area and start an IV line. No one knows anything or tells us anything.

A guy is brought into our area, and I have a difficult time containing myself over his endless whining to his wife and daughter about how cold it is. He just goes on and on and on and never shuts up. Here is Olwen, nearly twice his age, stoic, dignified, courageous, and uncomplaining about *real* health problems that portend the end of her life, and here is this overindulged man behaving like he is the center of the universe.

I manage to be very attentive, calm, and reassuring for Olwen, holding her hand, talking quietly but close to her ear. At the same time, I am watching her heart rate skip around on the monitor. She knows I won't leave her except for moments to try to get information and get something moving. I speak with a nurse about the guy carrying on a few feet away. I again request a room as soon as something becomes available. She nods on both accounts.

They find us a little room in the early evening. It is not a patient room as it holds some supplies, but it is private, dark, and quiet. Exactly what a patient really needs yet the very antithesis of standard hospital rooms.

I control the lighting in this little room and put a sign on the open door to please not switch on any big lights unnecessarily. The nurse who comes to check on Mother and those who come for supplies abide by my request. We do everything in semi-darkness, and for the first time in days, Olwen is sleeping and not restless. Sometimes she comes up into a more conscious state, we say important things, and she drifts off again. I nap with my head on the bed, always in contact with her. Her heart rate has come down, but is still skipping around.

I am afraid to leave (what if she dies tonight?), but my stronger intuition is she will get through this round, and may be able to get the best night's sleep she has had in a long while. I leave sometime after eleven. The abysmal documentation for my new cell phone prevents me from retrieving messages from empathic friends. My frustration knows no bounds. I sleep surprisingly well.

Tuesday morning, Olwen is still in her little dark room so conducive to sleeping and to private conversations. She has slept well, her blood is more oxygenated, her heart is behaving, and our conversations show she is alert and tracking. I tell her I have something important to talk about. I take the ideas in small chunks and pause frequently.

"Hospice will come and see us tomorrow. Hospice means you will never have to go to the hospital again, and you will never have to go to that place with the weasy little room . . . No more treatments, no more hospitals, no more antibiotics, no more rehab. We are just going to be at home and keep you comfortable no matter what . . . You won't be hooked up to any machines. The air quality will be lovely and under our control. *You* will have privacy. *We* will have privacy.

"Hospice also means I will be staying with you most of the time. A hospice nurse will come every day, but not for too long. I will need to find other caregivers because I will need breaks and I will need help . . . We will all work together to manage your symptoms at home. You will never be alone . . . We can respond to your needs right away. If you are hot or cold or thirsty or need to go to the bathroom, we can help you right away.

"So, instead of pushing this tired old body to keep going, the comfort care route is simply to treat your symptoms and make you comfortable, make sure you have no pain, that you can breathe okay, that you don't get bedsores, and there will *always* be someone with you."

She lies there, listening. The first thing she says is, "You wouldn't be making any money for yourself." Quintessential Olwen! Ever pragmatic, and ever concerned about me even when we are deciding how and where her own dying will take place. Clearly she is tracking the practical implications of home care.

"I've let go of that because this is more important. There is plenty of time for me to make more money and get my book out, okay? This is much more important: your life, your dying process is VERY important to me. I want it to be as good as possible. I know you want that. So that's what we're gonna do."

"This isn't the kind of life you have been living."

"We're not going to be doing this forever."

"You've got your own home down the line there. What would you be doing—running back and forth? It would never work."

"I've got it all arranged. You are incredible! Here *you* are worrying about *me!* Even now! That's one of the incredible things about you!"

Undeterred, she stays on her own track and ignores how amazing she is being. "I don't think it would work. To begin with, there wouldn't be any money coming in."

"I showed you a big check a couple of days ago. I just got paid a whole chunk of money for the work I did. That work came along at just the right time. Now I can spend time with you and help you to do what you say you want to do, which is to let go of this life and let go of this body. But we'll do it at home, at your place, okay?"

"It sounds good but you wouldn't be living here, you'd be back and forth, it would be a miserable business, and you would get tired of it. You can't do this, dear. It's too much. It's too hard."

Here she is, almost ninety-nine, having now inflected into dying, and she is still thinking like a mother, trying to take care of me! And, once again, her words bespeak her grasp of the heart of the matter. The double meaning of "too much"—too much for me to do, too much for her to accept—is not lost on me.

Is she, as she so often is, right? Or is she "doing an Olwen"—removing the potential for future disappointment by pre-empting my decision at this great fork in the road? If I don't try, I can't fail her or myself. This morning I am so naively confident that failure seems impossible. I need that confidence to override her sensible caution.

"I hear what you are saying. It is an incredible response! Most people would leap at the chance. Here you are, thinking about me, and I'm very moved by that. I am thinking about both of us, and what it is you want, what you deserve. You've worked very hard to stay independent. You got yourself out of the hospital, out of rehab, and back home, and you deserve to end your days in your own home. That's what we want for you."

"I would say this. I think your idea was a good one to try and do, but it would be too much to really do it. No, it wouldn't work. And it's not a very clean job."

"Maybe not in a physical sense, but there are other dimensions. Emotionally and spiritually it is very profound. It is not easy, but it is profound and important. Some of us think it is a great privilege to attend the dying. I would like to give you this. It's so hard to give you things because it's so hard for you to receive things.

"I think we'll have to go the other way, dear."

"I don't think so. Besides, there *is* no other acceptable way. All other options involve hospitals, nursing homes, and going through more rounds of treatment, dragging out the process. You would be alone a lot of the time. People wouldn't come when you needed them." I detail how it would be. "We know that is not what you want. It is not what I want for you. So there really isn't any other choice. We've been a great team. This will be our last team effort together."

We talk quietly about all this for some while. I close the conversation by saying, "You think about this. You let it turn over in your mind. Tomorrow the hospice people will come and visit us here. I think you will find there is no alternative that is acceptable."

It has come to pass that I am about to embark on the heretofore unthinkable: moving in with mother. The choice is driven partly by logic. Because Olwen knows "it can't get great again" and that the longer she lives, the worse it will get, she does not want to keep going on and on. If we are to meet her twin goals of "finishing up" while also avoiding a nursing home, I have to get her out of the clutches of the fix-and-cure medical establishment and into palliative care, and have a lot more control over her situation than I do now. The only choice is to bring in hospice, and I feel blessed to have the choice, even though it means my taking on the monumental responsibility for her 24/7 care.

What really drives my choice is the profound love that knits together our tremendously complicated, intense, and challenging relationship. Through thick and thin, Mother has always been there for me, and I want to be there for her through this lonely, awesome, frightening passage into the unknown. She has never asked for much (at least directly), but I know how overwhelmingly important it has always been for her to have a good death and not end up in a nursing home. By choosing this hospice/home care route, I can make this possible. It will be my final gift to her. Now that her defenses are melting, I have some last chances to get across how much she is loved, how worthy she is of being loved, how much she means to me, and what a difference she has made. The die is cast.

Later in the day, Olwen is moved to the same room she had last time around. We are accepted by hospice the following day. Within hours, the answering machine I bought when this started begins to receive phone calls from hospice staff. The scheduler offers me two time slots for the daily visits by a licensed practical nurse (LPN). I choose 8:00 AM -10:00 AM which turns out to be an excellent choice.

I am now facing the sobering fact that I have forty-eight hours before I am tied to being there for Olwen on a 24-hour basis or finding someone else to be there and paying them. How will I use these last two evenings of freedom? What do I need to do for myself? See my father tonight and attend my teacher's award dinner tomorrow. I know it will be the last time I see him until after she dies, and who knows how long he has. Olwen understands and accepts my choices.

The drive to my father's lakeside cottage follows winding roads through rolling farmland and villages, roads I learned to drive on when I was sixteen. The air is superb on this beautiful June day. He and his wife are up for watching videos, and enjoy the kitten acrobatics, tour of my home, and birthday party tributes and folk dancing. When we go out for supper, she drives him to the door of the restaurant before parking the car. Last year he could still walk from the car.

For some years now, he has been held together by fierce willpower and his devoted family caregiver. Every time I see him, I think it may well be the last time. His blood sugar shoots all over, and he has had a couple of cardiac events. Every year, with increasing difficulty, they have made it down to Florida in the fall and returned to their cottage in the spring.

I give them a short summary of the past few weeks and the transition to palliative care we will be making when hospice takes responsibility for medical management on Friday. They listen with unaccustomed attention and seriousness. Usually her small-talk and his long-winded accounts about people I don't even know consume the space, blocking the possibility of being present to the moment and my hopes for meaningful conversation.

When we exit the restaurant to go our separate ways, it is dusk. Although it has become increasingly difficult for him to stand for more than a minute or two without squirming and leaning against a wall, he manages to stand there for many minutes without shifting his weight with nothing but his cane to lean on ever so lightly.

The expression on his face is haunting. All his self-mocking and loquacious masks have fallen away. Never has he been so present, so real, so grave, so quietly intense. Profound sadness, pain, awe, and apprehension flow together as one. This is not about him, it's not *his* pain or *his* sorrow. It's about us—the two of us *and* the three of us—and where our story has come to at this moment, the story that began so long ago when he begged Olwen to go out with him until she finally said yes.

It is as if the history of our story with all its pain and sorrow and losses and missed opportunities were synthesized from all three perspectives into his innermost being at this moment and is now pouring through his eyes into mine. His naked face *is* our story *and* it bears witness to it. Like some ancient tragedy, our story has inexorably brought us to this crossroad where the Daughter must take on the monumental task through which the last possibilities for healing, redemption, and closure may yet come to pass. Thus the awe and apprehension flowing through his being, his eyes, and his perfectly still and erect body.

This is one of his finest moments. I will come back to it again and again in the Olwen time that follows, and in the months that follow his own death soon thereafter.

※

I arrive at the awards dinner just as they are sitting down. The niece motions me over to my place at their big round table. I am expecting to see other former students like myself, perhaps someone I haven't seen in decades. None here. Instead, three of the women are her former caregivers.

Instantly, I know each of them would be acceptable to my mother and be able to relate to her. They are neatly and conservatively dressed, do volunteer work for their churches, have good social and communications skills, and two are themselves senior citizens. They are tall and strong, and I already know they are completely trustworthy, reliable, and became very fond of my teacher and she of them.

Jesse and Dory are interested in several hours of day work during the week. Nicole, who moonlights from her day job, could do some evenings and an occasional overnight. It's a good beginning. I stop by the hospital on my way home and tell Olwen about my unanticipated find.

※

Equipment arrives early on Friday. Oxygen can be continuously generated in a box the size of a small trunk. Tanks last only a couple of hours, but the guys leave us a couple in case of a power outage. The wheelchair is an improvement over the heavy, clunky one from downstairs, but soon we have an even better option.

When Mary discovers Olwen is now needing a wheelchair outside her apartment, she immediately offers to loan us the beautiful new one her husband used for a few months. Light, sleek, made of black naugahyde and chrome with removable foot rests, it is easier to push and much easier to fold up and put into and out of the car.

I bring Olwen home midday. She rests a bit, and some of the hospice team members come by for short visits. Neal, our social worker, brings two foam mattresses, the kind with the "eggcrate fingers" that help the skin to breathe and resist bedsores. I put one on top of her mattress under the sheets, and stash one under the other bed for who knows what purposes down the line. Dinaz, the RN in charge of the team, brings supplies, goes over the medications on the CHF protocol with me, and sets a long appointment for Monday. Within two hours, a pharmacy guy arrives with the lorazepam (or Ativan) and morphine sulphate (or Roxanol) for which I must sign, and about which we must keep careful notes.

The shift from the glacial pace and inefficiencies of the hospital/rehab system to the highly responsive and proactive hospice team members who communicate with each other is splendid. Already I am feeling much less alone.

My body is starting to feel the enormity of what I have taken on, however. I am now responsible for the life and dying of another human being who just happens to be my mother. I am supposed to be here twenty-four hours a day, seven days a week but my life centers in another city far away. Whenever I am not here, I have to find coverage for her. I have been here a week now, and have been running every minute while taking in and metabolizing Olwen's dramatic decline, the monumental fact she is not going to pull out of this, the drama of her rehospitalization and watching her rapid, irregular heartbeats on the monitor, and bringing in hospice. I know I need to catch my breath and regroup, even if briefly, before the Dance *really* begins.

Reluctantly, I press Sue (which I never have before) so I can take care of myself. Good that I did. At 3:00 AM on Friday night I wake up almost certain I am about to have a heart attack. Never have I felt so much constriction in the middle of my chest. I pace around the living room, and dig through my files to have emergency numbers handy. I will later learn panic attacks that simulate symptoms of heart attack are quite common among the many somatic symptoms that appear in those caring for their beloved dying.

―※―

During the thirty-four hours I am not in Olwen's apartment, I am driving for nine and sleeping for twelve. The rest of the time, I am buying and preparing whole foods, getting film and a boombox with better sound quality, selecting more audio tapes, taking a bike ride, going through mail and e-mail, pulling out bills, listening to my Celtic music programs, and making as many long-distance calls (or calls that would be long-distance from her house) as I can. I play with the cats and brush them, reorder their food, give them as much attention as possible, and talk with the cat sitter. I have a real dinner during the dinner hour and read something that helps to recenter me in myself. I take a wider range of clothes and more vases for the flowers I am always buying for Mother or that others bring. I type up notes to make them more legible for caregivers. I pull out my flexible ice packs for cooling Mother when she is hot, a cozy red robe (which she gave me one Christmas) for when she is cold, and my sleeping bag to wrap around her feet and legs which get especially cold because of her poor circulation.

―※―

On Monday morning, June 9, Olwen is awake by seven o'clock and thinking about getting up and doing things. I suggest we both try and rest until Christine, the LPN who will come every day at 8:00 AM, arrives. Olwen wants to get up and make her bed. I say No! She is not to make her bed under any circumstances. "You think you can do more than you really can." We go round with this. She agrees she won't make the bed, goes back to bed, and so do I.

Two minutes later I hear a thud, and she is calling for help. She was trying to make her bed and has fallen between her two beds, opening a three-cornered tear on the parchment-thin skin on her forearm. It looks nasty, but amazingly, as always, she has broken no bones. I help her up and back to bed, find some sterile pads, bathe the open area very gingerly, prop a pillow under her arm, and call hospice. We wait.

Part of me is already freaking out because Mother's strength, stubbornness, and not accepting that she can't do the things she used to do not bode well for her not harming herself or for her being an easy patient. You turn your back and she's into something. She will be difficult. I knew that, but now I am living it.

By eight o'clock, Dinaz and Christine are here. Dinaz is already getting fond of Olwen and soon takes to calling her "Mama" because she in some way reminds her of her own mother. She chides her gently for trying to do things she shouldn't and can't really do anymore. They check her out and dress the wound. Dinaz spends the better part of an hour. Olwen says nothing but her arm doesn't seem to be giving her any pain.

I don't know how much of what Dinaz says Olwen can understand because of her accent, but the authoritative, musical, caring quality of Dinaz's voice and the way Dinaz interacts with her physically communicates at a deeper level. Olwen knows she is in good hands. She is already learning this is a person who shows up, knows what to do, cares deeply about her patients, and always goes the extra mile for them. Despite her heavy patient demands, whenever she is needed, Dinaz will manage to come by in short order. Each time, she will listen, observe, and talk until she is comfortable that both Olwen and I are okay.

In the days to come, Mother will be absorbing the ease and mutual respect with which these two nurses work with each other and with me, and the enormous caring, gentleness, and consideration with which Christine gets her up and ready almost every day. Christine's daily ministrations manifest the spiritual path she enacts in every detail of how she touches, moves, speaks to, and relates to my mother whom she addresses by her last name.

Although my mother has always been an early riser, her sleep patterns are becoming erratic and she is sometimes still in bed when Christine arrives. Christine speaks clearly, letting her know what she is doing. Each day she checks her vitals and redresses her arm.

As the weeks go on, it will be harder to get Olwen up, but in the first couple of weeks, the transition into the bathroom goes pretty well. Because Olwen finds the bathroom cold, Christine runs the heater to warm it up. We put a thick towel behind her so the coldness and hardness of the toilet is softened. Olwen's fall did not break any bones, but it has bruised her back, and pressure there makes her flinch. I apply arnica for several days, and make liberal use of lotions I have given her over time but which she has used more sparingly—"saving" special gifts as her generation did. "Saving for what?" I always ask. "If you like it, I will bring you more."

I pick out clothes, get breakfast and meds ready. Often the phone is ringing by eight. I try to use part of "Christine time" to make calls, to think, and to plan. I always feel Olwen is safe when Christine is here, and so I can actually concentrate on what I am doing. After she wheels Olwen into the living room, she can write up her notes while I am doing breakfast and meds.

※

Dinaz comes for our "real" appointment on that first Monday around 2:00 PM. She checks Olwen's arm, spends a good while with her and then with me. We talk about CHF, the directions it can take, and markers of terminal processes. Like everyone from hospice whom I will ask about their estimates of time, Dinaz says she has experienced so many surprises with patients and has been wrong enough times that she would not estimate at this point. Olwen has such willpower and is so surprisingly strong that she could last the summer. And then again, Dinaz describes her as a "ticking time bomb" that could go off at any time.

Dinaz explains why she would like to take Mother off her blood thinner and hold off digoxin unless her pulse becomes rapid or thready; I agree. Lasix, on the other hand, is part of the CHF protocol for reducing fluid build-up. We can crush it in sherbet or applesauce. The potassium needed to offset the diuretic can be given in liquid form and mixed with juice to avoid the big horsepill to which Olwen objects and which she will have more and more trouble swallowing as time goes on. Within hours, liquid potassium arrives.

I take this opportunity to inform Dinaz of Olwen's high sensitivity to medications and show her the list. I recap her recent antibiotic experiences and do my stump speech on the mismatch between results shown in clinical trials and the deteriorating ability of old, failing bodies to move drugs through their systems. I make my pitch about tailoring drugs, dosages, and frequency to the individual patient, and continually calibrating their administration to observation of effects.

I am so relieved to discover I am finally talking with a medical professional who has a similar, conservative view of drugs to mine. As Dinaz elaborates, blood levels of drugs can build up to toxic levels in the elderly and dying because aging livers can't metabolize them properly while aging/failing kidneys cannot excrete them.

That conservative orientation informs our discussion of Ativan and Roxanol. Olwen has already had Ativan in the hospital and it appeared to be temporarily calming without other ill effects. I am concerned, however, about Mother's potential reactions to morphine sulphate. I would like to hold off on it as long as possible, and, for both drugs, try smaller dosages than the protocol's standard minimum and see how she reacts.

Dinaz agrees on all accounts. We know we may have to ratchet up the dosages and/or frequency later on, but we will take our cues from Mother. We agree not to use morphine prematurely or without checking with me.

Rounding out the standing orders are multiple dosages and forms of drugs like ibuprofen, nystatin, and Compazine so they can be dispatched immediately if needed. Dinaz will prepare a list of standing orders for medications, discuss them with Noyes and ask him to sign off.

For now, I neither know nor care how the details of the Noyes-hospice relationship work. Only later do I learn that technically, he remained Olwen's primary-care physician and was still legally liable for the medications while delegating decision making and medical management of Olwen's case to hospice. Empowered by the standing orders, hospice did not have to call him every time there was a small problem and waste precious time waiting for him and the pharmacy. Every fifteen days, Dinaz had to conduct an assessment, meet with the medical director of hospice, and send a report to Noyes. Instead of being the decision-maker on her care, however, he was kept informed. His responsibilities were completed when he signed the death certificate (an interface that is actually managed by the funeral home).

I recap my experiences with Noyes, his difficulties in working with the family, and his fix-and-cure-the-symptoms orientation. I express my desire to not have to deal with him and my gratitude that she can take this burden from me and be far more effective than I can.

Dinaz calls me back later Monday evening to tell me she has already spoken with Noyes. Although he has a certain reluctance ("I feel like I am signing a blank check"), he has signed off on the standing orders. He has also agreed to terminating Coumadin and using digoxin only on an as-needed basis.

From where I sit, Dinaz has performed a miracle on her first real day with us, doing what I could never accomplish alone: shifting the paradigm from treatment to palliative care, removing the barriers to the unfolding of Olwen's own natural dying process, enabling Olwen to be managed and supported medically at home, and relieving me of the struggle of having to deal with the heroically-oriented, medical establishment personified in our case by Noyes. Dinaz manages the dual interface beautifully. For me, Noyes' involvement becomes a background factor that does not intrude into the foreground. For him, power is not ceded to me, but to medical professionals who have a different orientation than his own.

Dinaz has a bee in her bonnet, however, about falls and the height of the bed, and she is already talking about a hospital bed. I agree that falling is the biggest hazard for elderly people, but point out, as I will again and again, that Olwen has remarkable bones. She has had over a dozen falls, including the one this morning, and never broken anything. I relay an incident when a new lawyer leaned toward her and said with some awe, "Pardon me, but are those your own teeth?" She was pleased by his query. Not even a root canal or crown! While I want to reduce the potential for falls, I am not paranoid on the subject because she does have such extraordinary bones, and I think we have to weigh ostensibly protective measures, like a hospital bed, against their downside potential.

I point out Dinaz has never seen a restless and "confused" Olwen climbing over hospital bed rails, risking much nastier falls or accidents than rolling out of her own bed onto a carpet. Olwen feels like a prisoner in these beds, they have lousy mattresses and support, and it is very hard for helpers to get close enough to the patient when sitting by their bedside, even with the rails down. At this point, I view these considerations as trumping any upside potential of a hospital bed.

I agree her own bed is now too high, and I am working on solutions. She is using her foot stool now to climb in and out of bed more easily. For the next phase, I will remove the box spring, stash it between the mattress and spring of the other bed, and add lots of boards running horizontally across the frame to support her excellent, firm mattress.

❧

After Dinaz leaves, I take a moment and savor what has happened and start gearing up for tomorrow. It looks like it is going to be a gorgeous day—finally! I have been hoping for such a day to take Olwen to the Grand Hotel. We had a perfect day there last fall, and it is the one thing she has mentioned several times during the past months that she wants to do again. I want to go as soon as possible because we have no place to go but down from here. As Olwen says, "We know it cant get great again."

Tuesday, June 10 dawns as splendidly as promised. I pick out one of her favorite summer outfits: khaki skirt, tan leather belt, and crisp white jacket. I get out the new white top with the sweetly gathered neck and sleeves, an elegant, paisley scarf, and an amethyst necklace. When I am later gathering pictures for her collage, I will see that, with a different blouse, this is what she wore at her eighty-fifth birthday party and I marvel at how young and vigorous our family matriarch was at that age. I dig out the needlepoint bag Ginny started and Olwen finished during one of those Florida winters, reminding her of its history. The beige background and floral design pick up all her clothing colors. With her beautiful, curly, finely-textured white hair that still has some dark areas underneath, she looks smashing, even at ninety-eight pounds.

Olwen is alert and interested in the scenery, and still enjoys the particularly hilly route I have chosen. The Grand Hotel features a stately veranda on the main floor overlooking the lake, and an outside dining terrace on the ground floor where we will have lunch. Olwen opts for fruit with sherbet. We settle down and drink in the view. The lake has the slightest ruffles today, puffy clouds float by, and the breezes tousle her hair slightly.

I have brought my camera. I create portraits of the dignity of her ancient, valiant being, looking her impending death in the eye. I am delighted to capture a moment when she is looking at her watch. The angle of her head, her facial expression, her body language, and way of holding both hands at that moment are quintessential Olwen. This looking-at-her-watch thing has always been so exasperating ("stop looking at your watch, just be in the moment!") but now is utterly endearing.

We mosey around the grounds, sit closer to the lake, and ask someone who is also pushing a wheelchair to take a picture of the two of us. We both know it is the last picture of the two of us together, just as all of these pictures are the last of Olwen. I will be holding my breath a little until I see how they come out. As the afternoon wears on, we go upstairs and sit on the veranda, just enjoying this lovely day together. Eventually I fall asleep. She does not.

We take the route along the lake that has places to stop. When we get back to our village, I drop off the film and buy some rum, something I have not had for decades. On the veranda, people had been enjoying summer drinks, and the idea of piña coladas is suddenly appealing. Pineapple-coconut is one of the many juices I have brought to Olwen for variety, but it is too thick and she does not care for it. Cut with rum and ice in the blender, however, it might be refreshing on a summer evening.

I make supper and piña coladas, and Olwen asks for a small glass. I think, why not? There is little enough that entices her. She complains now that old favorites are too sweet or too salty. But her piña colada she relishes. She assertively reaches for it, picks it up, savors its flavors and texture in her mouth before and after she swallows, puts it down again, and repeats this cycle until it is gone. Does she want more? No, not right now. We will enjoy our piña coladas two or three other evenings in the next couple of weeks.

One of those evenings is Thursday, the twelfth. Hugh, my mother's friend since childhood, died on Monday. Olwen wants to go to the calling hours which are on Thursday. She opts for the outfit she wore to the Grand Hotel.

An entire wall of the reception room holds gorgeous floral arrangements, and the reception line is long—one of the perks of having been a pillar of the funeral business. I am annoyed no one is making way for Olwen in her wheelchair. I am also very protective of her arm whose bandages, bruising, and tenderness are invisible under her jacket. I run interference so the family members won't grab her arm or even that hand.

When we get our turn, Olwen is wonderfully "on" for what turns out to be her last real public appearance. She speaks of the old days when her family and Hugh's were neighbors who spoke Welsh and missed the old country. I take the opportunity to ask Hugh's sister if she can remember whether Olwen's family lived in a yellow house, but she was too young to remember.

Hugh is lying in an open casket by the far wall under the cascades of flowers. I am hesitant about Olwen's going over for a last moment with him because this has got to be very, very hard for her. She wants to go over. What is going through her mind, seeing Hugh like this, the last vestiges of her childhood, her last link to Mama, and a harbinger of her own fate? It is a good summer evening for piña coladas.

Seven

Building Our Own Family of Caregivers and Our Private World

> *We live in a world that is terrified by death and hides its dying. We know the vacuum that forms around the dying.*
>
> —Marie de Hennezel, PhD, palliative care psychologist

Starting the day with Christine gives me more confidence in getting Olwen up, especially as things get dicier. It demarcates the beginning of another day and asserts that there really is a rhythm to each 24-hour period, a rhythm that is already starting to dissolve into fluctuating, repetitious episodes punctuated by short rounds of sleeping and talking. I soon realize that part of the exhaustion of attending the dying is the withering of the macro-rhythms which silently underpin our normal lives.

When Christine is here, I feel Olwen is safe and so I feel safe. Christine is easy to be with and work with, even first thing in the morning. Although she has a lot to do (some days much more than can be done, and yet she magically does it all; I try to help), she never seems rushed. She is always in the moment, taking her cues from us, sizing up the situation from the moment she opens the door, and responding appropriately. No two days are the same. Christine aligns with Olwen *and* with me *and* with the totality of our situation at that moment, and moves everything forward as a unitary whole, leaving us in a better and stronger place than when she came. In her daily ministrations to the dying, Christine truly lives her spiritual path.

Having Dory or Jesse for here a few hours after Christine gives me a larger block of time to optimize all of my/our needs for the next twenty-four hours. Mother quickly becomes comfortable with them. Both are adept at interpersonal spatial relations, sometimes giving her space from across the room, sometimes sitting next to her but still holding the space quietly while she sleeps or they talk, sometimes leaning in to listen and talk, and sometimes being physical containers of her restlessness and repetitive movements. During "naps," Mother occasionally opens her eyes as if to check that Jesse or Dory is still there—and, I suspect, absorb the fact they are there just for her, and she is not alone.

I want Olwen to build connections with caregivers while she is more herself, able to talk, and semi-ambulatory. As her abilities continue to fail, I want her to *feel* the familiarity of her regular caregivers. No more "big house" full of strangers who are "not *our* family." No vacuum will isolate Olwen. We are building our own family.

By having multiple caregivers, Olwen will receive a broader spectrum of attention and care overall. None of us can see everything or do everything, and each has her own predilections and styles of attending, assessing, and responding. Each of us will suppress or bring out different dimensions of her self and her needs. It's good to have others who create openings I might close off. Because none of her caregivers will be here every day, I can also calibrate my sense of changes against their observations from visit to visit.

In addition, I want to give myself a block of time to do my own work on the roofdeck, in the solarium, or at the village library. By getting outside, recentering in myself, and doing a bit to move the rest of my life forward, I am in better shape for my 18-hour, solo shift and can focus on Olwen when I return. Doing "Olwen stuff" squeezes that hope, however. At most I can salvage an hour or two, and sometimes none at all, even during the first phase of home care.

Within days, sleep deprivation also undercuts the paper plan. Finding ways to get sleep will soon become my top self-care priority, competing for the same, few, precious hours against doing a bit of professional work, and eventually superseding the possibility or fantasy of doing work at all. Increasingly, I will only be able to sleep well and uninterruptedly during my nights in my own home, and to lesser extent, when someone else is keeping an eye on Olwen all through the night while I sleep in the next room.

When I am alone, part of me is always on guard and listening. I check on her several times in the night and get up at least once to help her to the bathroom, after which she often likes to talk, or one or both of us is too restless to go back to sleep. She is most alert, lucid, and talkative between five and seven in the morning when I am blotto. I am torn between having these critical conversations and coveting sleep. Dawn after dawn, I listen to her, we talk about what is uppermost for her at the moment, and then try to get her to go back to sleep until Christine comes. Sometimes I succeed, and sometimes I do not. Sometimes I can catch another twenty or thirty minutes of sleep during the middle of Christine's visit.

Increasingly, Olwen will nap and doze during the day, and her blocks of night sleep will rarely be for more than two hours, often less. I try to gather most of her sleeping into the nocturnal spectrum in order to maintain some semblance of day-and-night rhythms, and to get some sleep during the hours my body craves sleep and needs to go about its restorative, maintenance, and learning functions.

The real challenge is to find caregivers who can do overnights and commit to being part of a 24-hour, continuous care schedule. Sue's time is limited by competing demands. She can come during the day and stay overnight on Fridays, so that becomes my anchor in trying to develop an "away schedule." Caregiver leads are not panning out during the first days of home care, however.

I drop by to visit Mother's friend Helen to thank her for her note and cards to Olwen. She tells me about a team of caregivers who took very good care of a friend 24/7 for a year or more; her friend died a few days ago. I call Frieda, the one who does the scheduling. Frieda's propensity for talking is bothersome, but she knows a lot about end-of-life care and CHF, and can bring two colleagues over to meet with us tomorrow.

Dinaz wants to meet them to assess their understanding of palliative care and caring for someone in end-stage CHF. She is comfortable on both accounts, but is also put off by Frieda's know-it-allness. Olwen, sitting in her lift chair, says little during this meeting in her living room.

I like the way Rosanna goes and sits beside Olwen and how she initiates contact.

By Friday, the thirteenth, I will have been home only one of the last fourteen nights. At this early phase of the final Dance, my sense is Olwen can sustain my absence for three days. By handing off to Sue, I could transact business on Friday afternoon and Monday morning *if* Frieda can put together a schedule for the forty-eight hours after Sue and Christine wash Olwen's hair Saturday morning. She can. Jesse and Nicole can pick it up from there on Monday.

⁂

Scheduling for 24-hour care is a big deal. Overnight coverage is the hardest, but getting all the pieces to fit so there are no gaps is also difficult. No one can be late, and no one can not show up. Having someone who can handle continuous-coverage scheduling is a tremendous help.

In the kitchen I post the schedule, phone numbers, and key things I have emphasized to each of them, such as, "Call me immediately if there is a problem or significant decision to be made." I spell out my agreements with Dinaz about drugs and dosages. I describe Olwen's changing food and beverage preferences and organization of refrigerator contents. "Do not force or push food or drink; offer or invite it, and make small portions so she is less overwhelmed and more likely to finish it." In the bathroom I post information about her preferences in personal care and location of supplies. "She likes to comb her own hair and brush her own teeth."

I also iterate, "Wash hands after arrival, and before handling food, drink, or meds." I never stop being stunned when friends, strangers, and especially caregivers don't wash their hands upon arriving at one's house, before eating or handling food or meds, or before contact with a patient. I link hand hygiene to the fact Mother and I rarely have colds while those all around us are sniveling, blowing, and coughing. The importance of hand hygiene is being affirmed in studies showing how deadly infections are transmitted in hospitals.

Each weekend, I write a new set of notes because of changes in Olwen's situation. The notes, which I date, become a record of changes in Olwen's preferences and abilities. Three years later when I articulate the idea of the "3 Cs of seamless patient care," I see more clearly what I was intuitively trying to achieve through my notes and conversations with caregivers.[1]

Continuity of care means each shift hands off smoothly to the next so they are informed about what has happened, how the patient responded, and what will need particular attention. All our caregivers did this automatically. They came early so as to be let in and brought up to date, and during their shift, wrote in the log Jesse had set up. Hospice had its own log for observations and recording the administration of controlled substances. Both logs were left on Mother's dining table which served as our workstation.

Coordination of care means everyone is working together rather than at cross-purposes with respect to objectives, plan of care, drugs, and interventions. Everyone needed to be comfortable working in a palliative care paradigm and to understand the CHF protocol. This protocol was operationalized through standing orders which set broad limits within which judgment was exercised. Dinaz and I had established we were in sync about how we interpreted the protocol and tailored it for Olwen. Early conversations with each caregiver were geared to eliciting where they were coming from and communicating my expectations for Olwen's end-of-life care. Dinaz was doing the same thing by meeting with Frieda and her colleagues.

Consistency of care means low variability in care from day to day, caregiver to caregiver. Here my focus was on standardizing routine things while encouraging each caregiver to bring her own gifts and skills to her time with Olwen. Many notes were geared to consistency regarding medication dosages and use, Olwen's preferences in self-care, food, and beverages, and standardizing towel use by color coding. Caregiving is all about paying attention, and my notes helped direct that attention to salient details that can seem trivial, but mattered to Olwen, and made things easier for everyone else. Abiding by them entails seeing oneself as part of a fabric of care to which one is responsible.

I was highly conscious of building our own world and our own family of people who did not turn away from death or from her. The caregivers from hospice and whom I hired privately were respectful, patient, attentive, and responsive. They were struck by Olwen's dignity, her dearness, and her astonishing strength and gutsiness despite her growing frailty. Nothing in their body language backed away from her. By their presence, body language, and ways helping and handling her, they communicated her worthiness and created a context of safety. Even when she was "dozing" or "napping," she was aware of and absorbing their presence. Their patience and attentiveness were soon colored by real affection.

※

The June 13 weekend goes well for Mother and for myself. I call every morning when Christine is there, speak with a caregiver in the afternoon, and another in the evening. Each time I talk with Olwen briefly and remind her when she will see me again. Olwen and Rosanna have several outings and Olwen wants to show off Village Grove, including the penthouse floor—a sure sign Olwen likes her. They listen to music, talk about music and Wales, and look at photos. Olwen eats a substantial lunch on Sunday, and later, Angela reports, rejects cottage cheese and fruit in favor of going downstairs for a real dinner of ham, baked potato, and string beans, eating a good bit of it. Frieda describes nightly cycles of sleeping for about two or three hours, going to the bathroom, talking, and repeating the cycle.

I am able to work, go to the library, and prepare my remarks for an event I hope to participate in next weekend. I replace the cassette/radio in my car and buy a new, professional quality microcassette recorder because both quit on me this week. I exercise, get lots of sleep, and talk at length with three friends about their mother's dying processes. I am able to dash off an e-mail to an extended community of friends for the first time since this started seven weeks ago. I recap what's been happening, what I am juggling, how I am feeling, ask for support, tell them the best times to reach me, and spell out the kinds of physical, emotional, and spiritual support that would be most welcome.

※

During the week of the sixteenth, I take Olwen out every day, running part of the time because she likes going fast. We go to the village, or the shopping center, or sometimes stay closer to her apartment. We often go out in the early evening because it is such a lovely time of day and she is so acutely aware that, "They're all down there now" having dinner. Although the impending dinner hour makes her antsy and interested in going downstairs or outside, she doesn't show a strong urge (at least with me) to actually join them.

For Olwen's sake, their sake, and my own as well, I also time many of my outings with Mother to coincide with the dinner hour because we are least likely to run into residents. Before and after dinner, up to ten of them gather on benches and chairs outside the front door. When Mother and I pass by them, I move along to minimize the amount of time we all cohabit this awkward, painful space. They fall silent, or keep looking in another direction, or continue with their conversations. If someone does look in our direction, I nod to them and look away, sustaining Olwen's special, private world.

Through temporally segregating our use of this shared space, I am navigating unspoken parts of what I infer my Dying in Place agreement with Kate means with regard to protecting the sensibilities and defenses of all parties in an intimate apartment community. I want to protect Olwen from any embarrassment she would feel if her dying body were not clouding her mind. Her attention is withdrawing from the world, and she is not always doing "socially appropriate" nods or even turning her head to notice other people. This is not lost on her neighbors. As they edge closer to their own slippery slopes, they recoil from signs of deterioration or dying, wondering what their own fates will be, how it will end for them—and, in too many cases, who, if anyone, will advocate and care for them.

The residents sitting outside the front door sometimes see me coming and going by myself, carrying things or doing things. When I am by myself, I move a little less quickly, open my body language, and acknowledge them with a nod, but otherwise take my cues from them.

Before long, one of them engages me, and others turn their heads and listen. Gradually, others are emboldened to speak to me. When they initiate, I engage in a public conversation with them, but do not overstay my time. Their eyes and body language suggest they sense what is going on, but we do not speak of it directly. They speak obliquely, commenting, for example, on all I am doing.

As we delicately demarcate the fragile boundaries, the tension that had marked my passing among them dissipates. It is succeeded by an ease and a sense of their witnessing and approving what I have undertaken. One of the women will engage me in the lobby when no one is around and tell me how she wishes there would be someone there for her as I am for Olwen.

One evening I wheel Olwen up to the roofdeck. That requires our going through the solarium where her neighbors are playing cards, and helping her up two steps that put us on the roofdeck. I exchange nods with those she knows best, and, with a slight nod in her direction, they go on with their playing.

Olwen shows little interest in their activities, but I feel anguish for whatever may be going on within her far below the level of speech. She no longer dwells in their world, and they are terrified of her world seeping into theirs. With my words and protective body language, I make our private universe a special place where only we can go: out on the roof to watch the setting sun and the rising of the moon and stars. She really enjoys this evening, just as she has in the past. This becomes the last time she is strong enough to manage the two steps, our last time looking at the sunset and the stars together.

⚘

Frieda is pressing me to commit to next weekend because she and her colleagues must get more work than we can give her, but they will work around hard commitments. I am torn between, on the one hand, repeating one more time a schedule that took so much work to put together and that everyone has been through once, and, on the other, my doubts about whether Olwen can sustain my being away for as long as three nights again.

My home visits perch on a see-saw between my assessment of where she has come since yesterday, the day before, and a week ago and trying to pace myself for all the great unknowns into which we are headed. My body is already sending strong messages that its needs are not being met. I tell the recorder:

> It's about quarter of seven in the morning on June eighteenth, and the last time I looked at the clock it was just before three. So I've actually slept the last four hours, and I don't feel as if I have slept at all. I just talked with my mother, and she was fiddling with a battery compartment piece of the clock which had come loose. She doesn't think she slept all night. It's so exhausting—it's unbelievable.

After hedging a day or so, I uneasily go forward with the same schedule, albeit leaving later on Friday and returning early on Monday after my Sunday event. All spring I have looked forward to an event honoring the woman whose groundbreaking work in another field made it possible for me to have the breakthrough that transformed my work in social theory. I will speak briefly about her contributions and see friends I haven't seen in months. I have been hoping against hope I will have this one precious evening on June 22. It is now looking likely.

On Thursday, however, we start making use of the wheelchair in the apartment and run two liters of oxygen some of the time—the first since she left the hospital two weeks ago. The hospice scheduler is able to send us a night nurse.

Night nurses are a scarce resource shared by different teams and allocated according to urgency of need. They work from eleven to seven. They stay up all night, sitting in Olwen's bedroom chair, reading with a tiny light, and seem never to fall asleep or doze on shift. Although the presence of another person makes it harder for me to get to sleep, when I *am* sleeping, I sleep more soundly and for larger blocks of time because I know they are "on guard." But I also have to stay up until eleven to let them in and orient them to the situation or fill them in briefly since their last visit. I impress upon them Olwen's bad history with medications, the agreement about half-dosages, and the no-morphine-yet rule, and do my stump speech about tailoring meds and dosages to aging and dying bodies.

I usually have at least one conversation with the nurse in the middle of the night when I ask for her observations and for her to relate them to her experience and thus what may be portended here. The night nurse may speak to me on her way out just before seven. Sometimes I can go right back to sleep until Christine arrives, and sometimes Olwen is restless and I have to be with her, or my own mind starts racing, and I get little or no sleep in that intervening hour.

At 5:30 AM on Thursday, without consulting me, our first night nurse gives Mother the standard minimum dose of Ativan, twice the dose Dinaz and I had agreed upon. The log reads: patient was restless and anxious. She does not follow the drops with the ordained juice chaser. Two hours later, Olwen throws up some awful, bright orange stuff. I express my dismay to Christine that our agreements have not been followed and that my mother has been subjected to this unnecessary assault on her body. Olwen is feeling weak and lousy in its wake.

This incident heightens my continuing uneasiness about when I should leave to go home. My intuition continues to say three days is too long now, but I feel locked into the schedule and obligated to the caregivers. I do not want to jerk them around. They are counting on this income, have committed this time, and might disappear if I cancel some of their time and don't leave until Sunday. I consider leaving on Saturday, but that would virtually erase Sue's 24-hour block of work. Also troubling is the fact that Christine will be off this weekend, and there is a choppy quality to the actions of the LPN who will be filling in.

On Friday morning, I simply do not want to go. I am distressed by the orange vomit and Mother's getting a little weaker. Yet after Olwen spends time with Christine and myself and we get her bathed and dressed, she is amazingly centered and quietly lucid. I do Reiki with her and we have a beautiful, fluid, healing time. I want it to stay like this forever. We are very, very close. She is very, very receptive to the energy. Now I don't want to leave because I don't want to miss any of this intimacy and healing.

When Sue arrives midday, I am going all around the barn about what to do. I want to stay, but the schedule has been set up. I feel trapped and caught by the schedule.

It is always hard to leave, and there is really never a good time to leave. Every day there are things that make it worrisome to leave at that particular moment, or something lovely is happening that I don't want to break away from because I don't know how many more moments there will be. But if I had left only at times when it felt right or "safe" to leave, I would never have left for any of my trips.

The only way I manage to leave so that I can return somewhat rested and recentered for the next round, as well as keep my own ship from sinking, is to leave at the times I have spent hours setting up in advance. But it is impossible to know in advance how and when to schedule my comings and goings in an optimal way because we never know how things are going to be from one minute to the next, let alone one day to the next, let alone many days in advance. Besides which, any schedule reflects the conjoint availability of many caregivers that has been put together in a way that provides continuous coverage.

Olwen did not stay in the mellow mood in which I left her. Would it have been any different if I had stayed? Or is just the highly erratic, unpredictable disease course that CHF follows? That afternoon, Sue describes Olwen as weak, dozing a lot, and having episodes of restlessness and picking at her clothes. Mother tolerates a half-dose of Ativan, and later eats a little salmon, potato, and mushroom. At some moment, Olwen reaches out to pat Sue's arm—a very old Olwen gesture of caring and assuring the other person while reassuring herself, a gesture that always goes along with the sweetest of smiles.

Dinaz visits in the evening and is satisfied there is no bladder, bowel, or other problem behind the stomach distention. She gives Mother a bit of Compazine. Sue finds Olwen restless in the night, runs two liters of oxygen, and later gives her three more drops of Ativan. Around 2:45, Sue hears a noise and finds Olwen on the floor in a sitting position. No injuries noted. With Sue at her bedside, Olwen sleeps a couple of hours around dawn and pulls out her oxygen.

Olwen says she feels weak and has a lazy day with Rosanna and Angela. Later she perks up and I receive a sweet call from her around five o'clock. Before I can get to the phone, her message begins, "Mother here. I'm wondering—there's a group of us going, I guess, and I was wondering if you want to go down to dinner with us . . ." Our space-time structure is collapsing for her.

Sunday morning, I get a call from the LPN and Frieda. I put together the story from their nervous and disjointed accounts. Around 6:30, Olwen had fallen out of bed. No broken or cracked bones but Olwen hurts all over. Frieda called hospice. The on-call nurse told her to give Olwen both morphine and Ativan, using the standard doses. Frieda protested because she is aware of the agreements. Rather than calling me, however, she did as she was told by this nurse who has never even met Olwen.

I am furious. Furious with the on-call nurse for prescribing in a case she does not know and violating my agreement with hospice. Furious with Frieda for doing what the on-call nurse said to do rather than calling me *before* she acted.

I tell Frieda and the LPN that under no circumstances are they to give more morphine today. If there are problems, Frieda is to call me. Despite my conversation with the LPN, I am later told she left instructions for caregivers to continue giving both drugs every four hours. My private caregivers all refuse to comply with her instructions.

I ask the LPN to ask Dinaz to call me this morning if she can. In considerably less than an hour, Dinaz calls and I run through the incident. I am not upset with her because the behavior of shared resources is not under her control. While communication within her team is outstanding, these two incidents suggest that quasi-autonomous players are not as tightly linked to teams and patients as they could be—or, as I would like them to be.

What to do next? Shall I go back today and miss my event and seeing my friends? Frieda says, no, "Your mom is fine." A little later, Rosanna says, "Don't come, she is fine. Stay, do your thing." But even at this distance, even though Olwen has never had morphine, my intuition tells me she is not going to have a good reaction. She is not going to respond the way the protocol predicts. She is not going to follow the medical party line I sometimes hear, "Oh, don't worry, it'll be out of her system in four hours." Part of me says, the damage has been done. What can I do for Olwen now but wait? Why should I blow the rest of my pricey weekend?

❧

I drive back on Sunday, arriving in the late afternoon. Angela is sitting next to Olwen, reading quietly. My intuition was right. The morphine has had a devastating effect. It is dreadful to see her like this—very different from the weakened, semi-conscious mother I first encountered at the hospital. That was a natural state that comes to the very ill and dying, and I can cope with it. This is an unnatural, drug-induced state, and I am horrified by it, feel helpless to do anything about it, and angry that it happened.

I left two days ago interacting with a whole human being who, although weak, was still capable of interacting at a profound level. Now I do not know if I will ever see the likes of her again. Mother is so out of it right now it doesn't really matter that I have come back—or so it seems at this moment. I spend time with her, but it is hard to tell what she is able to take in. Somewhere in her foggy consciousness, I can tell I have registered with her, but beyond that, it is hard to know if anyone is at home.

It feels like I have compounded my original tortured choice to leave on Friday by coming back when I needn't have. I have now thoroughly blown the weekend for which I am shelling out rivers of money. I feel I have come back for nothing. What can I do for her now except to wait, be a presence, and see what happens?

Olwen falls back into her stupor and I bring my stuff upstairs. I add new food to "my shelf" in the small frig and to Olwen's. I see another jar of cranberry juice has been opened even though one is already open, and that the controlled substances have not been put back in their proper place. I am guessing it is Frieda who has not replaced the drugs properly and opened too many bottles of the same juice. I don't associate that kind of sloppiness with Rosanna or Angela, and the drugs were used only on Frieda's watch.

When I add new kinds of juice to the hall closet/pantry, I find trash there, including an empty ginger ale bottle. They all know where to take the trash. Why was some left here? I find another empty ginger ale bottle next to the garbage under the kitchen sink. Back in the pantry, I look at the six-pack of ginger ale I bought for Olwen this week; it helps her nausea, and sometimes she just likes it—icy cold like every other beverage. There are only two bottles left. No way Olwen has consumed four bottles of ginger ale in the last few days! If she has drunk one or two, that would be a lot.

The idea of someone taking ginger ale from a dying woman puts me over the top. It is hard to imagine anyone but Frieda doing this, especially since she is fond of ginger ale. The caregiver who succeeded her found the TV turned so it could only be watched comfortably while lying down on the sofa. Ginger ale missing, TV watching, sleeping on night shift, a fall that leaves Olwen in more discomfort than any fall ever has, and other "small" and careless actions point to something troubling that Frieda apparently cannot control and which undercuts her caregiving. Whatever it is, it, along with countermanding my standing orders, is unacceptable.

I am gone for forty-eight hours and *this* is what I walk into! I am angry with hospice, angry with Frieda, and angry with myself. Will

Olwen ever come out of this morphine stupor? I don't know but I do know we need more time of loving and healing and I am afraid we may be cheated out of it by the damn drugs.

Yet now that we know how our larger story turned out, it is possible to see the "weekend from hell" in other lights. Although devastating at the time, its events were things from which we could and did recover, and from which I could and did learn. The weekend renewed and intensified my adherence to my first principle—following my intuition—especially with regard to assessing Olwen's situation and its implications for my care and timing choices. Consequently, I made the right calls at the super-critical choice-points—the ones from which, had I taken different forks in the road, neither Mother nor I could have ever recovered.

Although I had hesitations about Frieda from the outset, I brought her on board. If I had not, I would never have found Rosanna, and Rosanna turns out to be an absolute gem. Disconcerting as she was, Frieda was able to put together a weekend schedule, and her gift to us was Rosanna.

The difference Rosanna would come to make is incalculable. Not only does she have an extraordinary gift for connecting with the elderly and dying, but she can also enter gracefully into a household at a very difficult and delicate time and become a robust presence without being intrusive. She is drawn to serving elders, and raises caregiving to an art form that is at once physical, emotional, and spiritual.

Part III

Rhythms of the Dance

Always the years between us, always the years.
Always the love. Always the hours.
—"Virginia Woolf" in "The Hours"

Eight

Peaks and Valleys: When a Heart Can No Longer Do Its Work

> *You die in episodes. Dying is an irregular process full of mountains and valleys. It chews away at your life while consuming hers.*
>
> —a friend, June 15

I sleep three hours, spending much of it going over and over the last three days, checking in on Olwen, helping her to the bathroom, and listening to her. By the time Christine arrives, I am in a meltdown state. All the uncertainties, dilemmas, fears, anxieties, pressures, grief, and losses of the past two months—indeed, of the last five years—are erupting in an unending stream of tears and overwhelming sense of having unnecessarily screwed up the one thing I really counted on for myself, and of having set the weekend on a course that might have unfolded differently for Mother had I held to my intuition. The weekend has blown everything open and I have come apart.

Christine is extraordinary. A long vivid moment stands out: Olwen already dressed and in the living room seated in her lift chair, me a basket case across the room sitting on the sofa, and Christine kneeling beside me saying awesomely comprehending things so I feel totally seen, and me saying to her, "but you're supposed to be taking care of Mother."

Hospice actually takes on the whole family—not just the patient—as their client, and this is the morning I am to viscerally experience what that means. Christine offers to call Dinaz, and I say not to bother her, she has done enough, but the next thing I know, Dinaz is in our living room.

Christine stays late, as she will each of the next few days, and soon Neal, our social worker, arrives, as does Dory.

The morning is a blur as to what was said—except for two things. I remember saying I could just walk out the door, keep walking, and never look back. This is called "burn-out" or "compassion fatigue." And I remember Dinaz, Neal, and Christine all telling me it is rare for one person to be "the family," and do it all. Hospice usually works with a family whose members relieve one other. Even through my fog, it is clear there is nothing happening in our living room that they do not already understand all too well.

The hospice team is here for Mother *and* for me *and* for us. They work together seamlessly, fluidly. At all times, at least one of them is tending to Mother while at least one of them is attending to me, and, somehow, they are each and all are attending to the entire situation as a dynamic whole. They do not say anything stupid. They say wise and insightful things, and they know they need to repeat them to penetrate my current opaque state. Dory sits quietly on the sofa, getting a sense of what is going on, being a containing presence, and moving next to Olwen when there is more space there to be filled. Singly and collectively, they create a safe context in which I unravel. They wisely do not press me to move out of where I am but support me in that place and allow me to evolve into the next phase on my own. Only then does Neal leave, while Dinaz stays longer, and Dory stays for her shift. In the meantime, with perfect timing, hospice chaplain Sister Mary Elizabeth, calls.

We have never spoken before. The contradictory tensions tearing me apart come tumbling out, as do my discouragement and despair during the last few years. Far too much of our precious time together got chewed up with Olwen running through her litanies, our having non-conversations, and just doing "stuff." I had became more patient, but nothing new seemed to happen, and the moments of insight, resolution, or validation never seemed to "take." So I had come to feel we were done, and had been done for a long time. Yet she is still here. Yet we both hang in there. Yet we both keep trying to find each other, and often do, having moments of great intimacy and connection.

Sister Mary Elizabeth listens to all that is churning within me and draws out a question. "Do you think something new can still happen? Do you think you have anything more to learn from each other?" Her question catches me. The churning stops. I stop. I do not answer for a long time. I am fully engaged with her question and also in observing myself. The immediate response that comes to mind is, "no." Just as immediately, I know in my deepest being that "no" is the wrong answer. It is this simultaneous juxtaposition that causes me to be silent for some while. Sister Mary Elizabeth wisely holds my silence with her stillness.

I know in my soul the right answer is, "yes," but I simply cannot imagine how it could be so. Yet I know amazing things do happen, often out of "nowhere," as people get closer to death. In fact, Olwen's old litanies have already stopped. New things are already happening. Olwen has become the moment and says extraordinary things that go to the heart of the situation at that moment. It is *I* who need to catch up. It is *I* who need to stop imposing the pattern of the last few years on the last few weeks.

Sister Mary Elizabeth's question and her capacity for holding the space in which I find the answer stops the implosive downward spiral into which I descended this morning, and opens a window in my consciousness that pulls me out of our past and into the present. I sense this conversation and its question are a pivotal moment in our Dance of Death.

In hindsight, I will realize this opening was born out of the cauldron of weekend events in which I had become so caught up and imploded in despair. The weekend triggered a meltdown, without which the hospice team would not have converged in our living room to surround, support, and hold the crisis and Sister Mary Elizabeth would not have called at just the right moment, midwifing my opening to another realm of possibilities for The Conversation. The weekend from hell can be seen in a new light and reframed as a catalyzing element in a larger story.

⚘

Dory strongly encourages me to get out in the sunshine. I run errands and take a book to the roofdeck, but cannot stop the tears from flowing. My head frequently snaps back as I start to fall asleep. I come downstairs around two o'clock with the intention of sleeping. Foolishly, I let Dory go, and *then* Olwen comes to from her morphine grogginess and goes into a restless period. She keeps trying to get out of her chair and I keep begging her to stay put, but she cannot. Having gotten up eight or nine times to settle her down, I give her three drops of Ativan around three o'clock, to no avail.

"Terminal restlessness," I am to discover this week, is common in late-stage congestive heart failure (CHF). The patient engages in repetitious behavior that has (from our perspective) no apparent goal. They may pick at their clothes or bedclothes, button and unbutton clothing, or engage in physical movement or actions that don't lead anywhere. The behavior has a compulsive quality; the patient cannot stop doing it. One of the night nurses says, "it's like they are claustrophobic. They can't stand being in their own body, they can't stand covers on, they can't stand clothes on. They just have to get out, they have to move."

Poor circulation means less oxygen for the brain, while declining renal function means more toxins are circulating in the blood; both can contribute to restlessness and/or confusion. Thus giving oxygen is the first intervention one tries.

But terminal restlessness may be implicated in a more complex web. Some researchers, I will later learn, view terminal restlessness as an expression of delirium as well as the underlying CHF. Urinary tract infections can also generate restlessness while presenting as confusion or delirium. I wish I had known about potential linkages among these symptoms, and how one may mask another.

My mother's primary form of terminal restlessness was getting out of her chair. Over and over she would reach for the lever on the side, the lever that for decades had to be released to put the footrest down so she could get out of the chair. The new chair had no lever, however, just a button. For hours at a time she would try to climb out of her new chair, half-succeed and fall back again, rest, and try again, or, succeed, get tired, and be helped back to her chair.

Terminal restlessness is heartbreaking to watch and exhausting for the caregiver. We wonder if this repetitive behavior is driven solely by biochemical and neurological breakdowns, or if our failing parent is experiencing turmoil and torment that has no other outlet. Certainly she is not at peace, and one imagines that her own out-of-control behavior must be confusing and frightening to her. She is caught in some awful cycle over which she has no control, and which responds poorly, if at all, to most of our attempts to soothe, divert, or help. The combination of attending to this driven, repetitious behavior so she won't get hurt, feeling so helpless to stop it, and witnessing such apparent torment is emotionally devastating and draining.

About five o'clock, I give Olwen four or five more drops of Ativan. Rosanna calls and asks if she can help out. Yes! *Then* Olwen starts to nod off! Rosanna takes Olwen for a long outing. But now, even with the apartment all to myself on this gorgeous June evening, I cannot fall asleep.

Olwen looks amazingly bright and upbeat on her return. They toured the entire shopping center, and seemed to have especially enjoyed looking at dresses in the windows of a bridal shop. They finished up with ice cream in the dining room.

Olwen is in a playful mood, and for a couple of hours, we enjoy a lovely, three-way flow of playful energy. She starts trying on my sun hat, putting it on and off, and trying it at different angles. I bring in her hats and a mirror, and we all start playing with hats and admiring her wearing them. The great Welsh bone structure of her head, chin, and jaw has always carried off hats extremely well. The phone keeps ringing, so I flow in and out of our play time.

By 8:30, Olwen is tiring and we get her ready for bed. It is so helpful to have two of us helping her in the bathroom and getting her into the center of her bed. Last week at ninety-four pounds she seemed lighter than this week and transfers were not that difficult because she could help. With direction, she readily pivoted in place, and, with help, she could push herself up from a sitting position. This week she is still responsive to directions like, "we're going to do this on the count of three," or "now, put your left foot there," but she becomes more difficult to move.

Christine calls the transfer process dancing or hugging, and I have adopted those words. "We're going to dance now. Put your arms around my neck and hold on. Let's have a good hug! That's it. Now you're going to follow me." Olwen embraces and hugs me and holds on securely. To turn ninety degrees, we take several tiny steps with our bodies pressed together, "Turn, turn, turn, that's it, turn. Yes."

This week, she begins pulling down more often when we are trying to get her up. She is starting to become dead weight and her response time to directions is increasing. There are long delays in trying to get her to let go of the arms of the wheelchair when she is transferring to the toilet, or in letting go of the arms of the commode frame (that fits over the toilet, reducing the distance for getting up or down) when I am trying to get her up.

During those delays, I am holding her half-way up but she is too terrified to let go of the commode arms which she must do to stand up further so I can pull up her Depends, get her skirt or nightgown down over their high-friction bulk, and pivot her back to the wheelchair. During those long agonizing delays, I am holding her body up with one arm and using the other to arrange and smooth her clothing while she is pulling my lower back muscles and ligaments at horrific angles. During one of those transfers, my lower back and sacro-iliac muscles and ligaments get strained, and the torquing and misalignment of my lower back ripples upward into my neck and shoulders. It becomes difficult to find any position that is comfortable enough to go to sleep.

Over the course of the week, the transfer process shifts from our helping Mother, to her helping us, to her becoming less able to help, to her becoming a dragging force. Yet as with everything else, this is not a linear trajectory. Wednesday she can pivot and help more than on Tuesday, and then Thursday there is another drop in her ability to help us to help her.

As she becomes a "two-person transfer," I am beset by a new set of worries. How am I going to be able to manage her transfers? How can I try and schedule people to reduce the number of times I have to transfer her by myself? As she keeps going down hill, what is going to happen to my back? I have already hurt myself, am in pain, and we are just getting started.

Hospice sends over a night nurse, but I am unable to sleep while waiting for her. After a six-hour block of sleep, I talk with her at dawn for over an hour about observations, terminal restlessness, and CHF patterns of dying. I press her for her best sense of timing. She says, "less than a month." I nod, because that is my best guess as well. And then again, no one knows. As the other night nurse says six days later, "The stronger the will of the person, the longer they can go on." I respond, "She has the strongest will and the greatest resilience of anyone I ever known. That's what makes this so terrifying."

Tuesday, it is a little harder to get Mother up. She hardly touches her cereal so I take it away and give her a small bowl of raspberries, blackberries, and blueberries. They sit in her lap for a long time. The bowl tips at an angle, but she seems oblivious. She eats a few berries, but makes no move to right the bowl. Neither her attention nor her eyes are focusing. Jesse arrives and immediately notices the change from Thursday. Five days is a long time, but it is during the course of this day that I notice the most significant deterioration of any day so far from the day before—a tricky assessment given the volatility of late-stage CHF.

Mother is quiet this morning and I have difficulty hearing what she says as well as making sense of it. Although deteriorating overall, her ability to form words is variable. Sometimes I can hear much of what she says and we have a fairly lucid conversation in which her words are audible and relate to one another and my responses. Other times, she utters a few words after a silence, and the poorly formed words whiz by before I can even try to catch them. Sometimes she tries to repeat her words for me, but usually she cannot. Even when she can, they often have no syntax or relationship to what preceded them, giving me few clues about what words she may have uttered. Her words are quantum mini-moments flashing out of her inner kaleidoscope that is otherwise unlanguaged. This morning there are long silences punctuated by such moments.

Olwen has an upsurge in restlessness today. Despite Jesse's efforts to contain her efforts to get out of her chair, she manages to fall once again, this time on her bottom, but has no complaints. She also starts shredding napkins and does this on and off for a couple of days. The uptick in restlessness seems linked to intensification of her feeling that she is burning up inside. All of these behaviors and sensations are common in late-stage CHF.

The strength she exhibits in her restlessness co-habits with being tired and wanting to rest on the sofa. She wants fewer clothes on, so we help her take off her blouse, shoes, and stockings. I apply flexible cold-packs to her armpits and groin. Every day, she will ask for *icy cold* water several times; her voice remains clear and loud on this critical point. I find an undershirt in a drawer and pull out the smallest of my tank tops. From here on, she will wear tank tops, and we will add a blouse or shirt if the surge of overheating passes and she feels cold.

The overheating characteristic of late CHF is produced by the heart and circulatory system trying to work extra hard to protect core organs, and help them do their work. The wisdom of the body gives those organs top priority for oxygen, nutrients, and removal of waste. This concentration of the heart's effort cheats the circulation in the rest of the body, however. Not surprisingly, it is during this week that Olwen's feet begin to turn purplish at times, especially when her legs are down—a sign that circulation to and especially from the extremities is getting to be a harder job for her heart, particularly now that it has taken on this heroic effort to save her core.

Michael calls this afternoon. I put the phone to her ear, but she does not know who "Michael" is or what a phone or phone call is, and she hands the phone back to me. Yet when we go out later for a drive, she expects Michael will be down by the car.

It's as if cotton wool were filling up more and more of her brain, yet she struggles to make the neurons fire and produce a trail of synapses that link back to the life she commanded for so many decades. Somewhere, Michael and his attempts to connect with her have registered. But the Cartesian time-space restrictions separating her from Michael are evaporating for her, much as they did on Saturday when she called me at home to invite me to go downstairs to dinner. She seems to inhabit a nonlocal, quantum world where there is no elapsed time, and people are present to each other despite being separated by spatial distance.

❦

Later than afternoon, Mother is extremely antsy to go downstairs, only too aware "they" are gathering for dinner. Surprisingly, no one is there. We sit, absorbing the rustling and swaying of the grove of tall, elderly trees next to the apartments. One of the tenants, bent over her walker but getting her exercise, makes her way from the street toward us, leans in, and asks directly, "How *are* you, Olwen?" Olwen does not really look at her or respond in a fully audible or appropriate way. The woman wheels around and goes back up to the street.

Back upstairs, Olwen propels herself around the living room in her wheelchair, rolling back and forth but edging ever closer to me while I am trying to make supper. In the midst of her agitated movement, she says clearly, "I don't have very long . . . You deserve everything . . . I'm very slow today." I stop and sit with her, acknowledging what she has said. Her restless movement prompts me to ask if she wants to go for a drive? Yes. I put food back in the frig and leave the place in semi-chaos because she cannot wait.

We tour the grounds of the country club where she made new friends and played golf in her fifties and sixties. She remembers none of it. I take a leisurely drive on a winding country road. She never turns her head and her eyes have a glassy look.

Although she is not actively tracking the ever-changing scene, she is fully alert and not at all restless when we are out and driving around. Her head and upper body are erect, extending forward slightly, poised and highly attentive. Her body language and facial expression suggest her mind is trying to make connections between her current sensory input and old receptor sites in her memory banks, but the synapses cannot form a path through the fog.

When we get back, Sue is there with her son-in-law to get the living room sofa and move Olwen's bed into the living room so we can make way for the hospital bed tomorrow. With all the movement of furniture, and unmaking and making of beds, Olwen gets mildly upset. She doesn't remember Sue's son-in-law and wonders what this strange man is doing in her living room taking away her sofa. Is this really okay? I try repeatedly to reassure her. After they leave, I finish making supper and put Olwen to bed. She laments, "I can't find anything, I can't do anything."

※

Because of Olwen's incredible bones, there have so far been no devastating consequences from her numerous falls during the past few years and even the last few weeks. Prevention of falls has, therefore, never been at the top of my priority list. Now, however, although I no longer have to worry about a fall that suddenly changes a high quality of life or leads to complications that could chop good years off her life, I still have to worry about a fall that could lead to a hospitalization that undermines everything we are trying to do with home care.

Until Friday and Saturday nights, she had never fallen out of bed in her life. Her prior falls have stemmed from either a momentary vascular insufficiency to the brain, or trying to do something that she can or should no longer do (like trying to make the bed a couple of weeks ago).

It has never been possible to prevent that type of fall. You can be ten feet away and, out of nowhere, down she goes. Or you turn your back for a moment, or go out of the room, and she goes ahead and does whatever she was bent on doing. No one can control her every move every second. To try to do so, as hospitals and nursing homes attempt in their crude ways (because they are so worried about liability), is oppressive.

The risk-benefit tradeoffs of a hospital bed are shifting. I have held off and pushed back against everyone's advocacy of such a bed because I know she will hate it and always feels imprisoned by the rails. She has been too strong not to try climbing over the rails and possibly injure herself more than by rolling out of her own bed. To defer this day, I not only lowered her bed, but also removed the nightstand that was between the beds (so she couldn't hurt herself on it if she fell), moved the two beds together (so there is only one open side), and used the second eggcrate foam to fill the valley between the beds. But now, the probabilities of her climbing over the rails are diminishing. Although Olwen is still stunningly strong at moments, she is weakening overall and cannot sustain her strength for long.

I've arranged for delivery at 11:00, but the guy doesn't even call until 1:30, fails to follow my excellent directions, clashes with Kate's trying to visit with Olwen before she heads off for three weeks, and competes with tenants for use of the elevator for a lemonade social—which is precisely what I was trying to avoid with my scheduling. Oblivious to the problems he has caused, he brings the hospital tray up first. Has the equipment been sterilized since its previous use. No, it hasn't. What!!?? In addition to coping with all the physical and emotional horror of a hospital bed, I now have to worry about who knows what germs being carried into our home!!?? He threatens not to bring the bed upstairs. Kate smoothes the situation. While he goes down for the next load, I start washing equipment as best I can in the hall, sweating profusely and flooding with tears. I get rid of him as soon as possible.

※

Only after Jesse has left do I realize Mother's bed is still only half-made, and we have another load of laundry in the dryer upstairs. Olwen is too rambunctious to leave long enough to finish either. She wants her skirt off now because it is too hot.

Her dear little body is just bone and hanging flesh. Given what she has eaten in the last eight weeks, it's a wonder there is anything left. Her muscles have atrophied or been consumed in her body's fight to hang on. What is even more amazing is how strong she still is, how fiercely determined she can be, and how able to persist in her desire/need to climb out of the chair with the footrest up.

I pull up a chair right opposite her and make calls for the next hour. I am facing her, watching her do this activity over and over, not interfering but ready to intervene if needed. Sometimes I hold her hand with my free hand, and it quiets her briefly. When she finally succeeds in freeing herself completely from the chair and stands up, I am standing right next to her, just in case. I am superfluous. She instinctively bends her knees, thereby lowering her center of gravity, and grasps the floor with her bare feet. She is moving in a more grounded and secure way than she has the last couple of years when has become a bit tip-toey. She of the perfectly erect posture is shedding her inhibitions and instinctually taking care of herself with her chimpanzee crouch. I applaud what she is doing, and tell her how smart her body is being.

I talk with Neal about her restlessness, my exhaustion, my difficulties in transferring her, and the growing potential for serious harm to my back, and trying to find ways I might get more relief. He will try to get us a night nurse tonight. He raises the possibility of "respite care" which hospice can offer to overextended caregivers. In the ideal situation, the hospice would have a residential facility that could take patients in for up to five days a month while the caregiver recuperates. Our hospice has to use a nursing home, however. The patient can still be followed by their regular hospice team, and Medicare pays for the respite.

Dinaz calls, we explore the same territory, and she suggests another option. Put Olwen on a regular schedule of Ativan every six hours to maintain an optimal level of the drug in her blood so she doesn't become agitated in the first place. Then perhaps both Olwen and I can get more sleep.

Dinaz had come by this morning to investigate the urinary tract infection (UTI) I learned about at 4:00 AM. when Olwen told me she had burning and itching but couldn't give me a sense of when it had started. And why didn't she tell me before? Because she didn't want to "bother" me, and she thought it was just something you have to live with. This just kills me. I tell her emphatically we CAN help this problem. "We have a whole army of people who are here to help you, who *want* you to 'bother' them whenever you have *any* problem or *any* need. Just tell us, and we will do what we can to help you, to make you more comfortable, okay?"

The night Olwen told me about the UTI followed the day her restlessness became significant and she began having trouble transferring—the *same* day she began seriously overheating, and we noticed the biggest drop in her functioning. How I wish I had known that UTIs can also present as delirium or as restlessness, as well as be linked to various failing systems. No one mentioned this or proactively checked to see if this was causing or contributing to her delirium or restlessness.

The risk of a urinary tract infection is one of the many reasons Dinaz and I have agreed not to consider a urinary catheter. Although it would greatly reduced the transfer problem, Dinaz believes Olwen would pull it out (so do I), putting her at greater risk of infection, particularly in its more serious forms. Furthermore, Olwen is continent and able to tell us when she needs to go to the bathroom. The ability to control one's bladder is such a pivotal and emotionally charged issue in human dignity that neither of us want to take that away from her despite the transfer burden it imposes.

※

Another night nurse comes for the first time and shares her views. Terminal agitation is not permanent but a phase. It foreshadows the end rather than being the end itself. It is typically followed by more sleeping, and sometimes a coma. Ativan can relax the patient and help them and their caregivers get past this difficult phase. After an Ativan schedule is introduced, families sometimes think their dying person is drugged because they sleep so much, but she believes it more likely the patient is exhausted and can finally get some rest. Our conversation dovetails with my earlier conversation with Dinaz, and we start an Ativan schedule at dawn on the twenty-sixth.

Olwen is barely swallowing a few berries today, so we crush her pills in sherbet and spend a long time encouraging her to eat it. During the middle of the day, I write at Mary's. Being at her computer is centering, and writing about this week helps me digest some of its turbulence and anguish.

Our hospice volunteer, Becky, comes by for an hour or so. It is a lovely, crisp, sunny afternoon. Olwen is in a quiet and sleepy place, and I use Becky's time to nap. I play a tape of a choir singing polyphonic overtones in a French cathedral. The music, breezes, the two of us drifting in and out of sleep, and the third quietly holding the space all form a gentle, seamless whole.

Later, doing Reiki with Olwen, I find that standing behind her chair and leaning over is not only helpful for my back, but also allows me to speak right into her ear, and to hear what she says. Out of "nowhere" comes another stunning quantum moment in which her words concisely crystallize the undercurrents of our situation and the dilemmas of her care: "You do what you have to do, and I'll do what I have to do."

―――※―――

With Rosanna and Sue doing the lion's share, a two-day schedule has come together easily for this weekend. Christine will be on, so even with Dinaz away at a conference, I am comfortable. I suspect this will be my last trip home before Olwen dies, and I do need to make a trip. Better to go before her birthday than after, when all bets are off.

Still, Olwen's trajectory this week has been disturbing, and she felt lousy yesterday. Because there were new symptoms during the pre-dawn hours on Friday, I decide I cannot leave. I am leaning this way at the moment despite the fact that only yesterday I was counseling myself that I cannot turn myself into a pretzel trying to schedule and reschedule around every uptick and downtick. All I can do is trust my intuition about her birthday, and try to trust her process and timing overall.

An on-call nurse points out at dawn that I already *am* doing the dying process with her, but, deep down, that's not enough for me; I want and need to be here for her transition. The signs I am describing suggest death is drawing closer, she says, perhaps less than a week. The RN substituting for Dinaz points out that patients often sleep for three days after they begin either an Ativan or a Roxanol regime. Juggling their inputs, I am glad Christine will be here shortly so we can assess the situation together.

I fill Christine in on the last forty-eight hours, and she asks good questions. She suspects bowel impaction may be the primary culprit in why Olwen has been feeling lousy. She attends to that, and within a couple hours, Olwen is no longer moaning or miserable. She is peaceful and almost smiling. I feel immense relief. It is not the Ativan! It is not her organs or systems collapsing! It is not the end—not yet anyway! When Jesse and I take her into the bathroom around three o'clock, she can push herself up, and she is not as dead weight as yesterday.

All of these temporary improvements fit with my sense that she will make it to her birthday before the Final Dance begins. I begin to feel I *can* safely be gone for two days.

Fortunately, I took a nap after Jesse came so I won't fall asleep driving. Unable to get away yesterday, Kate comes up for her real farewell visit with Olwen, and Jesse and I make ourselves scarce. After more Reiki with Olwen, I leave around four o'clock. Saturday, my chiropractor arranges to see me and relieves my neck, head, and shoulder pain.

Over the weekend, Sue and Rosanna experience increasing difficulty transferring her. They find Olwen tired and weak, dozing off more, and talking less, but her restlessness is much better, she is responding appropriately, and enjoying her outings where several residents speak to her. She is swallowing well, especially relishes ice cream with blueberries, and is also drinking milk, Ensure, juice, ginger ale, and asks several times for ice cold water. She wants to wash her own hands and face as well as comb her own hair.

When Angela cannot come for her six-hour shift, I arrange for Mary to come for two hours, Sharon for two hours, after which Rosanna will come back for a couple of hours until Sue arrives for the overnight. Not only are Mary and Sharon the "right" people to be with Olwen this afternoon, but each of them has also been a primary caregiver herself. Neither is freaked out about attending the dying. Each has known Olwen all her life, and each of them has become a friend and sometime helper in these last few years.

Before I found Sue, Sharon had taken Olwen to numerous appointments and errands. She is very fond of Olwen, and Olwen is one of her last links to her beloved mother whom she attended in her dying from CHF a few years ago. Our mothers had been next-door neighbors who had their first (and in Olwen's case, only) child late in life. I never forget the incredible generosity of Sharon's parents who loaned their log cabin in the mountains to us for an entire season when I was five.

There, Olwen pulled off one of the most awesome accomplishments of her life, one which the doctors and everyone else deemed absolutely impossible: saving my father's life by getting him well from tuberculosis outside a sanitarium. She made fires on chilly mornings, and we often went canoeing while he had his afternoon nap. Most strongly imprinted on my child-self is the still vivid image of her boiling his sheets and his dishes, and constantly sanitizing the bathroom we all shared. It was a staggering achievement, all the more so because neither of us ever became ill. I am so thankful for having her constitution!

As soon as Mary gets home, she sends an e-mail. "Olwen dozed or slept in her chair the whole time I was there. She didn't want any water or fruit juice and seemed to have no needs. She smiled a couple of times as if she might have recognized me. I sat right near her the whole time. Brought a book but didn't feel like reading it—as if some energies might have been flowing back and forth between us and reading would have shut down those circuits."

Sunday, I send an e-mail to a large network of friends, pick up a chocolate-almond cheesecake, and a slice of key lime cheesecake for Olwen. My last stop is at the home of my friend Brigit who has picked a wondrous bouquet of wild and healing flowers from her garden, and written thoughtfully on a card about what each is for.

The card itself reads, "Being alive requires of us a relationship with the mysterious lifelong experience of letting go. May grace guide you as you gently let go." Absolutely perfect. But gently? Oh, if only it were so!

To be sure, Olwen and I do go to the far end of gentle at times, but there is also much turbulence and angst. Her dying ain't like in the movies. Or those annoying books that paint lovely, peaceful, fully conscious scenarios leading to death and portray its spiritual dimensions antiseptically, devoid of their grounded richness and complexity. No way! In her cataclysmic struggle to let go, the spiritual, emotional, and physical are intimately fused.

When I arrive back in her apartment, Olwen looks at me and announces sweetly, "I see somebody's face." Yes, "somebody" is here, and she won't be leaving again.

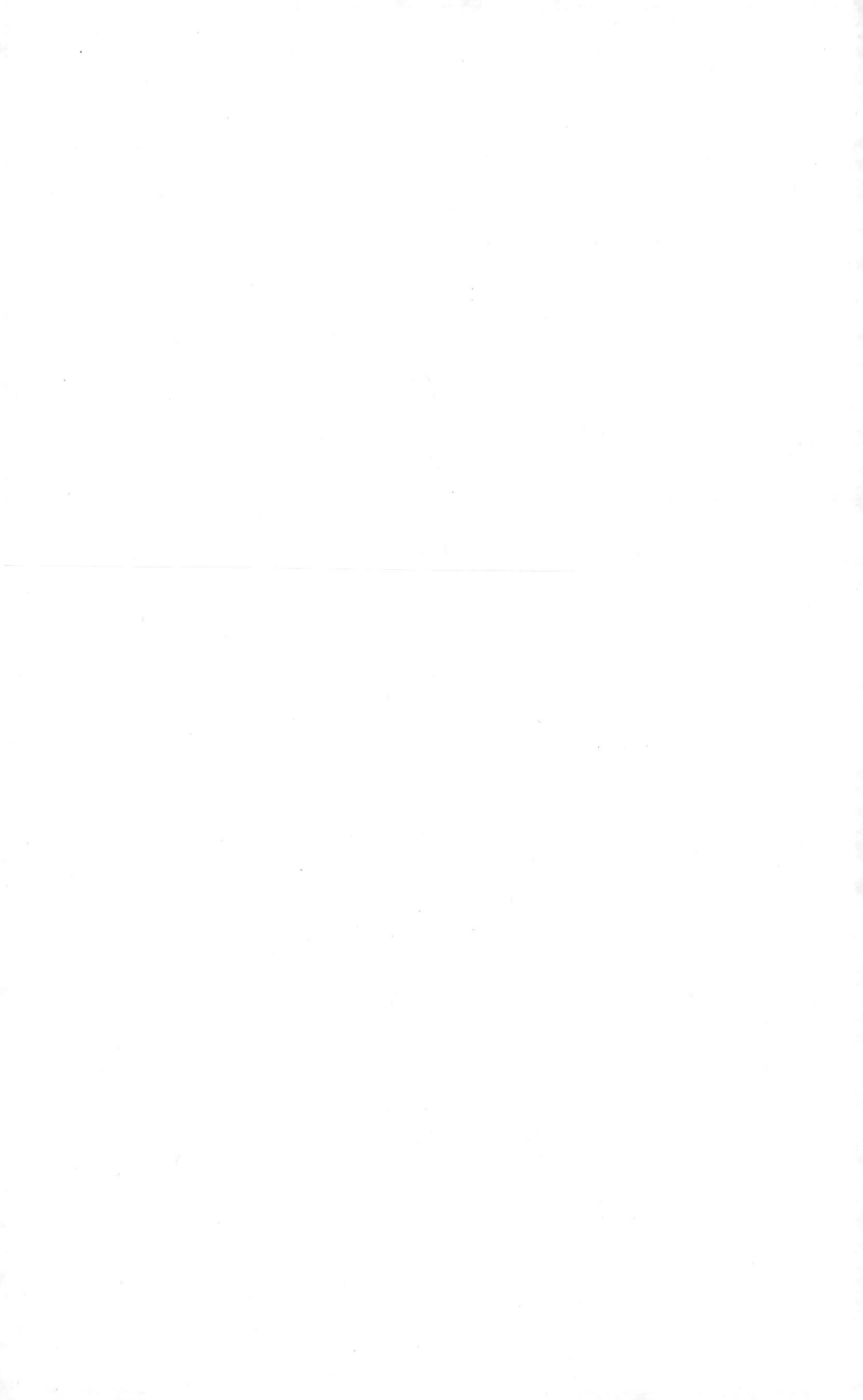

Nine

How Do You Let Go of Your Life?

I don't know what I'm doing, and I don't know if I'll ever finish it . . . It's the last thing I am doing, and I can't do it . . . I want to let go. I'm trying to let go.

—Olwen, June 25

A day or two after our Grand Hotel moment, Mother begins talking at five in the morning about *wanting* to let go, *trying* to let go, and her distress that she just doesn't know how. She wants help. All kinds of people have taken a crack at this, but they are usually in the clouds with their ethereal abstractions. Our situation is urgent and real, however.

Mother has rarely asked for help, and now that she is, she is asking The Question. I am trying to absorb this stunning fact while reaching for answers. I suspect the biggest barriers are the "unfinished business" of one's life, and uncertainty about its meaning to others and one's place in their hearts. As long as we are still here, something more can happen, something might get fixed, finished, clarified, made more certain, resolved, or even healed. Yearning for greater completion is perhaps the most powerful inducement to hang on. In her own way, Olwen has said as much many times: "I think I'll stick around a little while longer to see what happens," or, "I'd like just a little more time to finish some things."

So, what is most unfinished for Olwen? How do I come up with suggestions on the spot that connect for her? How do I move through this unfamiliar territory, and offer immediate, grounded answers her slowing mind can catch and hold, answers that give her a sense of progress toward her goal of going Home?

I take my cues from her. The question is being asked by a woman who has been a doer and a problem-solver all her life, a woman who doesn't know the meaning of procrastination. How then can I translate this open-ended, amorphous, awesome process of letting go of life into a manageable project? How can I shrink its infinite size into elements that feed into letting go, and make them concrete enough to seem doable? How do I help her see that she is already on her way and thereby reduce her frustration level?

"Your body is very wise and knows what to do. You are eating less and less because you are listening to your body. By eating only what appeals, your body wisdom is already helping you to let go." As we talk about the heaviness of meat and the appeal of juice, the body/food piece registers for her. She persists, "how do I let go?"

I point out she has been doing her mental and emotional work all along. "You have always looked death in the face and talked openly about your own death. That's a really big deal!! You've done that very, very well!! Many people can't look at death and so they lose out on having the conversations we can. You've already done a very big—and very brave—part of letting go."

Is some of this affirmation sinking in? Does she see her courage and lifelong pattern of looking at things straight-on have already done an important part of the work for her?

When she starts going around with her perennial issue of needing to "get things all taken care of," I remind her that her paperwork is all set, and that, "You don't have to worry about the money piece because you took care of that, too. You are the best money manager I have ever known. Now there is still enough money to take care of you right here in your own apartment. That's what your money is for. You won't run out of money."

Finally—I think, I pray, I hope—we are at the point where I am confidant we will not run out of money before she runs out of life, at least as long as I am doing the biggest share of caregiving.

After some iterations, I feel we can move on from what she has already done to what is still undone. The unfinished stuff I have been trying to chip away at for years, often feeling I am having no effect whatsoever.

The hard stuff is what will help Olwen find as much resolution as possible so it becomes easier to let go. I normalize the situation: "A life is always unfinished. It doesn't tie up neatly with a bow. Yet we all have to do the best we can to resolve unfinished stuff—the losses, the wounds, the if-only's, the roads not taken, the missed opportunities." I let that sink in—or, hope it registers.

"The big issue is: what do you need for a greater sense of emotional and spiritual completion of your life? What would help your heart and soul to let go? That's a hard one, isn't it?" I try to take the pressure off her. "It's hard for any of us to answer, and hard to put into words."

Especially hard for Olwen perhaps. She has rarely been able to tell me in a straightforward way what is distressing her. If she names a fixable issue and I fix it, it has no lasting effect on her distress. She does not dig into her interior and bring her excavations into words the way my friends, colleagues, and I have learned to do. Olwen belongs to the pre-psychological era when there was little language to talk about interior life and issues. Nor was there a cultural or familial context that made such expression possible and permissible, and enabled people to practice these skills.

Consequently, I have tried to figure out what is really going on with her. I believe the anxieties and sadness that have become more prominent in recent years represent a convergence of end-of-life issues with her oldest losses which had such life-altering, devastating consequences. As if that weren't enough, the fact my "real work" is not yet out—and thus my own life neither "settled" (as she would say) nor realized—always weighs heavily upon her.

I keep asking myself, how can I bring to bear some payoff from my vast education (in which she had invested and had always supported) and all the time spent with friends and colleagues exploring inner landscapes? What good is all our fancy talk if I can't help my own mother come to terms with the end of her life? How can I cut across our life-paradigms and reach into her world so as to connect up with the nameless fears and wounded places in her? Perhaps relieve some pressure points, or facilitate something coming unstuck?

I have tried over and over to name the nameless within her, giving it form and dignity, and pulling it out of the amorphous reservoir at the bottom of things. I give shape and visibility to the story-beneath-her-story, bear witness to it and to her struggles, and validate the largely mute anguish at the center of her Story, while addressing her perennial concerns about doing the right thing and doing a good job. My hope is to relieve some of the anxiety and sadness and move her closer to finding some measure of resolving the unfixable.

On this morning when she is lucid, intensely alert, pressing me on how to let go, and relentless in pursuit of answers in a conversation that lasts over two hours without her attention ever flagging, I tell her once again as I have for some years, "I know it must be hard for you to come to terms emotionally with your life because there is no way to undo the dreadful losses you had. Losing Mama so early and suddenly was terrible, and there were so many losses in its wake."

I disentangle this, beginning with the suppression of her anguish and grief—which I have deduced from her coping strategies and her father's emotional blockage. "You couldn't talk about Mama or show your grief because there was no permission to grieve, no way to bring it out in the open so it was shared. When grief is not shared, it isolates you. There was no one to help you grieve or work things through." I wait.

"So you had to cope by yourself. You did it the way people have always done it: by locking things away inside yourself so you didn't feel the sharpness of the pain. But it's always there underneath."

But buried grief doesn't explain it all. I don't know why it took me so long to figure it out. "Not only did you have all that ungrieved, unhealed loss and grief about Mama, but you also had to protect yourself against the traumatic events surrounding her death. How do you do that? You do exactly what you did. You separate the painful images and memories from each other, and from their meanings, and from your feelings. You had to park them all in different places so they couldn't hurt you so much, do you see? You couldn't let them all come together, it would have been too overwhelming. You needed to protect yourself from experiencing feelings that are too awful to feel and knowing things too awful to know."

I wait and I reiterate. Does any of this register with her pre-psychological mode of thought?

"What I now see—and it took me a long time to see this, honey—are the consequences of the trauma you suffered, the consequences for you, for me, for us. When you separated things in your mind so they wouldn't be so painful, it made it harder for you to get your feelings out and take good stuff in. It is so sad because you often got the opposite of what you wanted and what I wanted. The ways you protected yourself would drive me back when I had tried to come forward. Then I felt I had to protect myself, and I did stupid things that hurt you. I am so very sorry for all the ways I hurt you. I didn't know any better, and my own stuff was in the way."

Although I am craving sleep, I know we may never have this opportunity again. She is so eager, so energized, so alert, so open, and searching for help. "How do I do it? How do I let go?" she entreats over and over. Maybe, just maybe, more is getting in today than during all my other attempts. Or, maybe, all those other attempts are having a cumulative effect in this precious moment where she is open and reaching. Possibly more rather than less can seep in now because her protective layers are peeling away, and she is coming from her core rather than her periphery, her true self rather than her adaptive selves.

"I want you to understand this: It wasn't a *bad* thing how you took care of yourself. *It wasn't wrong.* You *had* to take care of yourself. But it's a *sad* thing because it got in your way and wound up hurting you. I find that excruciatingly sad." I walk a dicey line here because her paradigm tends to convert everything into "right" and "wrong" even though I try to keep her out of that place.

Nothing I have said to Olwen this morning about the emotional substrate of her Story is new for her. As her mental processing has slowed, I have found repetitions are needed for something to sink in. It may not be clear whether it is sinking in at the time, but, if it is important, it often shows up down the road, having apparently taken a subterranean journey.

I can only imagine the valiant struggle she is undergoing now to process my efforts to witness, validate, and frame her Story, and somehow absorb them into her being so that it becomes easier to let go. She is doing the hardest, most important work of her life. No wonder she sometimes tells us she has to work now, and in the same breath, that she has to go to bed.

As always, I am trying to assess what she is taking in and processing, how many repetitions are helpful, when we have reached a point of saturation, when it is time to move on or to stop. Today, it's not time to stop.

It feels imperative to go to the heart of the matter, the unnecessary nature of her mother's death.

"We can't change the past. But there is one important thing I can do to help you now, one thing you must hear and take all the way in. Listen to me now: IT WASN'T YOUR FAULT!! I've told you this over and over. It wasn't up to you to save Mama. It wasn't *your* job. *You* did not fail. Other people failed but you did not fail. Are you hearing me? This is the one big thing that has to sink in now. This is the great truth that is still alive and still matters. *It wasn't your fault!!* You did all you could, but you still couldn't save her."

Her entire being is alert and actively listening. I am hoping against hope this injunction is somehow miraculously penetrating to her core. No small thing because I am asking—no, insisting—she let go of the false guilt around which, I have come to surmise, she framed her edifice of self-negating, protective structures.

After we have worked that defining issue for a while, I think it's time to move forward to my own place in the unfinished business in her life. "I have such anguish about your not seeing how things turn out for me because you have been there from the beginning, always believing in me. I absolutely believe it's going to happen like we've talked about, but. I am so, so sorry I couldn't get my work out into the world faster so you could see how my real life starts to unfold."

A year later, I read Hillary Johnson's book, *My Mother Dying*, which captures this same excruciating reality permeating her relationship with her mother.

> My mother and I knew by then that she would never live to see the jacketed, bound version. Yet she recognized, as did I, that her peaceful death, and my peaceful life, depended in some part upon our unwavering faith in its promise. My unfinished first book had become, in a sense, our private religion. It was our ladder into the uncharted future, and the altar upon which we quietly laid our sacrifices and our love for each other. Completed, it would stand as the lasting monument to our bond. More simply, the book belonged to Ruth as much as to me, and therefore its completion would signify not just my success in life but her own. After all, I was nothing if not my mother's creation.[1]

"I have told you many times how grateful I am about all you have done for me. You never gave up on me, and that's amazing. It says a lot about you."

"Uh-huh."

"I've asked you to forgive me for the stupid and mean things I have said. I am so very, very sorry for things I have said, and the ways I missed seeing you."

"Umm-hmm." Ever pragmatic, she eventually comes back to her core question, "How do I do it? How do I let go?"

Well, I say, I think it is less about "doing" and more about "being." I add that it is much easier for everybody to *talk* about "being" than actually "doing" it. "You have been an excellent, problem-solving doer all your life, and it has taken you through a lot, it has gotten you this far. But, maybe now your very strengths are getting in your way. Maybe your strengths as a doer and your never putting off until tomorrow what you can do right now are making it harder to shift into just being, and trusting that it will all work out."

Maybe, I suggest, what gets in her way of just being or of letting go is her trying so hard to "do" it, and to do it "right." "Maybe your trying so hard clouds the process. Maybe the fact that it is getting harder for you to think and to talk is a spiritual gift forcing you to go to a deeper level of your being—into your soul. Your soul knows what it is doing, honey, and it is doing just fine."

Not only is this line of thought emerging with ease, but I find myself really believing it. I reiterate the idea that her body knows what it is doing, her soul knows what it is doing, and it is just her mind that hasn't gotten on board. Rather than being distressed at the loss of (conventional) mind, maybe, I find myself saying, we can see it as a gift that is actually helping her to open to something deeper.

"What we both need to learn is to trust your soul's wisdom and its process. I know it's hard. It's hard for me, too. But remember when I told you about the rainbow I drove toward for way over an hour? And how the full moon emerged out of a tiny opening in heavy clouds? I took all that as a good sign for us, for your process, for our process. I took that to mean we should trust the process."

She presses me for more clues about how to "be." I dig for answers. "Music," I finally say, "is kind of a bridge between worlds. If you can just go with the flow of it, music carries you, it transports you. To really be with the music, you have to be in the moment because music happens from moment to moment. Music is a movement of notes and sounds. So maybe when we are playing music, you can try to let yourself just flow with it, melt into it."

She is relentless in her appeals for help in letting go. After a long silence, I find myself speaking of something I have never voiced in my life. "Well, I think letting go has something to do with grace." That, I soon add, doesn't really tell us too much because, "What *is* grace? I don't pretend to know. It is a mystery. Does grace come to you? Or do you come to grace? I don't know how we come into grace. But I do have a strong sense that the mystery of grace is the ultimate key to surrendering and letting go and finding peace."

Having said this, I feel our conversation has found the answer it had unknowingly been seeking. Her body language says we are done.

The following Tuesday, I am tucking Mother into bed. When her "worry face" comes back, I ask, "Is there anything you are afraid of? Anything I can help you with?

"What do you mean, 'afraid of?'"

"I don't know. Sometimes you've said you are scared. I don't know what you are scared of, and I don't know if there is anything I can help you with. You have mentioned being scared of being alone. Now someone will always be here with you. So you are not alone in that sense."

I try to normalize her fears because she is not of a generation that shares them easily, and is thus prone to privatizing them—thinking she is the only one who feels this way. "I get scared, too, we all do. Everyone has fears, even though they may not talk about them. Most of us are scared of dying. Any fears you may be having are very, very common."

She does not name her fears or what may be troubling her. After a bit, I ask her about the most fear-erasing thing that could possibly happen for her. "Do you have any sense of your mother's being close to you?"

"Umm-hmm." I should have asked her to tell me what she sensed.

"Know that I love you very much, and I have always trusted your mother would come to you when the time comes, that you will see her again. I do hope so."

After I let that sink in, I remind her that, "We already know her spirit has been active in my house, turning her picture these last years. If Mama knew how to find me so far from where she had ever been, then she must know how to find you, right? We already know she knows how to come to us and be active in the space between the worlds. So she'll know what to do and when to come to you," I state with more confidence than I thought I had. "Do you think you can go to sleep now?"

"Umm-hmm."

My faith about my grandmother builds around a vague hope I have held for as long as I can remember. It took an enormous leap a couple of years ago when I realized her picture was turning on its own. When I had first noticed it was out of alignment with pictures on each of the two shelves below it, I thought I must have accidently moved it. I repositioned her picture, but a few days later, it had again turned counterclockwise, so I lined it up again.

After a third round, I said to myself, "Okay, I am not making this up. Something really is going on here. What will happen if I don't intervene?" I realized that if this pivoting continued to about 120 degrees from where it had started, Mama would be facing a picture of her three daughters. Her picture did exactly that, at which point it stopped for several months before resuming its movement.

In experimental mode and tired of looking at the back of the frame, I brought Lizzie's picture back to its original position. There she was looking majestic in long white dress and full-length gloves, with an elaborate hat on the bench next to her. The occasion: a picnic in a lovely city park. I didn't get to look at her for long, however, as the entire process repeated itself, and, once again, Lizzie stopped when she faced her daughters.

Somewhat apprehensive I would mess up whatever was going on, I made copies of the picture. To my relief, its outing with the scanner didn't interfere with its own energetic processes. The turning repeated itself yet again.

Who or what was turning the picture? All things considered, one answer made the most sense: who but Lizzie would be turning her picture to face a picture of her three daughters?

So I had thought, "Okay, Lizzie, you've got my attention. What does this mean? What are you trying to tell me?"

My cautious openness about what may lie beyond the three dimensions organizing our material reality does not belong to any belief system or fit any trivializing category. Experiences such as those with Lizzie's picture suggest two things: that other dimensions and energies can be active in or act upon our three-dimensional reality, and that the short lives we lead between birth and death are apparently not the whole story, and may be part of a far more vast and complex web about which we understand very little.

My matter-of-fact ease with extraordinary experiences such as Lizzie's picture is consistent with my understanding that multiple dimensions, energies, and/or realities are co-present, flowing into and affecting one another. My understanding and language for talking about them draw from three, compatible streams of thought: experiential, earth-revering, wisdom traditions, such as those of the Gaelic Celts, indigenous North Americans, and indigenous "Old Europeans" who preceded the invading Indo-Europeans;[2] biophysics and vibrational medicine paradigms which have begun to explain the role of energy flows, forces, and therapies in maintaining and restoring normal health;[3] and the leading edge of quantum physics. String theory, for example, postulates eleven dimensions, most of them "curled up" inside our familiar, three dimensions, and operating on nonlocal, quantum principles.[4]

I suspect these dimensions operating on nonlocal or not-yet-understood (by science) principles—and evidently right here in front of us—could tell us something about how Lizzie's picture was able to move. Regarding what happens after death, belief systems make me uncomfortable, especially when held with the closed-minded certitude of many secularists and religionists. By instead allowing extraordinary experiences to flow through us without resistance, we may expand or transform who we are and act on our connectedness with all that is and was.

Lizzie apparently knew exactly where I was and how to contact me through her picture. She was very clever to do something physical, because my skeptical self would not believe something intangible ("I'm just making this up"). I need something I can hang my hat on as my doorway to accepting that there is something non-physical emanating from outside of me.

Turning to face her daughters suggested Olwen's time was coming and I needed to be acting accordingly. I took it as a sign to hold the faith that Mama would be there for her at the end.

Last summer, I told Olwen about the turning picture. Although she was not making many new memories by that time, this registered immediately and permanently. She asked me about it in subsequent calls, and I wrote it all down so she could reread it whenever she wanted. Although Olwen had given me Mama's picture several years ago, I decided it belonged with Olwen for the rest of her life. Significantly, Olwen, who rarely asks directly for anything, called to ask me to bring the picture on my next trip.

Our process of finding where the picture should reside was an amazing moment. Olwen actively led the process. She was completely present to the moment and attuned to the picture and its energies and where it needed to be. She knew immediately when it was in the right place—her small, marble-top coffee table. She tried the picture of the three daughters/sisters (the same as the one I have) in different places, and knew when it was right.

Her confidence was wonderful to behold. No second-guessing, no asking me (as she had been doing in recent years), just seeing-moving with complete ease and self-assurance. Her confidence was coming from the core of her being, and was quite different from the Olwen of prime years who did things right and did the right things and, without being asked, instructed others in doing the same. That older mode of being was, I thought, shaped in part by reassuring herself about herself. But the Olwen of this magical moment needed no reassurance because she simply *knew* and carried her knowing into action.

Something was moving through her and through me and throughout our space. The energies were palpable and guided us through a dance that took over and flowed through us. It was a three-way dance being orchestrated I felt by Lizzie in which we three were united in an organic, magical way. As Mother and I sat by the dining table gazing at Mama's picture on the marble table, I could feel a new center of energy radiating there, becoming the invisible center of the room.

※

After again viewing videos of the cat, the birthday party, and my apartment on the evening of June 18, Mother says she is pleased she is feeling better. Her breathing is also better than yesterday.

Out of nowhere she says, "I love you very much." I reply, "I love you very much, too." She continues, "Who else would be good at the job?"

"Who else would be good at what job?"

"The job for carrying on."

"Carrying on in my work? Or carrying on with you?"

"Carrying on with your work."

"Well, right now, nobody. I'm unique, and my work isn't out there yet. No one else can build on it yet."

"Yes."

"I'm going to make it happen. I've always had a strong sense I am here to do certain work. Staying with it all this time has been hard. I couldn't even talk about it for a long time because there was no language for what I was exploring or the new way I was seeing things. So I had to figure out what the parts were, how they fit together, create a language, and find a way to tell the new story. That's why it has taken so long. But it *is* what I am here to do, and I've done the lion's share of it. Now I have to get it out into the world."

"Yes."

"Thank you. Thank you for all your help. Without you I never would have been able to do this work and stay on a path that was invisible to everybody else. You have always believed in me, hung in there with me even though my life and work were so outside of the world that is familiar to you and your friends. I couldn't have done it without you."

"It's nearly done?"

"Yes, it's nearly done."

"Please, Heavenly Father, help this young girl with her work real soon. Have it be right for her." I am overwhelmingly moved by her sudden prayer for me.

"Thank you."

"I think it will be."
"I think it will be."
"I hope..."
"You hope what?"
"I hope it will work out well."

"And I hope it will work out well for you, too. What I want for you is peace and resolution. Sometimes you are so agitated and so restless."

"I need somebody to help me."

"You need somebody to help you. Do you know how they can help you?"

"Yes, I think they can."

"How?"

She cannot put into words (or words that make sense to me) what I or "somebody" can do to help her. I ask her again what kind of help she needs. She says, "I'll go back to bed how. Got to work for a while."

I interpret "work" to mean her usual "doing" kind of work, and tell her that her working days are done. On second thought, I realize she is referring to her end-of-life work. I am guessing such work is tiring as one moves in and out of different states of consciousness, and suspect that oftentimes the dying are actually doing their work when they are described as "napping," "dozing," or "out of it" because their attention has been withdrawn from our mundane concerns.

A couple of days later, I write, "She seems to have let go some since our conversation on Wednesday evening. I feel a shift, less resistance. It is so hard to know just what she is taking in and what is going on within her. Her processing is not at the surface anymore. It is at a very deep level and its rhythms have little to do with the surface of life or what was just said. She may be answering a question today in response to something I asked two days ago, and next week will say something connected to what we were talking about today." Spiritual work is not of this world, but flows between the worlds in its own time.

That same day, she announces out of nowhere, "I just think it's time for me to let go."

During the night of June 24 in which I sleep a total of four-and-a-half hours, we make a trip to the bathroom around 4:00 AM. I take a little flashlight so we don't have to turn on the bright lights. The flashlight hits the floor, and I hear batteries scatter. Cursing and feeling around for them in the dark is a ludicrous counterpoint to my discovery that she has a urinary tract infection and the poignancy of her despair about being unable to "finish it." The combination of her insight into her situation and her feeling that somehow she is not doing something "right" rips me apart.

"I don't know what I'm doing, and I don't know if I'll ever finish it. I can't help it."

"Honey, of course you can't help it! Try not to worry about what you need to do because you don't need to DO anything. You just need to be, and your body will do it for you."

"I'm just gone. I'm not myself. I can't help it."

"I know, honey. Of course you can't help it. No one but you has these expectations of you. You are at the end of your journey and everything is wearing out. You can't do things you used to. No one expects you to. But, hey, you're still coming in here to the bathroom and until four weeks ago, you never had a bit of trouble walking."

"I don't know where the end is, or where the beginning is. I'm no good, I know it. I haven't got much time."

"I know you don't, honey. We all know that."

"I want to get to the end of this."

"I know."

"I'm going crazy from . . ."

"What makes you crazy? The length of the process? The hardness of the process?" I kick myself for asking a double-barreled question."

"Yes."

"Both?"

"Yes . . . It's the last thing I'm doing, and I can't do it . . . I want to let go. I'm trying to let go." Her reference to "the last thing I'm doing" clearly says it is her life she is trying to let go of. She is also holding tightly to the arms of the chair which she must let go of to transfer. Her struggles to let go of the chair she is in to get to the next place is a perfect metaphor for her struggle to let go of this life in order to get Home.

Later, after I have helped her to bed and tried to position her in the middle without dragging her fragile skin or forcing her ancient bones, she continues with her theme, "I don't know how to do it."

"Honey, you don't have to know how. Your body is doing it for you. You don't have to figure out how to do it like an accounting problem . . . Are you warm enough?" She had announced that, "it's cold here," when we went back into the bedroom, so I pulled up the bedspread.

"I feel I must be doing something wrong."

"Oh, honey, you are not doing anything wrong! That's in YOUR mind. Nobody else thinks that. Nobody! Only you. You give yourself pain you don't need to have. It's sad for me to watch you hurting yourself because I can't do anything about it."

A fair bit of ice water later she announces, "Oh, "I'm sick."

"I know you are sick, honey. And that's hard because you've never been sick in your life. You've had some very serious things, but in between, you haven't felt lousy."

"Yeah." By now, she is pushing at the bedcovers and seems too warm. I move them for her. "Do you think that will cool you a bit? It's worth a shot, huh? . . . I don't think you ever thought it would come to this."

Her response is strong, clear, and immediate, "That's right."

✤

The "it" in her sense that she is not doing things "right" seems to be both not dying "right" and not being herself. I know I cannot change a lifetime's paradigm that sees things in terms of their being right or wrong. But I can try to get her to take in the fact that she is not doing anything wrong by her dying process, and that dying is not a right or wrong process, but a biological process over which one has little control. It doesn't belong in her "wrong" box.

On the afternoon of the twenty-fifth—the day of the hospital bed, a day of incessant agitation, low-center of gravity walking, and her burning up inside while I am introduced to the tantalizing idea of respite—I say, "Let me turn this fan toward you so it's blowing right on you. It is seventy-eight degrees in here, but that's not why you are burning up inside. You are burning up because of things that are going on inside of you, you see?"

"Okay."

"You can't help that. You get hot, and then you get cold.

"Ay-yuh."

"Your feet get cold because your heart doesn't work so well. *It's not your fault!*"

"Ay, I know." Would that she always knows and remembers this!

"What's going on with you now is not YOU, but a natural process. You're very sick, and the sickness causes behaviors that aren't really you, and that's just part of the process, okay? It's not good or bad. Sometimes it's beyond my capacity to cope with all by myself, but that doesn't make it bad. It just is.

"Ay-yuh."

"It's just your disease, and your age, and things in your body breaking down."

"Ay-yuh."

"You can't help it. It's not a bad thing. It simply is."

"Thank you."

'You understand that?"

"Yes."

"Yes. I love you very much."

"Okay."

❦

We are interrupted by phone calls, but I finally settle in with Olwen around five o'clock. Although her body continues to be hot, she wants something around her neck as day turns to evening. I get her a long scarf that flows from one tone of pink to another. She drapes it around her neck and experiments with how she wants to tie it. Wearing only underwear and her elegantly-tied scarf, she is looking incredibly chic. She settles back into her rose-colored, lift chair as if she were a queen on a throne.

I sit down close to and opposite her, and ask for her attention. It is a lovely evening, and we need to do some important things. She is composed and listening. I play a tape by David Hykes and the Harmonic Choir singing overtones in a French cathedral whose amazing acoustics resonate haunting yet comforting tones.

"You're somewhere in this dying process, and we don't know how long you have. It may be days or weeks, but it's not too long. Things are happening with your body that are making you very agitated and restless, and harder to move from one place to another. The sickness causes behaviors that aren't really you, and your body can't do what it used to. It's not a bad thing and it's not your fault. It is a natural process. Do you hear me?"

"Umm-hmm."

"What is needed to take care of you keeps expanding and expanding, and sometimes it feels like more than I can do to take care of you here and get the overnight help I need. They can give me a few days off and take you to one of the nursing homes for those days, but I worry you would feel abandoned and might die there all alone, and that would be just awful.

"I love you very much and I see your struggle. I see the pain you're in, and I've never been able to fix it. And I can't fix it now, I can't take it away. I can only try to be with you in it. More than anything, I want to be with you at the end. But it might not work out that way because I need to go to my house sometimes, and you may be getting beyond my capacity to take care of at home. Do you understand that? What you need to do is to let go, and I don't know how to help you do that. I've tried."

"We'll try . . . together." Her wisdom and generosity are staggering. While I am teary throughout this part of our conversation, she has become absolutely calm and alert since we sat down together. Apparently, she has become more lucid as well, and is once again taking in what is happening at a profound level, and responding from her greater self.

"There you are taking care of me when I'm trying to take care of you! . . . We have some very special things here to do together."

A while ago, I had brought a trilogy of Native American plants used for spiritual cleansing (sweetgrass, cedar, and sage), and now I put them on the small table. "This is sweetgrass—you can smell it. American Indians use it to purify themselves and clear the energetic space they are in before they consider an important issue . . . I got you some new flowers today, would you like to smell them? . . . Let's bring Mama's picture over here right close by so you can see her and feel her presence."

I also get out a tiny bottle of Angel's Trumpet, a flower essence that my friend Brigit had given me. I had first gotten it out on Monday when I felt we were getting to the time to use it. Just as I was holding it, Brigit, with perfect timing, called me, and we had a long conversation about the weekend from hell and my meltdown that morning. Brigit had also given me a little write-up about the spiritual intention of this flower essence, and I now paraphrase it for Olwen.

"These drops are the essence of a particular flower. They are taken from dew drops on the flowers in the morning sun. Isn't that nice? Flower essences work energetically, not physically on your body. A friend who knows about these things says the flower essence in these drops helps with spiritual surrender and transformation. It is about opening the heart and soul to the spiritual world so that the soul can experience death without fear, and even joyously.

"Umm-hmm."

"Surrender—that's what we need help with here. We are trying to find a path out of this maze we're in. Your body is failing you and you're sore from your falls, and you feel locked in, and you don't know what to do. It's hard and getting harder. And I don't know if this could help us both to surrender to this process, and for you to let go. A friend brought it to me shortly before Pandora died, and it was wonderful. She behaved like a little kitten again."

"Ay-yuh."

"You are supposed to put a couple of drops in water and sip a little, and then a little more. I am using that pristine water that we like. Let's put it in Auntie's pretty glass."

The brandy snifter glass is a rarely used antique that had belonged to Elizabeth's darling aunt whom we all called Auntie. I sip a little, and give it to Olwen to sip. Then I use my hands to put some of the water on her and on me, and in her hair, especially around her crown chakra. We sit with our opposing legs entwined and look fully and deeply at each other a very long time, two souls pouring into each other.

She is not wearing her glasses today, and her eyes seem larger than they have become of late. She is backlit by the setting sun. The play of light and shadow illuminates a radiant beauty never before visible to me. She is beautiful, luminous, glowing. I tell her this.

Perhaps it is only now that she is paring down to the bone that her innermost beauty and being has dared to shine through so nakedly. And perhaps it is only now when I am shedding layers of the past that I am able to see her or receive her on this level. She has never looked like this before, nor has she ever looked at me in the way she now is. It is as if we are seeing each other for the first time. We are each seeing and comprehending the other in new ways while at the same time saying goodbye.

The answer to Sister Mary Elizabeth's question (Do we have anything more to learn from each other?) is "yes." When I am able to think, I realize it's been "yes" since I first arrived at the hospital. Not only learn *from*, but learn *about* each other.

At some point I say, "I don't know how to do this either. I love you. We've been together a long time, haven't we?"

"I don't know."

"Well, yes, we have. Always remember I love you. You are never alone."

"Yes, I am alone." There she goes again—right on the mark!

"Yes, you're right. Each of us is alone."

"Yes."

"I've tried to bring you support so you wouldn't be alone in the sense of all by yourself. There is somebody with you all the time." We have several exchanges in which I can't hear her or figure out what she is saying. Some of her words are slurred, and some barely audible. Then she says suddenly and with energy behind it, "We've been through a lot together."

"We've been through a lot together, we sure have."

"Ay-yuh."

"And I appreciate all your help and all your love. You've always been there through thick and thin."

"Yes."

It is astonishing how our time together with the herbs and flower essences and music has brought her into such sustained serenity for so many hours following a day of such extreme restlessness. Around nine o'clock, she is still so peaceful and centered I dare to leave her alone and go upstairs and get the last load of laundry. When I get back, she is still sitting in her chair, as calm and composed as when I left her. She smiles at me sweetly, her head cocked a little to the right, looking almost like the ancient mother of these last years. She asks if she can do something to help!

"How about you come with me into the bedroom while I finish making up your bed?" I wheel her into the bedroom, finish her bed and the spare bed, and put clothes away. She watches me throughout, at the end of which she says, "Tell me how to get Home . . . I better come to it."

"Come to it? Come to what?"

"To know where I'm at."

"Well, you're a lot clearer and calmer right now than you've been, so there's a nice moment right there."

"Ay-yuh."

"I don't know how to tell you the way to get Home. It's something about surrender." We talk of other things, and then she says, "Well, I think I'd better get started."

"Where are you going to go?

"Started home." Or does she mean, "Started Home"?

"You want to get started H/home?"

"To your home."

"Well, my home is kind of far away. Right now, I'm staying with you in your home.

"I'm very tired."

"I know you are very tired. Can I put you to bed now?"

"Ay-yuh. Where are my glasses?"

"They're in their case in their regular place on top of the dresser. They're safe."

"Oh, good, they're on the dresser."

She goes off to sleep very easily. She also stays asleep for the better part of the night—most unusual.

Ten

The Dream versus the Nightmare

You do what you have to do, and I'll do what I have to do.
—Olwen, June 26

The birthday looms as the great marker of our future. I am convinced Mother will make it to Tuesday. For months now, she has said not, "I'm ninety-eight," but rather, "I'm going to be ninety-nine on my next birthday." She wants to be ninety-nine and fully intends to be ninety-nine. Given her immense willpower, I cannot imagine we have come through all this so she can die just before she makes her milestone of choice. Once her birthday is over, I anticipate a shift.

I draw on that intuition to turn down Neal's first mention of respite care on Wednesday, the twenty-fifth, when Olwen is extremely restless. He might be able to get a room tomorrow. "No, too soon. Not before her birthday. Let's get through the birthday and see where she is a couple of days after that."

Perhaps being able to articulate respite scenarios with Neal gives me some breathing room, an escape hatch, even though I cannot imagine acting on them. Or can I? Or, can I imagine respite in my own mind for my own equilibrium, but never carry it out in the real world?

Respite sounds reasonable on paper, but fits poorly with our situation. It strikes me as a viable option for the caregiver(s) of someone with a lengthy and reasonably predictable disease course, whose mind is still clear enough to comprehend a *temporary* transfer, who is not at great risk for disorientation or delirium, and who is unlikely to die alone during the respite.

Olwen, however, "knows" very well where she is, and knows the difference between her own home and a "weasy little room" in an institution. She has lost her sense of elapsed time and the idea of "temporary," her brain is intermittently cloudy and extremely vulnerable to disorientation, and, despite her amazing strength, she is increasingly fragile. Her disease course is highly unpredictable. Although the hospice team could follow her and ostensibly be in charge, the other twenty-two hours she would be on her own in an alien environment. Olwen would know the difference. Three days away is now too many. How can I possibly think about five?

I am terrified that if we do a respite, even with daily visits and ministrations by our family of caregivers, she will feel abandoned and won't know where she is. The image of her sitting or lying alone and frightened in yet another strange place as her body and mind continue to fail her is too horrific to bring into sharp focus. She could die all alone in an alien place. Respite could undo all the mountains I have moved and all I have striven to do these last five years and these last two months. It would be totally inconsistent with the goal we have shared forever of keeping her out of a nursing home. The likely or imagined consequences would haunt me for the rest of my life. I could never live with myself. My inner brakes screech to a halt.

The respite idea/fantasy gets recycled, however, when I injure my back transferring Mother on the thirtieth, her birthday eve. In the moment, I feel a tearing of muscles and ligaments in the same sacro-iliac area I injured the week before, but this wrenching is much worse. My neck is now out of alignment from behind my right ear into my shoulder and down through my back, and I can turn my head only a little. I have a headache that will last for days and develop right-side sciatica. Sleeping is now even more difficult because no position escapes the pain.

Not only am I paying out a lot of money, not earning money, and using up my savings to care for my mother instead of moving my real work into the world, but now my own health is also at risk. What if I should permanently injure my back? I am frightened in a new and unanticipated way. Where do I draw the line in terms of the costs being too much? How do I weigh risks to my own health and the realization of my dream against keeping her out of her nightmare?

The next day as I am watching Dinaz do a transfer, I see what is happening. Mother's feet are getting rubbery and dangly. Her right foot often hangs in the air. She can't put it down on the ground as a starting point for supporting herself and standing up. She cannot really hold herself on her feet even with support from her caregiver. Her legs and feet now slant towards the caregiver, almost sliding under her. From the side view, Olwen's upper body and legs become two sides of a triangle when she tries to stand up, thereby exerting horrific pull on the caregiver's lower back. As her legs become more rubbery, she becomes even more terrified to let go of the chair and try to get up. She grips the chair with ferocious intensity and won't let go. The result: she pulls down on her caregiver in a back-wrenching way that can last for the better part of a minute. This triangle is not a sustainable position for the untrained caregiver, and could do great damage.

What are the implications of Mother's becoming a two-person transfer? Or requiring a very skilled person to manage her transfers? It's no longer enough for me to be here twenty-four hours a day. Now I have to have someone every time she needs to be transferred! The scheduling and financial implications are daunting. But it's not just the money; it's even finding people to do the night shift.

How would respite work? Although I have been told hospice would oversee her care, my nitty-gritty conversations with administrators and nurses about the roles of Christine and Dinaz reveal otherwise. I am left feeling extremely dubious anything we negotiate would actually be translated into practice with any consistency at the bedside. I also become aware of more of the perverse rules in institutional care: private caregivers would not be able to do any hands-on work with her, but friends could. Obviously then, one sends "friends" over to be with her.

At complete odds with my intuitive resistance to respite is an heretical thought. If, by my mother's own account, she can't let go, yet wants so much to let go and to go Home, maybe this recurring proposal of respite care is an opportunity being offered to us to facilitate her wish? Her emotional experience of respite care might well shorten the dying process (how would we ever know for sure?) which is what Olwen keeps asking for. But at what cost?

Despite the profound maturity of her statement that I should do what I have to do while she will do what she has to do, I fear respite could interrupt and short-circuit all that has been flowing and healing between us and her own healing process. Now that her lifelong defenses are evaporating, I cannot imagine she would not feel abandoned (by me) and terribly alone. She might well shut down in the ways in which she has been opening to receiving from me and our family of caregivers in her safe and familiar environment.

Most of my energy has gone into creating a safe, attentive, healing/caregiving space for her Dance to unfold at its own pace and in its own way. Much as our ancestors evolved in interaction with foods, climate, and rhythms of their ecological niche, so also it is my sense her dying is evolving in relation to the physical-spiritual ecology I have created in her own home. And, it is evolving in relationship with me. *Her* Dance is clearly also *our* Dance.

I had said that her soul knows what it is doing, and we must try to trust its wisdom. If that is true, and if I really believe it, then I should avoid doing anything that might interrupt her soul's journey and how it is unfolding in her familiar, responsive, home environment. Given that she is not in pain, we are in a privileged position of catering to her heart and soul. Respite might short-circuit their struggle to complete her learning and bring resolution to her life's journey in the fullest way she can.

Are there reasons not yet apparent as to why her/our Dance is taking as long as it is? Are there reasons she is not making a quick, easy exit? Are there reasons her soul has chosen this hard exit strategy? Hard for her and hard for me? What are we here to teach each other? What haven't we each yet "gotten" that we need to get?

The birthday morning is a whirlwind. Bouquets arrive. Phones ring. Cards are slipped under the door (the custom among residents here). Sue appears with 99 daisies she has just picked from the field by her house when they were still heavy with morning dew. Michael calls, but Olwen can't handle a phone because she is still groggy from the tiny dose of morphine I reluctantly acceded to at midnight because the night nurse believes the restlessness is coming from soreness accumulated from her falls. Olwen wants to lie out flat, so Jesse, who has brought her a beautiful red rose, takes her into the other room.

By the time I get the dining table cleared off and set up for the party, it is afternoon and I haven't even had a shower yet. My headache is awful, and I am trying not to be devastated by her being unable to enjoy fully her last birthday because of the damn drug.

Mary and Jesse have brought their cameras. Rosanna tenders a coconut creme pie with the hope Olwen can imbibe a little cream. A steadfast friend from church who has taken Olwen to many appointments has chosen vibrant flowers from her garden. Dinaz and Neal offer gold and cream lilies from the hospice garden. The lilies are extraordinary, as is their artful arrangement with greens and little pinks—made possible by one of the hospice volunteers with a gift for flower arranging.

Dinaz and Neal are also bearers of a beautiful hand-made card in lavender tones and rich textures which has been signed with good wishes from many hospice staff. As morphine wears off and Olwen becomes more alert, she glances at her cards but it is this one that will draw her attention over the next couple of days. She will pull it out and keep handling it, turning it over, opening it up, seemingly absorbing its meanings or energies in some wordless way.

With the comings and goings of people's schedules and Olwen not cutting any cake, we forget to sing "happy birthday" when the room is full. But then Mary, Becky, and I remember and sing to her. Olwen likes that a lot. She smiles and really looks at us and takes it in. We sing to her again. I iterate that this is July first, she is now officially ninety-nine years old, and we have all come to celebrate that with her.

The most moving moment comes during an unexpected visit by her neighbor Jim. Though blinded by macular degeneration, Jim takes his walk every day and is part of the regular crowd that gathers on the benches outside the main door before dinner. When he encounters Mary in the hallway and learns what the singing was about, he wants to add his birthday wishes—if it's convenient. Mary comes in and checks. It isn't and I am having a frazzled moment, and yet Mary and I both sense the depth and sincerity of his desire.

Mary guides him in, and he stands facing Olwen who is seated in her rose chair. The sight is very dear: this sweet blind man speaking from his heart to the deaf and dying woman who is leaning forward on full alert to hear him. Despite their sensory failings, there is a connection between them that is real and tender. Deeper than any words he speaks, he has brought the gift of himself and she is receiving it. And, in her receiving, though she speaks no words, something is flowing back to him.

As Olwen becomes intermittently more alert on the evening of her birthday, we settle in for quality time with flower essences, Reiki, music, and more recapitulations and affirmations of her life story. We are surrounded by seven bouquets whose visual splendor, lovely aromas, and vital energies pervade our space. "My friend who picked these flowers [I gesture toward Brigit's profligate, wild flower bouquet] knows a lot about the subtle healing powers of flower essences. She says the one I have put in this water tonight is very good for sorting out decisions about when to let go. The drops in this water are about trusting there is some greater power to which we are connected . . . by which we are protected and guided . . . that can give us permission to let our guard down, to trust, to be in the flow . . . and help decide about when to let go. I am going to have a little. Would you like a little?"

"Umm-hmm."

"Here's our special glass we use for these occasions."

"You're dear."

"I'm dear? No, *you're* dear. You're very dear."

"Yes, but I'm scared." She can't elaborate.

"I love you very much, you know . . . You have such a constitution, such a will, such perseverance, such resilience. They have taken you so far. I am so sorry it has come to this . . . I do think you will be reunited with your mother and maybe others without whom life has never been the same. You won't be alone . . ."

"I got to decide."

"That's right, you have to decide. Because your body is telling you this is getting awfully hard. You need to make a decision about letting go. Well, not so much a 'decision.' It's more like allowing all the parts of yourself to surrender together to what needs to be surrendered to." We drift a while with the warm summer air.

"I am not sure what is holding you back. Whatever is unfinished for you may get in the way of letting go. There seems to be stuff going on for you, and I don't think it's just the soreness from your falls. Only you can find your own resolution inside of yourself." Later I will read how common it is for the dying to be in emotional and spiritual distress.

I segue back to the water which contains drops of Golden Amaranthus, and again describe its essence. I read aloud Brigit's card that says, "being alive requires of us a relationship with the mysterious lifelong experience of letting go. May grace guide you as you gently let go."

"'Grace.' That's what we were talking about three weeks ago so early in the morning. You asked me, 'how do you do this? how do you let go?' You sure do ask hard questions, Lady Jane! And you were relentless! I really had to dig for answers that might help you."

"I said to you, 'It's not about doing. I think it's about grace, and grace is ultimately a mystery. It is through grace we can let go, but I can't say what grace is or how you come to it.' This is really hard stuff we are doing now . . . Let's do a little more Reiki." In the background is Jennifer Berezan's "Returning," recorded in the underground acoustical and ritual chamber known as the Maltese Hypogeum, dug out by Neolithic people with nothing more than antlers to pick through three stories of rock. Talk about hard and patient and trusting the process! While I do Reiki, she glides into her expanding inwardness.

For years now during every visit and many phone calls, I have found myself taking on the role of witnessing and validating Olwen's life, her big choices, and her small, daily triumphs. I try to address her perennial concerns about doing the right thing and doing a good job, or, to use her phrase of late years, "doing the best I can." Friends and communities provide this validation informally for one another, but those with whom she made the life journey are gone.

My realization of her need for recognition and validation came late in both our lives. In her prime, it never occurred to me. She claimed her virtues for herself, irritating me because I didn't yet see through her veils. Only as I got older and wiser did I realize that this was her way of asking for validation and get past the resistance it set up in me. I was also coming to the view that being seen is arguably our deepest human need, and that it involves a two-way flow: manifesting who we are, and having it received and reflected back so the loop is completed, nourishing both the giver and the receiver. Yet most people waste their lives camouflaging themselves, and our culture does not value or teach us how to validate others.

In Olwen's late years, I took on her validation and recognition almost as a project, finally realizing how much she needed it *and* that she needed it most of all from me. When all was said and done, it was *my* view of her that really mattered—a fact that we, as adult children, both can't quite believe and try to run away from because it gives us too much power and feels too close to being responsible for our parent's happiness. Giving-recognition-to and being-responsible-for are not the same, but it takes growth on our part to know the difference.

The occasion of this, Olwen's last birthday, seems an especially appropriate time to recapitulate and validate her overstory once again, and sketch the arc of her narrative with its themes of resilience and independence, triumph over loss, making good choices, being wealthy in friendship, and building and rebuilding connection and community.

"I've told you over and over that I think you made good choices all your life. You always did the best with what you had, and you didn't have very much. You came out of your mother's death making healthy choices for yourself, and you pulled yourself up by your bootstraps. After Mama died, you had no family here or in the old country to help you. But you had good instincts for survival. You were smart and got noticed and were quickly promoted at work. You chose good people to be around you and put yourself on a path of trying to heal what was missing in your childhood. You made wonderful friends and were virtually adopted by their families."

"Umm-hmm."

Olwen found a new home with Elizabeth's family, living in the solid, double-decker house that Elizabeth's grandfather had built. The household no doubt revolved around him, yet Grandpa, a carpenter-builder by trade who was seventy-six when Olwen joined them, seems to have had a capacity for seeing things as they are, accepting family responsibility, and valuing women's often invisible and unpaid contributions. Fed up with his son's inability to hold a steady job and provide a stable home for his wife and daughter, Grandpa took on the care of his daughter-in-law and granddaughter (Elizabeth). His will makes his daughter (Auntie) his executor and leaves everything to her, "for the reason that she has always lived with me and cared for me, and in the belief that my sons are better fitted to earn their living than she is." Auntie, although a dressmaker who took in sewing, was, Grandpa seemed to recognize, at a structural disadvantage relative to men in making her way in the world. I suspect

Olwen's gifts and abilities did not go unnoticed or unacknowledged in Grandpa's house, to which she and Elizabeth brought income.

During these same post-Lizzie years, Olwen was virtually adopted by the family of her friend Judy. The older Olwen has become, the more she has talked about how wonderful the Andersons had been to her and how grateful she was for how they insisted she be a part of everything they were doing. In the days before Mr. Anderson, an architect, bought a car, they took the train to their summer house north of town. The memory Olwen fondly comes back to over and over with Sue and myself is, "We took the train right to the village. That was the end of the line in those days. Then we all carried our suitcases, food, and everything we needed up the long hill." The last half-mile of the one-and-a-half-mile trek is quite steep.

Olwen describes Mrs. Anderson sharing confidences with her, suggesting that even then, Olwen knew how to listen and be a trustworthy confidante. She recalls Mr. Anderson gathering everyone together to talk and tell stories. She depicts him as paying attention, listening to everyone, and letting them know how much they each mattered—observations that reflect how strongly these qualities registered for her, presumably in contrast to her own father's limitations. Warmth and emotional inflection comes into Olwen's voice when she recalls her life and times with the Andersons. I presume it reflects the warmth and sense of belonging they provided when she most needed it.

"You have always had a gift for friendship and your life was rich in life-long friendships. Even when someone moved away, the relationship continued. You wrote and visited one another. Remember all those trips to New York to see Charlotte, Judy, and Helen when I was a kid? We saw lots of plays and went shopping. You talked and talked and talked with your old friends, and I fell in love with The City."

She is smiling and more alert now.

"After Mama died, you became the center of your family. It was *you* who had been the closest to Mama. It was *you* who kept the connections with the old country. It was *you* who held this branch of our family together through the hard times. It was *you* who took care of Florence. It was *you* who bailed Peggy out of her scrapes."

Last fall, I took Olwen to the mountains and lakes where she had vacationed at every stage of her life, going there with every member of her family and many friends. She remembered almost nothing about it—except her earliest visits there with her older sister Peggy who was working at one of the resort hotels. When we ran through the good old days through photo albums last Christmas, it was Peggy whom Olwen recognized immediately and by name in every picture. That Peggy sticks at the core of things is another clue about the deepest layers of Olwen's psyche.

When Peggy's son Jack came back east for Olwen's ninetieth birthday, his stories illuminated what I had long surmised: Olwen was the reliable, stabilizing figure in the patchwork of living situations her siblings cobbled together for themselves and their children in the decades following Lizzie's death and abandonment by their father. His stories shared a common thread: getting through shared hardships punctuated by small pleasures such as berrypicking and picnics. Out of that period came Olwen's role as family matriarch, and deep feelings of admiration, gratitude, and love from her siblings and their children—spiced, however, especially in the case of her sisters, with a lot of bickering, and more than a sprinkle of resentment and envy.

Jack's stories revealed something else. I realized there *were* family stories but their events had taken place way before I was born. I had walked into a play in which all the parts had been cast long ago, and everyone knew their own roles and everyone else's. They didn't need to say things because they had lived through them. They shared a collective memory in which I didn't yet exist.

"You regrouped with Betty and Auntie after the divorce." (Elizabeth liked to be called Elizabeth so that is what I called her, but everyone else called her Betty. I think "Betty" is easier for Olwen's failing synapses.) "That was a smart thing to do. You reinvented your life as an independent woman at a time when no one was divorced. No one showed you how. No support groups. No talk shows on radio or TV. No Oprah. You did it *your* way. You really blossomed after that and came into your prime."

"Ay-yuh." She's very alert now, has more expression in her face, and seems to like this.

"You grew in many ways, but I can't see that my father did. He *did* keep his financial commitments all these years—and that's a big deal! Only an honorable man would never waver on such a difficult commitment. And he did mellow some on his moodiness and perfectionism."

In the days before grade inflation, my father used to give me a quarter for each A+ on my report card, but the reward dropped to 15 cents for a mere A, a dime for an A-, and a nickel for a B+. Our Elizabeth, who was gifted in being remarkably centered and non-judgmental in her astute observations of everyone, wryly recollected his checking with white gloves for dust in Olwen's house.

I remember the tension his moodiness generated at the dinner table: Olwen trying to please by getting this or that, my provoking Michael-of-the-perfect-manners by ostentatiously chewing food with my mouth open. Michael recently remembered a counterpoint moment when Mac, having just figured out some financial problem at the table, put down his pencil, and, leaning toward Michael, confided, "Your uncle is a pretty smart man," just as Olwen returned to the dining room and tartly rejoined, "That's a matter of opinion."

Olwen helped Mac learn to manage his anger at work where it was threatening his potential for advancement. His second wife, a warm and unpretentious person, learned how to manage his moodiness at home and make him comfortable by doing the emotional work for him and spinning a web of connection around him.

"But when it comes to you, he still seems stuck in the same old place. A half-century later, he still blames you." Yet for most of my life, he had said not a bad word about her. When, in later years, I repeatedly pressed him to tell me *his* story, he veered off-subject as long as he could. When he finally ventured near his own unhappiness, I was struck by how isolated he had been during that time, and by his perspective not having grown more complex with years and distance. He seems to have encased his raw experience within a self-protecting story, and locked them into a dark place he resisted visiting. They had never come up into the light and been brought into the kind of multi-faceted dialogue that generates interior movement and growth.

"But you, on the other hand—although you are stubborn and pig-headed and have always had to do everything your way—you did mellow, you did learn and grow. You did take some responsibility about your marriage. You did see how you might have done some things differently with me. We've been able to look at those times together and do some healing work with each other.

"When I look back, I see his leaving was a blessing in disguise. You came into your own, you became more self-confident, you expanded as a person, you were able to take in new ideas. Eventually you were even able to let go of the bitterness and anger, and that's a really big deal! You were able to move on with your life because you grew as a person and had a lot of support from family and friends."

"Yes." She is smiling and looking right at me.

"Do you remember—just before you built the house and we were still living at Betty and Auntie's—when we drove to Florida in the old Ford, and came back in that gorgeous car with the sun visor and leather seats? It was deep turquoise and cream and nobody had ever seen anything like it up north. What a statement you made! It reminds me of the young Olwen who saved her money and bought that car with the rumble seat.

"You didn't throw out your engagement ring or put it away in a jewelry box. You designed a whole new ring around it, filling it out with an oval of diamonds and two baguettes—just like you filled out your life when you were on your own again. I carved a ring stand for it so it would always be in the same safe spot when you were working around the house. Your new ring went with your new life and all those lovely winters in Florida with Ginny and her family. Those were the glory years."

Little smiles and nods and glints of recognition play upon her face.

"You knew the exact lot where you wanted to build your house, and you jumped on it when there was activity on the lot. You and Betty went right to the library that night and found the floorplan you wanted. You were up there on the site every day overseeing its construction. You got a great house with never a drop of water in the cellar, and you reigned over your neighborhood for many decades. You were an outstanding neighbor and had neighbors who wrote the book on what it means to be a neighbor. You sure did pick the right street and the right lot!" At her memorial service, I ask Colleen, her neighbor for twenty-five years, to speak. Coleen said in part:

> A major portion of her life was enjoyed upon a street that bore her name. It was some time before we realized the street really wasn't named after her . . . Olwen was the matriarch of her road. She set the standard for everyone. Her lawn was always manicured like a golf course. Her bushes, always

sculpted, perfectly. Her windows radiant, just like the smile she gave to everyone in the neighborhood. She took pride in her home, and pride in her appearance, and further pride in the neighborhood. She passed that special feeling about our road onto everyone. If we needed something done in our neighborhood, Olwen would get it done . . . She took her daily walk up and down our road, and you could always catch a glimpse of her working on her home . . . The neighborhood has changed since Olwen moved. Many new families, strollers being pushed up and down the street. Yet number 12—the cute, white, Cape Cod—is still referred to as her house. Olwen was respected and loved by her neighbors, both children and adults, and this will always, in all of our hearts, always be her road.

I get her to bed early. I move medical items into the closet or to the far corner of the bedroom and bring in all the bouquets that have been picked from the wild or from people's gardens and arrange them in a kind of protective semi-circle around her. Their subtle yet powerful energies profoundly affect the ambience of our space. Every morning, I will move the flowers back into the living room for the day and get things ready for Christine in the bedroom, and every night I will bring the flowers back into her bedroom.

Mother goes into a deep sleep during which I continue to do Reiki. I try to tune into my intuition and to Mama. My sense is that she will be appearing to her daughter, but not yet. We are getting close, but we are not quite there. A couple of weeks perhaps?

※

Olwen is a little feistier, a little stronger, and a little more able to support herself the day after her birthday. Yet she also tells me she can't see. While this is not literally true, her vision is deteriorating and may have dropped by an increment that is noticeable to her.

After going to bed, Mother becomes restless and keeps saying, "Take me Home, take me Home." I say, "I don't know how." Eventually I go to bed, but I am up and down checking on her.

At 3:48 in the morning of July 3, I hear something. She is moaning and calling me to help her. I dash in and there she is crumpled on the floor. She is stretched out, lying more or less on her left side and on her left shoulder and arm. I am horrified and fear the worst. Because of her position, I am imagining her shoulder and arm may be broken or badly hurt. I am afraid to move her, afraid to make anything worse, and I have no idea how to get her up. I am down on the floor with her, supporting any action she takes, but not forcing or trying to make her move in any way. Amazingly, she slowly pulls herself up to a sitting position. I start to breathe again. I figure if she can do that, nothing is broken, and she will be okay. She is shaking, however.

I drag her low chair close to her, hoping we might get her into it, but she hasn't the strength to get into it, and I feel my back pulling in the same injured place when I try lifting her. I call hospice to come, pull her blanket off the bed, sit in the chair myself behind her, holding her up against me. I wrap the blanket and my arms and body warmth around her, and try to keep her in a sitting-up position as her body wants to slide down again. She keeps talking about wanting to go Home, and asking me to help her to go Home.

I am pulled in many directions during our long wait. It is unbearable witnessing what could be the end-game of making things harder for herself. The more she tries to do what her body can no longer do, the harder for me to manage her at home. To give up now and move her to a place even for a few days where she may well die, and where everything I have tried to do may unravel—the oldest and deepest parts of me (which we might call my child-self and soul-self) would scream that I just utterly failed. Failed her and failed myself. I am ripped through with anguish that she seems unable to let go in this perfect setting.

Another aspect of myself stands back from the scene in a more dispassionate way. It says, "I am her witness but it's *her* journey, she has to do it. All her life she has been willful, stubborn, done things her way, and made things harder than they need to be. I can't change her pattern, I can't change her paradigm. It's not up to me."

Another part of me, perhaps my adolescent-self, says, "So? Isn't this a repetition of what you have experienced with her all your life? She can't take things in. She can't take in love. She doesn't take in the joy, the beauty, the good stuff all around her." So I am also feeling anger, frustration, and "okay it's her choice. *I* can't fix it."

Yet if I "abandon" her through respite, won't I be replicating the "truth" she has taken away from her great losses: that she *will* be abandoned, that the other person will disappear on her at the critical moment, and that she perhaps deserves it because she couldn't miraculously and magically save her mother? Wouldn't it be her paradigm's ultimate revenge for her to die with her self-negating paradigm intact? Leave me to wrestle with the guilt the rest of my life? She—or it—would thereby have succeeded in defeating us all in the end.

This is old, old stuff. This is *her* defense structure, now ossified for eighty years, giving her less than she should have had and exacting a toll on others. This is *my* defensive structure where anger shuts down the connection.

No, I don't have to respond to the Olwen who protected herself so well for so long, and to a fault. No, I don't have to respond to the only Olwen my father could ever see or elicit. No, I don't have to be stuck with the same narrow options he left himself.

I can to go a deeper and even older place in her. To the real Olwen who would go to the end of the earth for those she loves, most especially for me. To the real Olwen who loves me beyond all loving and has never failed me. I can see her through the lens a friend brings to the flawed beings around her: as a soul in struggle. It is absurd for me to see Olwen as the formidable yet sometimes manipulative or martyred being she was in her prime when she is now a fragile, frightened little person facing the end of this life. Her defenses and barriers are eroding, and it is ludicrous for me to project them back onto her.

I can go to a deeper and even older place in me. My maturing soul-self can reach back to what my child-self yearned to do and couldn't, to what I have tried to do many times in my life and always failed. I *can* fix it. I *am* going to get through to her. I am going to break her pattern, her paradigm. Of course, *she* must be the one who does it, but there is something I must do that allows her to do it. She can't do it alone. This is about us, the two of us, and it goes way back.

Traditional therapists and many self-help people would say no, no, no, but they tend to come at things from the level of the personal self and the position of the still-young, adult child trying to define herself and set boundaries. But the daughter must mature and move to a deeper level. There is also the soul-self and what we are here to do with and for each other.

What ultimately is my work with Olwen? Why did I choose her—if indeed we choose our parents? Is it not to unlock her from her paradigm—or enable her to unlock herself, to open her heart, to free herself—and somehow heal our lineage? And in the doing, becoming the full self I must become to externalize the work I am here to do? Is it not here that we are to find the deepest and ultimate answer to Sister Mary Elizabeth's question?

We wait for forty-five minutes with me wrapping my arms and the blanket around Mother and holding her up against me until the on-call nurse gets here from her last house call. In one swift motion, she gathers Olwen up, and Olwen is asleep before she is fully in the bed. The on-call nurse disappears as quickly as she appeared.

By now it is five o'clock. I sleep for an hour, and come in to check in on my mother. She is thrashing around, gripping the bars of the bed, a bed she describes to Rosanna and myself as "that jail." She hates this bed just as much as I do. During my previous, late night check-ins, I had forgotten to put the guard rail back up. I forgot to put her back in the prison she hates, and within an hour or two, she broke free of her prison.

Is the prison bed a metaphor for her paradigm? Is she telling us she really wants to break out, not only of her failing body, but finally of her life paradigm? Is she really ready?

※

I am zonked by the time Christine arrives. On three hours of sleep, I attend the case assessment meeting with Dinaz, the medical director, and heads of all the departments. I make my pitch about the impact of drugs and their longevity in frail, dying bodies which can no longer metabolize and excrete drugs efficiently. I underline Olwen's bad experiences with a number of drugs and the need to tailor medications to individuals. I acknowledge morphine is an important tool in their arsenal and is supposed to clear out in hours, but it knocks Olwen out and does not clear out of her system for a couple of days. I don't know if any of this is registering, but I think it important to keep hammering away and add another voice to the more conservative drug orientation of people like Dinaz.

I inquire about end-stage scenarios and dehydration and its effects. End-stage dehydration is not painful, they say, and the dying body cannot really handle food or liquids. Fluids only prolong the dying process, and can pool in an immobile body as well as increase respiratory secretions. No one ventures a timetable. Although Mother has had hardly any solid food for a week, she is still drinking Ensure, juices, and sherbet. Despite her rubbery feet, restlessness, and bouts of intense overheating, she could go on for some weeks or she could go at any moment.

The medical director offers the three most likely scenarios for the final days. Mother could be going along okay and then, bang, become short of breath and cyanotic. We could use nitro for shortness of breath, inject Lasix to reduce fluid retention, use Compazine for nausea before giving morphine which will reduce the acceleration in breathing while opening the airways. She could have a sudden cardiac disturbance that leads to a quick death. Or she could slowly withdraw and fade over a period of days. In any of these cases, indications of approaching death are rapid pulse, lower blood pressure, more rapid or slower breathing, and hands or feet turning blue.

After the meeting, Neal explains more about the mechanics of respite. My intuition and everything in me balks. Tomorrow is too soon. Besides, we've got all these beautiful flowers, and they shouldn't go to waste. I am going to stick it out these next several days and then we'll see. No, the time isn't right. I keep pushing the "in a few days" forward. A parallel track is always running in my head: she needs to be at home and she needs me to be with her, and there's just no way we're going to do respite.

After the hospice meetings, Thursday is consumed with phone calls and errands. Exhausted and feeling dreadful for even thinking about respite, I drag myself upstairs to the apartment. When I open the door, an entirely different universe greets me.

Music is playing. Olwen is sitting in her chair, alert, really looking at her cards, especially the one from hospice. The morphine residues have vanished. She and Rosanna are playing. Rosanna has a gift for touching into and igniting dimensions of the dying that one would have to see to believe. Olwen looks right at me when I come in and smiles. I instantly say to myself, "okay, get with the program," let go of where I have been all day, and enter into their magical space.

Mother's voice and words are amazingly clear, and her mind is intriguingly lucid. She is exhibiting a dry humor, and Rosanna and I are cracking up. (Why didn't I get this on tape?) I make her a fruit frappe in the blender, and she practically grabs the cup out of my hands and drinks it all with gusto. When we take her into the bathroom, she can almost stand by herself.

In the midst of all this, Olwen says, "I'm going Home this weekend." Later in the hall I ask Rosanna, did you hear her say she was going Home this weekend? Yes, she heard it, too. I also ask if what she is witnessing here today fits with what she had described to me a few days ago as an "awakening" that sometimes happens to people shortly before they die. Yes, it does. Those attending the dying often mistake the "awakening" for their person's getting stronger and better (perhaps that is what happened with Elizabeth the day before she died?) rather than being a temporary uptick that is actually a harbinger of death.

※

This evening Mother goes to sleep rather easily and sleeps quietly for a while, her hands folded across her chest. After I bring in the flowers and sit down next to her, I feel such peace in the room and with her. I play the extraordinary music of Hildegard of Bingen, musing on her new popularity so many centuries after her death, and the serenity her music can still bring to so many. I sip the Angel's Trumpet, putting a little in Mother's hair after she becomes a bit restive, and it seems to quiet her. Hours tick by.

I sense we are no longer alone. I have never felt anything quite like this before. It is as if "they"—her spirit guardians?—have come to be with us and let us know we are not alone. The peacefulness and protectiveness exuded by their presence is palpable. I whisper a prayer for her. "She said she is going Home this weekend. Oh, please, may it be so! May I have the grace to know and to help her. May grace come to her."

She awakens around midnight and we talk quietly. "I think they're here getting ready to take you Home."

She says "yes" in a strongly affirmative and knowing tone.

"You keep saying you don't know what to do. But you don't have to do anything or know anything. They will take care of it. They know what to do. They will help you. You just go along for the ride."

"Yeah."

"You're safe, you're not alone."

A little later she says, "She's known for a long time I've been trying to get Home." I don't know who "she" is but it may be the girl in white whom she tells me she sees.

Olwen can't give me any clarifying answers to my questions: "Do you know her? Can you make out her face?" Could it be Mama whom she sees (who surely would know she is trying to get Home) even though Olwen has said "girl"; age has become extremely labile in her world.

Is it herself she sees—or that sees her? Has her wise, soulful young-self separated from her ancient, failing body, and become a witness or guide to her transition? Has the beautiful young girl who lost her Mother so traumatically and became lost to herself now returned as they prepare to be reunited?

Mother floats off to sleep and then wakes up wanting to know more about what she is going through. "You're going through a process of making a transition from this world to a far larger world that we don't know very much about."

"Umm-hmm."

"Your guardians or angels are here to help you because it is a transition we earth people don't understand. We don't know much, so we need help from the others. Remember you are surrounded and protected all the time now by your guardians. You are safe. You're safe enough to go with them when you are ready. You won't be alone."

In speaking to Mother, I am affirmative. I leave my questions and uncertainties parked in another room. In this moment, I completely believe and trust what I am saying. Perhaps I am coming from the most trusting part of myself that I have never fully trusted before. Perhaps by trusting I can help the reality we want to actually come to pass.

"We're getting together quite a team to help you with this transition. You and I have been a team for a very long time, haven't we? We've been doing a lot of healing work going through this together, step by step.

"We have a team of caregivers to support you on this side of things. It has always been so hard for you to ask or to receive, so maybe our caregiving team is helping you to do that, to experience that, to learn that.

"Now we have guardians from the other side who are here with us and will be there with you. We can learn from them you are not alone, and you will not be alone.

"And now we are waiting for Mama to come and help us with this transition. It's not yet time, but I know she will come to you."

After a while and out of the blue Olwen says, "July first." "July first—yes! What happened on July first? You entered your hundredth year! You are ninety-nine years old now. Wow!" July first, which is as much Lizzie's day as it is Olwen's day, the birthday without which I would not be, or I would not be me. "How about we try to get a little sleep, huh?"

Then she asks if we've lost her glasses. "No, we haven't lost your glasses. They're in the case on top of the dresser. Just where they always are every night." Her glasses, which I had always assumed would be one of the many things I could toss out when she died, will be impossible to part with after her death.

Eleven

Weaving a Path Through the Shadows

*I've lived a good life really, but I know I worked at it.
I had to do a lot of things, and I was able to do them.*

—Olwen, October, 2001

Olwen asks to go back to bed soon after Christine leaves on Friday, July 4, but doesn't sleep. She is working her tank top as if it had a button, and at one point tries to work my hand the same way. The ferocious strength of her grip is uncanny. I bring her flowers back into the bedroom and sit with her, sorting years of cards, showing her some and throwing out hundreds along with old makeup. It is a quiet day punctuated by fireworks and calls from friends.

Although Olwen's restlessness has diminished since we introduced an Ativan schedule ten days ago, it still comes and goes and varies in intensity. Yesterday she had a round before her lucid and charming "awakening." Today she kneads or picks at whatever is nearby and pulls out the oxygen cannula from her nose at least twenty times, playing with the tubing and rolling it up. She rejects water, chocolate Ensure, bears I gave her years ago. The only thing that vaguely passes muster is a frappe blended from ice, berries, and butter pecan Ensure.

The twelve-hour gap between her midnight trip to the bathroom and the first time she needed to go today suggests she is becoming more dehydrated. She seems more removed, more remote, and less animated today. She does become absorbed, however, in playing with the flexible bear Sue's granddaughter gave her, inserting it into and out of the bars of "the jail."

Many words or phrases are barely audible or intelligible. Some are important and I am frustrated I can't give her better responses so she feels more fully heard and less alone. I keep jumping up, crouching over, leaning in, and asking, "What? What did you say?" Sometimes I don't know if I can straighten up again because my sacro-iliac joint feels as if it will lock or has already locked. Then again, audible phrases and moments of interaction reveal she is still tracking the meanings of her situation and what I am saying. We are—and have been—having The Conversation in ways I had never imagined.

> *It is the image in the mind that links us to our lost treasures; but it is the loss that shapes the image, gathers the flowers, weaves the garland.*
> —Colette, My Mother's House

In a stronger and more certain tone than I have heard all day, Mother announces, "that little girl—she's still here."

"Do you know the girl?"

"No, I don't know her name."

"You don't know her name. You never saw her before?"

"No."

"Is she a young girl? Eight? Ten? Fourteen?"

"She ate a lot of food."

I crack up with laughter, "She ate a lot of food!!??" In the middle of the night recently, Olwen announced she was terribly hungry. I couldn't get her to name anything or respond to any goodies I offered. It is the only time she has expressed a desire to eat. Is it possible the girl in white is eating vicariously for her? And that she can do this because she *is* an aspect of Olwen?

"I am . . . pretty good for . . . coming from . . ."

"You're pretty good for where you're coming from? I guess so! I guess you are! For one thing, you can still tell us when you want to go to the bathroom, and you don't go until we get you in there. That's a really big deal at this point! And now you are officially ninety-nine. That's a pretty ancient age."

"We'll talk about it a little later."

"Okay. What would you like to do now?"

"I don't know. You've been a very good helper." Interesting tense. Not "are" but "have been."

"You think I've been a very good helper?"

"I think you better sleep." She's aware I haven't had much sleep, still worrying about me, still being a mother! "She's right side of us."

"She's right side of us? The little girl?"

"Yes. She just moved."

"Is she talking to you? Or gesturing to you?"

"Not too much." This thread of experience/conversation fades out. The notion to which I am most drawn continues to be that this girl in white is Olwen's young-self or whole-self who became lost to her through her mother's unnecessary death and the consequences that followed.

> [W]herever I traveled, I carried within me a sadness I couldn't leave behind . . . Someone dies, you cry, and then you move on: this was no mystery to me. What was far less clear was how the effects of this loss were likely to appear and reappear throughout the rest of my life . . . My mother's death ha[s] been the most determining, the most profound, the most influential event of my life.
> —Hope Edelman, *Motherless Daughters*

Olwen's accounts of Lizzie have always been sketchy, as were her accounts of her childhood and early life. She relayed incidents and glimpses, but not narratives that located them in a context, or connected them to her emotional experience or the meanings they carried for her. I have always known she has intense and complex feelings and that some of her storied bits have deep emotional roots, yet her telling of them was for the most part emotionally flat. I was puzzled by this most of my life until I conjectured that trauma had fragmented her stories and produced freeze-frame pictures with little flow, context, or emotion. When you dissociate, you are pushed outside of your own experience and see it happening outside yourself so you don't know it or feel it from the inside.

Despite the sketchiness, it has always been evident to me that the death of her mother was the pivotal, life-shattering experience of Olwen's life. As a child, I was struck by the fact that neither she nor Florence could speak of Mama without crying. It had been thirty years and more since Lizzie died, and yet it was still raw and unhealed. This, it seems, is not unusual for women who have lost their mother in their teens or earlier. Of the 154 motherless women in Hope Edelman's study, 80 percent were still mourning their mothers although, on average, they had lost them twenty-four years ago. Even for most adults, the loss of a parent is a life-altering event.[1]

When still a child, I was picking up two things: that Lizzie's death was the key to understanding Olwen (and Florence), and that unhealed grief endures forever; one cannot "get over it." My child-self's experience would come to inform my adult understanding of grief and loss, one not shared with other members of my natal household or American society generally. When I brought up Lizzie's death with my father late in his life, he hadn't a clue about its significance in shaping his first wife. Florence's son Michael, who lived with my parents for eight years during which time I was born, thought the past was past and that Olwen and Florence should move on. These differences in perception marked a chasm between my interior world and theirs.

Olwen's overstory of resilience, independence, friendship, triumph over loss, building and rebuilding connection and community, and doing the right thing did not come out of nowhere. Her encounters with, and avoidances of deep currents flowing through her consciousness formed the overstory in which she created herself and wove the fabric of her life.

> *The loss of the daughter to the mother, the mother to the daughter, is the essential female tragedy.*
> —Adrienne Rich, *Of Woman Born*

The deepest currents were the life-shattering loss of her mother and all the losses in its wake: her home, her family under one roof, her sense of place in the world, the fabric of assumptions holding the meanings of family and safety. Her remote father was incapable of seeing the needs of his grieving children or of giving them a sense of place. When he remarried and sent them packing, they felt "thrown away."

Yet Olwen's good instincts for survival helped her find new homes for herself and a sense of place. She gravitated toward surrogate families that functioned better than her own and gave her things missing in her father's house. She expanded her friendship networks, and earned a place of respect, admiration, and affection in her work environment.

Her life-pattern of being the Weaver of multi-generational quilts was thus established early. She began reweaving the fabric that had been ripped asunder, using different colors and threads than she otherwise would have, but reweaving it nonetheless around the great hole at the center. In the long run, she herself would become the new center of her fabric.

> *[Shadows are] the darkness that is ours, which we cannot escape and which is most difficult to contact . . . To encounter the shadow, we must be willing to go into the dark, for that is where it lives.*
> —Deena Metzger, Writing for Your LIfe

Yet there were also shadows haunting her life and they took up permanent residence. These nameless, unrecognized, unvalidated currents of loss and grief shaped and informed not only Olwen's and Florence's lives, but also mine. I absorbed them by osmosis from before birth and became their silent carrier.

At a conference in the spring following Olwen's death, I encountered someone who had given a name and incipient shape to such currents. Peggy Whiting's concept of *shadow grief* clicked with my experience in a powerful way that enfranchised my quest to understand Olwen's story by finding my way through our shadows and bringing them into the light.

When loss disrupts the assumptive continuity and coherence of our inner world, *shadow grief* may flow out of the loss(es) in the form of an enduring, permeating, isolating sorrow. Shadow grief is not highly visible to others and may not be conscious for the griever. It is often heightened by anniversaries, objects, sights, and smells that temporarily sharpen our losses, but, unlike such particulars, shadow grief is always present. Whiting summarizes shadow grief as the layered, unfolding ramifications of a loss or losses after which life is and can never be the same. It transforms our narrative in ways that keep unfolding over time.[2]

As I have worked with this lens for giving form to some of the nameless currents within Olwen and myself, I have come to think of shadow griefs as taking up permanent residence in the gap between what is and what might/would/should/could have been. Whereas losses are about the past in contrast to a bereft present, shadow grief is about two contrasting futures or two contrasting selves, the one that is unfolding or has unfolded, and the one that "should" have or could have. Whereas losses—of meaning, of the irreplaceable person, of the self one was in relation to her—may attenuate to the degree that one can reconstruct a full and meaningful life, shadow griefs may become even more powerful with time because the ramifications of the loss keep playing out, layer after layer, and become more clear, revealing the full scope of what has been lost.

Shadow grief carries a haunted quality to it, a yearning for something nameless, loss in the mist, the shadows of what might have been and can never be. We hear its sound in Celtic music—the wail of pipes, the fiddle's lament, the dirge of the drum's slow march, the exile from the holy ground of the homeland. Shadow grief exudes an aura of unfixability. It is that sense of hauntedness and unfixability that I absorbed from Olwen. With it came the need to get hold of its amorphousness and understand it, so as to do two seemingly contradictory and impossible things: fix the unfixable and release myself—and perhaps both of us—from it.

The longest and deepest shadow in Olwen's life—and mine—was cast by the nature of Mama's unnecessary death. It could, in all likelihood, have been prevented by timely medical intervention. Olwen tried and tried and tried but got no response. If Olwen could have saved Lizzie, then perhaps *none* of this would have happened. There would —presumably—have been no alternative future, only the one that "should" have been.

Self-tormenting questions must have spun round and round interminably. "What else could I have done? There must have been something else I could have done. Somehow, I should have been able to do it." This terrible burden haunted Olwen her entire life. It must have contributed to her overwhelming need to "do the right thing" and to "do things right." Certainly it must have fed doubt about her worthiness, her being good enough.

Her own shadow grief becomes visible in a photo of her high-school graduating class. When I took it to a scanner and kept enlarging the tiny image of her face, what had seemed with the aid of a normal magnifying glass a great picture of her fabulous facial bones revealed something else. Olwen's entire face is a study in grief, and she is holding her mouth and chin the way she did when she was either crying or suppressing tears. Her celebratory moment is instead a time of devastation and mourning for all that it is not and never will be again.

Not only is her mother not there, but the graduation itself was to usher in a new phase in their relationship. Lizzie and Olwen were to make a greatly-anticipated journey together back to Wales when Olwen graduated high school. Lizzie, who had never viewed her American sojourn as permanent, would finally see her mother again. This is the daughter Lizzie would bring back to her family, this one in whom she had such pride. In contrast to the unpleasant tribe hatched by Lizzie's self-centered sister, this is the daughter who was the true heiress of the lineage, the one who already carried the dignity, backbone, and "stuff" apparent in the faces, bearing, and hard-work stories of my great-grandmother and great-grandfather.

Olwen's shadow grief sometimes manifested in undigested anger on behalf of Florence and her brother Emlyn. Her brother, fifteen when his mother died, quit school during the next year or two and bounced around from one living situation to the next, even joining the cavalry. Olwen was forever angry their father never made him go back and finish school. Although Emlyn made his way into lower management, Olwen was certain he could have gone further with more education. Her anger on this account was easily focused and expressed, probably because there was language and cultural legitimacy linking education and career success for men.

Florence, twelve when Mama died, was a darling, beautiful child who had been doted on. After Lizzie's death, Florence was farmed out to eager, smiling families who turned out to be abusive and piled on the work. She also spent a fair part of her teen years with Papa and her stepmother who was mean and off-loaded her own work onto her stepdaughter. Olwen frequently recalled how one of Florence's friends often had to wait on the steps until Florence finished her chores to her stepmother's satisfaction before the girls could walk to school together. Where was their father in protecting his youngest daughter from his new wife and these abusive foster families? Oblivious, as usual.

Responsibilities of fathers to daughters were ill-defined, and what we today would consider abusive treatment—especially of girls—had no language or cultural visibility. Yet Olwen saw only too clearly that Florence's life and potential were derailed by Mama's death, that her teen years set her up for making poor choices in husbands who drank, and that Papa had failed his youngest daughter. Florence rarely complained about anything, but Olwen carried Florence's buried anger and the painful disparity between what Florence's life could or "should" have been and what it became.

> Shadow grief . . . *is the enduring and permeating aspect of grief that causes us to pronounce "I will never be the same."*
>
> —Peggy Whiting, PhD, and Elizabeth James

If anyone could have exorcised Olwen's own shadows, it was Walter. As I told Olwen several times, his photographs reveal a young man who was at ease in his body, present to the moment, and not at all self-conscious. He appears to connect easily with others, and, I suspect, made other people feel almost as confident in themselves as he was in himself.

My "reading" of his photographs will later find affirmation and illumination when I get together with his niece after Olwen dies. She says repeatedly, "My father admired Walter so much." Unusual for the eldest brother to admire the youngest. Why?

"He was so strong. He could do things no one else could. And, he could always calm the horses. He had a way with them." Ah, so Walter was gifted in working at a deep level with those high-strung creatures! His aptitude had apparently been appreciated and developed since childhood, leading him to evolve into a self-assured young man.

In an extraordinary conversation in October 2001 during which Mother finally gave me the missing pieces about her mother's death, she also offered a slightly fuller glimpse into her courtship with Walter when I asked, "Tell me again how you met Walter. Was it through Judy Anderson's family?"

> Yes, he was just down the hill from their summer place. I met him, and then he was asking me—oh, maybe two or three weeks later—asking me to go to a dance with him. That's how I got going with him. I met his family, and they used to invite me to dinner. His sister was married and lived up in the next town there, and oh, she was wonderful to me. She would invite me up there to stay with her the weekend, and then of course he'd come over. Dancing was the thing you did a lot of in those days. There was always a dance. I was a pretty good dancer.

Michael has always said Olwen was an excellent dancer and so light on her feet. He adored dancing with her, and, in his younger days, was himself quite a ballroom dancer.

Walter's nephew remembers his dazzling uncle who sent tin cans up in the air with fireworks on the Fourth of July. He describes Olwen as "a very beautiful girl" who "didn't change much over the years." When I show him the picture of Olwen in her first car, he says, "I remember when she looked like that."

He says, "They were really in love. Olwen and Walter had something special. They would have been a great couple." When I tell him I have always loved the cedar chest Walter gave Olwen as an engagement present and will be keeping Olwen's best things in it, tears come to his eyes.

When I refinish the chest (as I told Olwen I would be doing), I will come to appreciate more fully its excellent workmanship and perfect blend of elegant yet clean and classic design and pragmatic choices of woods: walnut on top, cedar on the back, bottom, and inside the top, and maple sides and front. Walter not only had good taste, but he also seems to have known that if Olwen herself were a cedar chest, this is the one she would be.

Was Walter able to see and elicit the most authentic Olwen? Did the young horse whisperer reach into and begin to heal the unarticulated, wounded places in her? Bring to her that same perceiving, attuned presence to which the horses responded so readily?

Olwen's relationship with Walter emerged on the intuitively self-healing path she had followed in the aftermath of Lizzie's death. Having a sense of place amidst her adoptive family and a supportive community could have been solidified by their marriage. Life with Walter would, it appears, have been seamless with Olwen's new fabric, exorcising some of the shadows and narrowing the gap between her life had Lizzie lived and what it was becoming in her absence.

One autumn afternoon, however, Walter, his father, and middle brother had finished their work for the day and were headed into the house. Someone turned, saw smoke coming out of the barn, and called the fire department. Walter dashed into the barn where he freed the four big horses who pulled the plows and released all the cows from their stanchions.

The story, as I had always heard it from my mother and others, was simply that Walter had "saved all the horses." After meeting with his niece, I realized how limited my image had been. I had run a black and white movie in slow motion with sounds blocked out. I was watching the movie, staring into the barn, waiting for him to come out with yet another horse, counting horses, counting minutes and seconds, silently screaming, "get out of there now! now!!" I hadn't thought about how terrified horses become in fire and how difficult it is to get even one of these creatures out of a burning barn and prevent them from running back in again—let us not speak of four.

The insights of Walter's gentle niece open up my slow and silent frame. My new movie is in technicolor, action everywhere, men's voices yelling to each other over the sounds of the terrified animals. Horses rearing, eyes rolling in panic, yet doing as Walter's hands command. Hands that know every stall, every latch, every stanchion. Body that knows every square foot of the barn, moving quickly, firmly, confidently through ever-thickening smoke, dashing through openings as the flames creep ever closer. Walter, the horse whisperer. The only one with the strength and gifts to get four terrified horses and scores of cows safely out of a burning barn.

His nephew recalled, "the fire got going very fast." Once Walter had freed all the animals, he came out of the barn by himself. He was not burned, but he had inhaled a great deal of smoke which, in his nephew's words, "scorched his lungs. He lived about a year after that."

Olwen has always been vague about that year, no doubt never wanting to bring it into sharp focus, and I was always reluctant to press for more. In our conversation sixty-some years later, Olwen fuzzily recalled, "I think he just sort of—he got TB, and then his sister took him up to her house, and he lived on her porch—out of doors so he could get the fresh air—and I used to go up and see him. I don't know, he was quite a while."

It is painful to make the images in my own mind of the nightmare of her coming to realize, whether gradually or suddenly, that he would not be getting well, of her coming up to be with him and having to go back down to work, of seeing her dreams slip away, of once more being helpless to save the person she loved most. More painful yet are images of its becoming ever harder for the strong-yet-gentle young horse whisperer to breathe.

When a friend of Olwen's who knows Walter's family gives me pictures of Walter and shows me where his house was and where he is buried, I am startled by the cemetery's being virtually across the street from the teacher I visited since high school, the one whose caregivers we inherited. Olwen sometimes came with me to visit my teacher, or sometimes drove her own car, dropping me off there while she drove on to visit her friend from the old days. Only now do I know she would have driven right by Walter's house on the way to her friend's house.

I will wonder why, although she told me over and over how she used to take the train up there with Judy's family and how they carried their stuff up a long hill, she never pointed out it was *this* hill. Nor, in all the years she talked so fondly about her home on Elm Street, did she ever point it out when we went by it—and we must have gone by scores of times when we were living three blocks away at Betty's.

Why did she never link her stories with real places that we passed many times? These houses might as well have been artifacts of a lost civilization on a lost continent. Why didn't I ask her? Was I too young? Afraid it was too painful? Did her distancing also distance me from asking? Did something tell me to leave the shadows alone, not try to visit the lost continent?

During that stunning call in which she suddenly had access to her memory banks and the missing pieces poured out, I said, "I can only imagine how unbearable it must have been that you could not save Walter any more than you could have saved Mama. Probably today they could have saved him and they could have saved her, but they couldn't back then. And that has got to be so hard to accept!" At the least, they could have helped him breathe and made him comfortable, but I do not want to raise that dreadful spectre with her.

Then and since I have said, "I think Walter was part of your healing process after Mama died. Walter brought joy into your life, and joy is healing. When he died, I think the joy went out of your life. Whatever had begun to reopen for you closed down again. I think you had to lock away *all* the pain after Walter died."

Parts of Olwen died with Walter. The dream gone. Joy crushed. Her practical, risk-averse side took over. I do not know these things as facts. I have always known them in my bones.

> *Life can only be understood backward, but it must be lived forward.*
> —Niels Bohr

Although Olwen married my father several years after Walter's death, retrospectively he claimed she had married him on the rebound. Rebound is an odd claim since he went after her, begging her to go out for months before she said yes. Perhaps his claim is part of his pattern of not taking responsibility and instead putting the onus on her. Yet perhaps it does hold some emotional truth. He was perhaps always competing with a shadow that could not be erased.

Was "rebound" his way of framing something he resented, something he couldn't get from her that he sensed belonged to someone else, or had died with someone else? Is that why I saw no pictures of Walter? Did Mac need to erase any signs of Walter, just like he later would need to erase and simplify the complex reality of his first marriage? Or did Olwen choose to put pictures away because they were too painful? Or tear them up because she just had to close this chapter of her life? Or because she believed a married woman didn't keep pictures of the other man she had loved, a man who may have elicited feelings that her husband never could?

Was Olwen's refusal to go out with her new admirer for months just about their age difference, or did she sense his being "too young" (her words) was about more than age? Did she intuitively sense, however vaguely, it was "too soon"—for him, because he didn't know himself yet and was projecting his romanticized needs onto this "older woman" in his department; for her, because she sensed there might be parts of herself not yet or no longer available? Was "too young" her interpretation of something more fundamental—not right—that she couldn't access now that her radar was impaired?

Two bright, ambitious, handsome people each disconnected from themselves, each needing what the other couldn't provide—surely a recipe for heartache and even disaster.

Did she get worn down by his flattery, his determination, his hitching rides to the mountains to see her when she was up there, his willingness to walk over to Betty's from his side of town, take Olwen to whatever dance or event they were attending, walk her back to Betty's, and walk home again? Was she worn down by his persistence, attractiveness, dressed-for-success appearance, his eagerness to rise in the company, her belief (she later shared with me) that he would be a good and responsible father? Did he seem dependable and consistent in contrast to the financial ups and downs of her musician father? Did she factor in the thought, "I'm not getting any younger and I do want a family"?

Although she repeatedly expressed her sorrow about not having been able to go to college, she never once spoke of having sacrificed her career for marriage and family. Perhaps she did not see herself as having a career but as having gone to work out of necessity. What she did tell us many times was what the president of their company said to her while dancing at her engagement party.

"If you think enough of Mac to marry him, then we'll see that he goes places." Olwen's tone in telling this was matter-of-fact, but colored with pride that she was so highly regarded in the company where my ambitious young father-to-be had also come to work. I, by contrast, am appalled that she was being told, "We think so highly of *you* and trust *your* judgment so much that we'll be looking for great things from *him* and expect to move *him* up. We hate to lose you but of course *you,* as a woman, will be the one who has to leave the company after you are married."

As she saw it, "I got out, you see, so Mac could work there. We couldn't both stay there. Oh, well, that's a long time ago . . . They felt very badly about my leaving them, they really did, but we couldn't both work there, so that is the way it worked. Isn't that funny?"

"No, it's not. It's outrageous, it's discrimination against women." My mother never had a good job again, or one where she was part of a department that valued her and had an interesting work environment. Instead, she did only part-time bookkeeping. In keeping with norms of the time, my father did not want her to work full-time after they were married and even after the divorce. He said he did not want me to come home to an empty house, and preferred to pay modest child support and alimony to make that possible.

When I later look up my parents in city directories, I find that in the years before I was born, she identified herself as a bookkeeper while he identified himself as an accountant. He, who had started as a messenger soon after high school and learned from and with Olwen as they poured over old books to figure out how to handle new problems, became treasurer and chief financial officer of her old company, active in professional accounting associations, and got his picture in the local paper from time to time.

When Mac developed tuberculosis, Olwen's motivation in taking on the monumentally heroic and dangerous task was ostensibly to save her marriage. He promised he would give up the young woman he had been seeing if Olwen would keep him out of a sanitarium and do this impossible thing of getting him well, thereby putting herself and me at risk. A Faustian bargain, perhaps, but that was the deal.

I see a deeper and an even more powerful motivation. Olwen could not save Lizzie and she could not save Walter, but she could perhaps save her husband and her marriage. She could make it possible for him to breathe again and thereby *herself* exorcise at least some of the long shadows that haunted her.

Yet, even when she succeeded at getting him well, the outcome was the same: she lost the person she was trying to save. The message was crushing: even when she succeeded, she "failed." This loss carried another brand of devastation because of his betrayal.

During the five months at our neighbors' cabin, my father's mother carried messages back and forth from the young woman, taking the bus up and back weekly on the day we came down to do our errands. During my father's evening walks taking the air when we got back, neighbors even a mile away observed his meeting up with his girlfriend—and, Michael recalls, they sometimes called to inform Olwen.

Even decades later, Mac, an otherwise honorable man, never owned up to these actions (at least to me), or expressed gratitude to Olwen for all she did for him. Through my sorting and sifting of their lives and deaths only months apart, I finally understood why he had such difficulty acknowledging these things. One loose thread could have unraveled the cocoon he spun around himself back then. His self-image and comfort with his second life rested upon his black-and-white account of the first. The price he paid for his self-protective mythology is that he became its prisoner, and that impaired his growth.

> *The goal of the journey of grief is not to escape, but to travel well within the shadows.*
> —Peggy Whiting and Elizabeth James

I have for a long time intuited the third great loss in Olwen's life as different from the first two, perhaps because it ultimately had a liberating rather than debilitating effect. Now I see more clearly why that is.

First of all, her husband's betrayal enabled Olwen to feel rage at him, a rage which I suspect gathered into itself the cumulative anger she would have repressed about Mama's "leaving" her and Walter's impetuous nobility, and, most of all, her fragmented and partially blocked rage at her father. Her anger in the post-Mac era was, in contrast to any "negative emotions" she had experienced earlier in her life, fully enfranchised. She had the support of all her family, all her friends, all "their" friends, all the neighbors, her church congregation, and even his family except for his mother. Indeed, the divorce was the last straw in his already difficult relationship with his own father. When my grandfather read the riot act to Mac about the impending divorce, his son cut off from him completely, never seeing or speaking to him again. My father's aunts and his brother's family withdrew from him.

The outcome of Olwen's "getting in touch with her anger" was both cathartic and mobilizing. She got up off the mat after this third altering of her life trajectory by reinventing herself. In contrast to the deaths of Lizzie and Walter which shut her down and filled her back rooms with shadows, this time *she herself took up residence in the space where new shadows might have formed*. She built the life she, in her own mind, would or should have had as Mac's status in the company rose.

She began by selling the house and regrouping again at Betty and Auntie's where we all worked together to "spruce up" their house. I still remember scraping layers of old wallpaper, and that bringing our refrigerator to replace the ice box was a big deal.

I had come to enjoy the frequent rhythms of the ice man, however, when Michael and I spent the May and June weeks of "TB summer" at their house until his school term was out. I had witnessed the cooking miracles Auntie performed with the coal stove, her daily ritual of winding the clocks, and nightly ritual of getting up to shake the coal embers. Although I had always known Elizabeth had a magical ability to play and engage with children, I, not yet in school, now had hours to absorb her artifacts and photographs. They weren't like the dead objects I saw in stores or "decorating" some people's homes, but wondrous entities that had a history and a meaning, and made the house feel alive. I felt free to ask about them and she told me their stories.

During the post-divorce years at Betty's, I had two, built-in "babysitters," which freed Olwen to create an active life for herself, something I encouraged her to do. Olwen explored another line of work, began painting and taking other courses, became more involved with her church circle of friends who had already been together for fifteen years, joined the country club, took up golf, made new friends, redesigned her engagement ring, and bought the flashy car on our trip to Florida.

She also had her bedroom furniture antiqued. She did that right off, between the time she sold the old house and we moved to Betty's. I remember the day the furniture was delivered. I had no idea what "antiquing" was until then. They did a beautiful job with it, white with gold, but even as a small child, I preferred wood to be stained rather than painted. Perhaps it was all those months in our neighbor's log cabin with (what my child-self heard as) its "naughty pine" interiors that set this preference. (I did wonder how pine could be "naughty.") Olwen was so thrilled with her "new" furniture that I can remember her delight even now and my deciding not to say anything that would dampen her pleasure. It was *her* furniture and *her* life after all, and I hadn't seen her this happy in quite a while. But even at that tender age, it struck me as curious that Walter's trunk was not spared from the antiquing. I did ask why she had included it. She had no answer.

Now, so many decades later, I do. She was closing the chapters on both Walter and Mac, turning a new page, and reinventing her life. The symbolism is transparent in her choosing her *bedroom* furniture and the *hope chest* from her fiancé and turning them from dark to white.

Olwen carved out a new life that was not partner-dependent well before the women's movement would ratify such a path. Despite the downward pull of her shadows, she pronounced to me in that unique conversation just before her hospitalizations in the fall of 2001, "I've lived a good life really, but I know that I worked at it. I had to do a lot of things, and I was able to do them." Do them she did. Resurrect herself three times she did.

Although Olwen began the post-marital half of her journey by building the life that the wife of a company officer "ought" to have (the club, the golf, the ring), she branched off in her own way, creating an independent life around her family, friends, neighbors, home, travel, and volunteer activities. By acceding to my father's preference that she not work, she was able to create the life she did, yet retrospectively she had some regrets about not returning to work.

What she created was also more adventurous, less confining, and presumably more stimulating than running a farm with Walter. Yet, if she hadn't had the life she did ultimately have, she might never have missed it. Especially if life with Walter had unfolded into the journey of healing and personal happiness that it was promising to be.

Marriage to Walter would have faced its own crisis within a decade, however, because his mother was as proud of her German heritage as Olwen was of her Welsh roots. Olwen could not abide Walter's mother rooting for the Germans to bomb the British. She did something virtually unprecedented for her: as war clouds gathered over Europe, she stopped visiting his parents.

What if Walter's mother had been Olwen's mother-in-law? What if, even though she and Walter had built their own house, they were still working the family farm he was expected to inherit? How would Walter have handled the situation? Even if he had sided with Olwen, they would no longer have had the support of his sister, who had obviously been such a champion of their match, because she died just as the war was starting. Walter's mother lived a decade after that, and such a breach would not have been easily reconciled even after the war.

The path taken and the paths not taken may in the end lead to the same and not the same place. If Olwen's were a mythic tale, Walter might be her Twin, and Mac, the Stranger. The Twin and the Stranger bring different gifts, different challenges, different ways of meeting oneself.

What of me? I would not be the me I am if Mac were not my father. I have always been haunted by Walter, however, and for a time I explained it to myself by the fact that if Walter had lived, I would not be, or I would not be me. So Walter's fate and my own are indissolubly linked. But the linkage is more than that.

It's also that I brought the joy back into Olwen's life that "died" after Walter died. I see that clearly now in Olwen's body language in pictures with me as an infant and small child and in the most extraordinary letter she wrote the day after I was born, a letter that will find its way to me in the weeks after she dies. And, there is some other connection that does not seem to be of this world or this lifetime.

My sense is that my soul-self (whatever that means; I don't pretend to know, it is simply a sense I have) is linked not only to Lizzie and Olwen and Elizabeth, but also to Walter, while my personal self is linked to my father. The gifts of this Stranger, including his conflicts with the Queen, produced a Daughter/Priestess whose journey requires restoring wholeness by going to the underground and finding greater truths that release and complete something for all of us.

Olwen's way had been to stay in the conscious upper world, look its challenges straight in the face, do what has to be done, and get on with it. Her learned pragmatism served her well. Having tried to exorcise her deepest shadows by saving her husband's life, she reinvented herself, traveling well within her shadows by choosing a path on which she did not engage them, and herself filling the spaces where new shadows might have formed.

My way has to been to journey to the unconscious lower world to engage our shadows on behalf of all of us. Intuitively, I have long known that it is I, the last of my line, who can and must become Inanna and journey to the underworld to encounter our shadows, heal our lineage, and restore our wholeness.[3] I have long known that it all comes down to me.

In the earlier stages of my journey, I foundered over and over on the same dilemma: I can't bring Mama back and I can't bring Walter back. I cannot undo the past. I cannot undo the legacy of their loss and their shadows in Olwen's structure. I cannot erase the shadows that took up residence in the deepest, silent levels of myself so long ago. I cannot erase what it has cost us.

Yet since childhood, I have longed to fix the unfixable. If only I could take her pain away, if only she could feel whole again, then—what? Then she can find her way to peace and I can find my way to completing my own journey to wholeness—which, I have come to realize through this transformative journey with Olwen (a journey which will, in turn, ripple into a healing process with my father), is necessary to bringing my work into the world.

So, what is it that can still be fixed? And how do I do it? I must draw upon my child-self's longing and, as an adult, become my fullest priestess-self to do what I am here to do on my long journey with Olwen and Lizzie.

Twelve

Retrieving the Understory

"When I go way back, I'm glad sometimes I didn't know—not the answer, but what did it mean?"
—Olwen, June 13

Saturday, I ask Olwen's pastor if he would like to come for a final visit, and what he has learned about letting go of life. He allows that he has limited experience with those nearing death; he is more likely to be called in to offer prayers with the family. I am startled as I thought he was in the death business, but I appreciate his candor.

Forewarned, and knowing how challenging it is to enter a dying process, I facilitate their getting started. Mother knows who he is and makes "socially appropriate" responses. I take laundry upstairs, and when I rejoin them, she is saying poignant things and stating them clearly and audibly. *She* has put *him* more at ease because she, as she has always done, has risen to the occasion and is behaving graciously—her last performance.

Sue arrives midafternoon. After seeing the pastor out, I go hunting for white, light-weight pants in fine cotton that breathes, and an all-cotton tank top for Olwen. I have been dismayed to realize how many of her summer clothes are what I call plastic, and what Olwen would call easy to wash and care for.

When I get back, Olwen and Sue are returning from a short outing. Mother looks a little blotchy, and her nailbeds are somewhat blue ("cyanotic"). Something tightens in my gut. On Thursday, she had said, "I'm going Home this weekend." We give her a nitro tab, increase the oxygen flow to four liters, and Sue goes home.

Mother settles into her rose recliner chair. We sip flower essences and I do Reiki with her, but soon I sense her life force ebbing. At low volume, I play Hildegard and Berezan's "Returning," and sing softly with the music. Mother quietly states, "I'm going Home before dark."

She needs to be more comfortable and in her own *real* bed. In her listless condition, I dare not try to move her by myself. When Sue returns, I am doing Reiki from behind Olwen's chair. Sue wordlessly merges with our energy, holding and directing energy around Olwen's legs. Using gestures, I ask Sue to bring over my little pendulum which gives me an external check on what I sense but don't quite trust. The pendulum barely moves when held near any of her energy centers—except over her crown chakra which some say is connected with a greater Consciousness. Sue and I exchange knowing looks. Much later, I will read that this energy pattern is a precursor to death.

We move Olwen across the living room to her bed. Sue gets pillows, changes tapes, brings water, facilitates the situation, and becomes a supportive presence without intruding. I sit behind Mother, cradling her; lie next to her; and sit facing her. I feel as if everything has already been said, scores or hundreds of times, and we are way beyond words now. Silent except for the music, it is a beautiful, peaceful, intimate, summer evening.

Her breathing is shallow, and, at times, she is breathing more heavily than she has to this point. Her nailbeds are variably cyanotic, turning blue and pinking up again.

Mother opens her eyes and looks right through me for a long time, focusing on nothing, yet all-seeing. Her eyes have been fading and have become less focused over the past couple of weeks. They have often been at half-mast with her attention drawing inward. But tonight she has opened her eyes more fully, or as fully as she now can. Then she looks at things in the air. No fear, no curiosity, no engagement, just an otherworldly seeing of what to us is unseen.

Eventually, her gaze fixes fiercely on me and is absolutely riveting. It is as if she were taking my measure in some final, summative way. The Day of Judgment of my soul. Her gaze is interminable, implacable, unrelenting. It is the Death Goddess. I hold her gaze and never look away. Her final statement to and about me is "yes."

Around 9:30, Olwen begins to fidget. Sue and I hold her hands and she grows calmer again and stares off into space. She begins coming back to us, almost joking with us. After forty-five minutes or so of this, Sue and I silently yet jointly conclude she has pulled out of this and is coming back to us. We take her to the bathroom and put her to bed in the bedroom.

Sue has never seen anything like this, and I certainly don't know what to make of it. Olwen went right up to the edge and was, we both thought, almost over. Had we been wrong? Did she not start to cross over and then pull back?

Sue leaves and I am suddenly hungry. I finish my lunch, leave a message with one friend, and talk with another whose mother died a year ago from CHF. A garden designer, she will later plant a lilac bush below my living room windows in memory of my mother. The on-call nurse tells me there were others tonight who almost crossed over.

I am confounded. Is this the beginning of the end? Or has Mother decided to hang on a while longer? Are we still talking about two or three weeks? Is the layered shell that began to form around the gentle, young girl after Mama's death still trying to force her into a death where she ends up feeling abandoned and alone—as Lizzie must have felt? We've come so far in these last weeks. Can we finally penetrate all the way through the shell, and really break the pattern? Is it still possible?

<hr />

I feel more dead than alive when I wake up on Sunday. Less rested than when I went to sleep, as if I had had no sleep at all. Christine's substitute does not notice any changes in Olwen. Mother, in her new summer clothes, is quiet and clearly wants to sleep. She won't be climbing out of her chair any time soon so it is safe for me to fall asleep. I awake more refreshed, explore my confusion and all the possibilities with an old friend and leave messages for three others.

Olwen continues to sleep. Rosanna comes over midafternoon so I can get outside, clear my head, and actually see this facility where rooms are available for Olwen if we do a respite.

The building gives me chills. All I can think of is a nineteenth-century asylum. No way I can image wheeling little Olwen up to this place! I shudder and recoil. No way!! Nonetheless, I go through the exercise of checking it out. Absolutely no question now: Olwen is never to come here. I should have come over and seen the place right away. I can't wait to get out of here. However long she has, we will find another way to care for her and give me relief.

Once in the car and feeling I can breathe again, I know what I need to do. I head straight to our family plot, sit on my mother's gravestone facing my grandmother's stone. I firmly state, "Lizzie, this is your granddaughter. I need your help. I need a timetable. Whatever you can tell me."

The speed and authoritativeness of the response leave no doubt in my mind that I am not making this up. "Hang in there. It's only a couple of days." I do not think Lizzie of the long white gloves and grand hats worn at picnics has adopted American slang. I think the mysterious translation process from energetic waves to verbal language is completed by the attuned receiver.

During a visit to Lizzie's grave about ten days ago, I wrote down: "The time is coming. We're not there yet . . . I *will* appear to her . . . Two weeks, ten and four." Puzzling at the time, ten and four soon make sense. In response to my lamenting my failures with Olwen, Lizzie insisted, "Olwen wasn't easy. You've tried to open her heart. You've done all you can." Yes and no. I could have made wiser choices along the way.

> *Like Innana I am called to go down deep to a place of darkness where I have no name.*
> —Apara Borrowes, "My Ear was Tuned to the Great Below"

I have seen about ten photographs of Lizzie. They affirm images my mother sketched. Erect posture, great dignity, stylish clothes for outings, spotless housedresses for daily work. Because Mama always stood straight, she never—so my mother admonished me as a child and recounted with pride—splattered food stains on her dress or apron as she prepared meals.

Lizzie's enormous presence shines through the photographs. This was a woman of substance. Her face fascinates me because it holds such silent depths and I can see each of us in her, especially Olwen and myself. Hers was a handsome beauty that ages exceedingly well because she, like her husband's mother, had fabulous facial bones Olwen will inherit and pass on to me.

Her marriage certificate shows that when Lizzie was just shy of twenty-one, she married John, then twenty-three, in London where he was studying at a college of music. Did they elope? Yes. Her sister's granddaughter, Gwen, says our great-grandparents disapproved three of their four children's matches, including Lizzie's. In two cases, they were right.

John's musical abilities were evident and encouraged from an early age. Both parents had exceptional voices, and his mother was reputed to have had the best voice in the chapel where she grew up. While studying composition, harmony, and conducting in London, John also began investigations into his passion: the human voice and the way vocal chords work. At the conclusion of his studies when he was twenty-five, he was made a Fellow by the college council, its highest honor, apparently uncommon in North Wales.

When Lizzie and John were young children, their families had moved to the same slate-mining, boom town, Pen-y-Dyffryn *(penn-uh-duff-rinn)*. I suspect they got to know each other through chapel and music. John was organist at the grandest of the town's chapels by the time he was in his teens, and Lizzie's father was an elder active in his local chapel, and also associated with the main chapel.

Chapels, which were run by the elders, were the primary centers of religious, cultural, and political life for Welsh Calvinistic Methodists or "nonconformists" who resisted English landlordism, churchism, and imposition of the English language. Chapels, nonconformity, the Welsh language, and Welsh culture (in which music, especially singing, was central) were especially strong in the quarrying areas of northwest Wales, a huge region known as Gwynedd *(gwinn-eth)*.[1]

Throughout the nineteenth and early twentieth centuries, Gwynedd was the world center for roofing slates, but almost all of Gwynedd was owned by English merchants and landed families. Indeed it was owned by a *few* families (thirty-five families controlled 75 percent of the land), the *same* few who also controlled the quarries, industry, and commerce, and built railroad links to send the slates to ports for shipping.

Lizzie's family was active not only in chapel life, but also, I suspect, in civic and political life. Quarrymen, as I will discover her father to have been, were keenly interested in politics and Welsh culture. Her mother ran a shop and was a member of the Women's International, while her older brother learned the printing trade as a foundation for starting his publishing business, newspaper, and retail newshop. Literacy rates among the Welsh were high and local papers such as his abounded, carrying the fight for antilandlordism and disestablishment of the church.

Following a decade of married life in Pen-y-Dyffryn, John decided to move to America. Why? The family story is that he needed to get more work. Once he came over, it appears John never looked back. He became an American citizen as soon as it was possible, and there are no indications or accounts he ever returned to Wales.

Her sister's grandchildren say Lizzie was not eager to come to America and did not see it as a permanent move. She had, they say, great affection for both of her parents and they for her.

One of Olwen's most vivid early memories is the ocean voyage. When told she would be going on a great trip over water, little Olwen worried her new coat would get wet. The adult Olwen emphasized that her family had a real cabin on the ship and had not come steerage. Mama was miserably sick and stayed in her cabin. Was it just her stomach, or did she already have a history of somatizing stress, disappointment, and sadness—as did so many women of her time whose corseted bodies bespoke the squashing of their lives?

During the crossing, the steward was memorably kind and helpful to Lizzie and her children. Olwen, already the responsible child, comforted her as best she could. Peggy, on the other hand, had a wonderful time exploring the ship and meeting people.

Before embarking for the States, John had secured a position at a conservatory of music teaching harmony and sight singing in an area with a large and flourishing Welsh community. He was chosen conductor of two major choruses, and began teaching voice privately. In the years that followed, he adjudicated competitions, led all-male and mixed choirs to prizes and victories in the eisteddfodau *(aiss-teth-vodd-eye)* and other music competitions that thrived in the days before radio and film, apparently becoming a star in the Welsh and musical communities. His choirs were cited for outstanding voice and tone quality, use of tone to convey feeling, as well as for grasping the meaning of the music and giving the most effective interpretations. His motto was said to be, "link the tone with the feeling."

Even so, Olwen's stories indicate family finances waxed and waned, and were sometimes iffy, while Florence asserted, "we weren't poor." The truth in both their memories is suggested by a small trove I will unearth from the annual reports of their Welsh church. Their parents' initially generous donations dwindled to nothing the year Florence was born. Over the next six years, donations slightly above average alternated with three more zero years. By the time Florence was old enough to have had a clear memory, her parents' donations had increased, stabilized, and exceeded the average.

Mother has always described her family's large flat on Elm Street as lovely and its furnishings as being of good quality. The up-and-coming neighborhood was comprised of well-built, double-decker houses owned by upwardly mobile Welsh, Irish, and Germans who rented out one floor, often to kin or people from the old country. Olwen's standout memory was of Welsh song, laughter, and story reverberating throughout the house when visiting musicians came for tea following competitions and musical events. Olwen pointed out there was no liquor in the house and none served at such gatherings; if a recipe called for spirits, someone had to go to the saloon and bring home a little in a glass or cup.

In Olwen's mind, Elm Street is the one and only home her family had in America. With the help of city directories, I find they actually spent their first six years five blocks away in an apartment on a square whose elegant homes were noted for their architecture and would later be deemed historic. John had immediately had a phone installed at a time when phones were the exception, and phone numbers had but four digits. Situated close to the Welsh church and bordering downtown, the apartment in the square suggests Lizzie and John began life in American with a little money behind them and optimistic expectations.

It is clearly Elm Street, however, that represents "home" to Olwen. If anything was a candidate for the "yellow house" she expected on her return from rehab, I expect it was Elm Street.

What these two apartments represented to Lizzie I cannot say. Certainly she had more space and light than attached cottages afford. The infrastructure of her small city was highly advanced for the time and ahead of many larger American cities. Lizzie had Welsh neighbors, attended a Welsh church, and the town was crawling with societies and groups. Her new city was on the upswing and thriving, underpinned by a diversified industrial and commercial base. I suspect there were many ways that life here was physically easier, but I do not think that Elm Street or America ever represented home to Lizzie.

※

Lizzie's first trip home was to be with Olwen when she graduated high school. Although Lizzie greatly longed for this reunion, it must have carried uncertainty and ambivalence. Did she still have a home where she imagined home to be, the image she had held on to through a miserable ocean crossing and all the years since? Given parental disapproval of her mate, had Lizzie in her letters felt a continuing need to prove her choice and not let them know of her own financial uncertainties or marital disappointments? Had Lizzie felt she had to keep validating her choice of husband by never seeming to need anything and never sharing her disappointments or concerns?

We will never know. Lizzie never did see her mother or her homeland again. She died in the summer of 1922 from the complications of a burst appendix—sepsis and peritonitis.

Olwen has described getting a phone call from the hospital telling them the news just as they all, including Papa, were sitting down to dinner. It seems as if the news was not what they expected. Were the children not being kept realistically informed? Probably not. Perhaps they weren't even allowed to visit at the hospital in those days. Or did the children need to think Mama was going to get better and would come back to them? Probably. Was John any better informed? And why wasn't he at the hospital?

What I do know from her death certificate is Lizzie had surgery but it was too late, and she was in hospital three days. She died there alone, probably in pain, and with who knows what going through her mind.

※

Twenty months later, John remarried. Irma was a voice student, a homely woman with no neck, bad hair, a wandering eye, and a powerful solo voice that, her granddaughter reminds me, could not be submerged in a choir. She was often the soloist for John's choirs, and she sang in our church choir for decades. As my child-self recalls, Irma mostly kept her eyes down on the hymn book as the choir came down the aisle toward us, but I think sometimes her eyes and Olwen's did meet. Perhaps I think so because my body remembers picking up Olwen's apprehension each week as the choir came in and sensed her anguish if their eyes met. I just stared at Irma wondering what on earth he had seen in her. What was wrong with him?

Quite a lot, especially when seen through a contemporary lens through which we understand the impact of parental behavior that, at the time, may have slid by as unremarkable. For a year after Mama died and Olwen graduated high-school, the family remained at Elm Street. It must have been ghastly with the silence and emptiness, Papa so unable to express emotions or relate to children, and the children each fractured in their own way by grief. Early in the second year, John told his adolescent children to leave because he was going to marry Irma and break up Elm Street. "Thrown away" is the phrase they used to describe their feelings.

John's abdication and distancing behavior is consistent with other fragments my mother related over the years. Papa would hardly have thought to change his clothes if Mama had not put out a change for him. Papa did not always collect his fees from his students. Who was sent out to collect them so that, as Olwen put it, "Mama could put food on the table"? His middle daughter. Before he had a studio downtown, the children had to be quiet when they came home from school because Papa was teaching. With the exception of giving Olwen pointers on breath and voice, it did not occur to him to give music or voice lessons to his own children, and Peggy had talent. She taught herself to play piano by ear. Even in her late years, Peggy was still the life of the party with her piano playing during gatherings at her senior apartments.

Florence was "allowed" to stay at times with John and Irma, but she had to pay board. Who paid it? Olwen of course. Perhaps the most quintessential of Olwen's tales, and certainly her most told, was that when she started working at $12 a week, she paid $7 to Betty's family for room and board, $3.50 for Florence to stay with her father and stepmother, walked to and from work and everywhere else, and spent the remaining $1.50 for fabric to sew clothes for Florence and herself.

Here we see the very practical Olwen, already managing a great deal on her small budget, doing what she can to take care of Florence. We see Olwen the seamstress, taught by her mother and tutored by Auntie, and

Olwen the indefatigable walker. We see her defiant pride, and her pulling herself up by her bootstraps.

Olwen has always concluded her short account by telling us with pride in her voice and posture that before long, she was making $28 a week.

Olwen did not frame her vignettes or comment on Papa's behavior but I do. My inferences have been borne out by conversations with members of his second family who tell me he was just as inattentive to his new son born a couple years after his remarriage. Irma, they say, doted on him and was content to revolve around him as his satellite.

I see the handsome, dashing, romantic, young musician morphing into a self-centered, entitled, middle-aged man who lived for his music and was oblivious to most everything else. Only the music could express all that was within him, the music he served to the exclusion of all else, the music that stole his being. In his time, people said he was aloof and distant. Today we might say he was relationally stunted and narcissistic. It seems evident he never really knew who Lizzie was, nor saw her in her own right as her own center of subjectivity.

How devastatingly ironic that his choirs were known for their ability to express emotion through tone and to interpret the meaning of the music. John had no idea how to move feelings or make connections with others except through the medium of music.

Somewhere in the aftermath of Lizzie's death, Olwen deduced that her mother's sadness derived from John's attentions having strayed to Irma. Young Olwen was reflecting on changes she had noticed and, as she told me long ago, did not really understand at the time.

Perhaps Irma was the first of John's wanderings, or perhaps there had been a string of temporary romantic infatuations reflecting his glory back to himself. Then again, his strong Calvinistic Methodism may have held him back from acting on feelings or even recognizing them. The spacing of his children suggests some kind of self-discipline. Were they already involved emotionally if not sexually when Lizzie died? Was Irma, as her granddaughter intuited, a "homewrecker"? Or did their relationship begin after Lizzie died, with the infatuated voice student, nineteen years his junior, comforting the widower? We will never know for sure, but somewhere along the way, Lizzie developed migraines.

It was not until October of 2001—when Olwen was having some health problems and fearing the worst—that we had a once-in-a-lifetime telephone conversation that gave me the final bits that allowed me to put her story together, and more fully understand her trauma and deepest shadows. Something had finally come unstuck or moved out of the way, and she was able to say things in a connected way that she never had been able to before.

Numerous other times Olwen had said, "Oh, Mama was so sick." I would say, "What do you mean? *When* was she sick? *How* was she sick?" Olwen couldn't tell me. The conversation would just stop, or she would say, "Oh, she had migraines," and that would be the end of it. I'd think to myself, "I don't think that's it."

This time it is different. "Mama was so sick," she says several times, and now for the first time in my life, she connects it to the days before Mama died, the days before she was taken to the hospital. Olwen allows the horrific images to come into focus: Mama so sick, Mama calling the doctor, Olwen calling the doctor every day, even several times a day, and he doesn't come, not the first day, not the second, nor the third, or maybe even the fourth. Olwen is desperate to get him to the house, but he doesn't respond. Mama is getting worse. Olwen goes to his office at least twice. Not until the fourth or fifth day does the doctor finally show up. With Welsh accent, Olwen repeats his words: "I'm afraid you have appendicitis and will need to go to hospital." And Olwen, eighty years later, crying to me on the phone, "I should have gotten the doctor there before that!"

For the first time I know the full horror of it. In firm, authoritative tones, I state, as I will over and over, "IT WASN'T YOUR FAULT!! IT WASN'T *YOUR* JOB to get the doctor. You were still a child. Was the doctor going to pay any attention to you—a child? a girlchild? No, he wasn't. The *doctor* failed. It was your father's job to get him there. Your *father* is the one who failed. *You* did not fail! You did everything you could but *they weren't listening to you.*"

But the damage had been done. Olwen, the sensitive, responsible, quiet child, silently absorbed the responsibility by herself and carried this heavy load all her life. By not stepping up to the plate, her father let her.

What kind of a man lets his daughter take the rap? The same one who lets her collect his fees.

And where was John in all this? I try to get a sense from Olwen, but beyond his not being off with his choirs somewhere, she cannot bring up any sense of his presence, let alone taking any action.

Her inability to do so even in this conversation where her closed-off rooms have finally opened to each other suggests his multi-leveled absence or worse. It appears it was still business as usual for John. Off to his studio every morning and back every evening. Certainly he could see this was no migraine. But he apparently did nothing to get the doctor there, or enlist another doctor, let alone move heaven and earth to get help.

Now we come to the very bottom of things, the key to Olwen's understory. It is not just that Lizzie died way too soon, nor even that she died unnecessarily. It is not just that four young people suddenly and unexpectedly lost their mother and their emotional security and were subsequently kicked out of their home, nor that they were emotionally and financially abandoned by their already distant and unavailable father. Nor is it that Olwen took on the responsibility and guilt for somehow not having performed a miracle and gotten a paternalistic doctor to pay attention to her.

Although factually we can never know if timely medical attention would have pulled Lizzie through her appendicitis attack, at the very bottom of things we have a stark emotional truth: John, as well as the doctor, let Lizzie die. Whether through self-preoccupation, or being so wrapped up in his music that his feet never touched the ground, or because he could not look reality in the face or deal with life-threatening illness, or because his attentions had wandered to one of his young students, or all of this and more, my grandfather is implicated in my grandmother's death.

His role in her death could have been a failure to be proactive in getting the doctor there. Whether by being passively complicit or his actively discouraging timely medical attention, the bluntest psychological meaning in John's behavior is that he killed his wife—physically in that last week of her life, and metaphorically and emotionally over the years. I doubt any of their four children ever allowed some version of those words—Papa killed Mama—to be spoken to one another, or even to come into their own conscious minds. It must have been suppressed along with everything else.

Yet significantly, the word "kill" did work its way to the surface. Peggy was scapegoated for "killing her mother." I have heard this phrase since childhood. What I, the youngest member of my clan, would eventually learn this meant was that she had gone to work in New York where she subsequently had her first child without marrying his father—a situation that was devastating to Lizzie. Peggy became the black sheep of the family, and Olwen, who held her family together in the post-Lizzie era, its normative, emotional, and communications center and its new matriarch. In contrast to Olwen who never smoked and drank only socially, her siblings all became heavy smokers who self-medicated by making alcohol a low-grade staple of their daily lives.

No wonder Olwen could not express anger fully and directly at her father on her own or Florence's behalf because any specific complaint was too loaded. It could open straight into the cauldron of rage that his neglect and self-absorption (or worse) had killed their beloved mother. No wonder Olwen split emotions, meanings, and events up in her mind and couldn't tell her stories in a complete way. No wonder she did not journey to the underworld where her shadows and trauma hid in the crevices, ready to strike if she came too near. No wonder she didn't remember what was too dreadful to bring into consciousness. No wonder that when she went "way back," she was "glad sometimes" that she "didn't know—not the answer, but what did it mean?"

※

After spending time at our plot musing on Olwen and Lizzie, I drive home. No longer in pieces and exhausted, I am clear, calm, and more centered than I have been in a long time. Olwen is still "sleeping" (or "reviewing" her life, or doing her end-of-life spiritual work?) and has done so for much of the afternoon. Rosanna is so relieved about respite being permanently off the table. "I knew if you saw that place you would never be able to take her there."

Olwen is quietly responsive to Rosanna today, with sweet little smiles and a hint of playfulness, but she is less responsive than usual and talking very little. She feels much better after a trip to the bathroom and a bowel movement. She drinks Ensure and has some sherbet. She is still wearing my cozy red robe with no complaints about being either hot or cold. Her nailbeds are pink. Rosanna and I talk a while longer, and she goes home.

I glance at my efforts earlier in the day to make a caregivers' schedule. It would not come together because it was not supposed to. It now seems like an archaic relic of another era. I experience a sea change. The chaos and having a million things to do and being pulled in all directions evaporates. All of me is now in one place. I am completely centered in my full self. I am calm because I finally know for certain that I won't be in the wrong place when she dies. I will be with her every moment until the end.

I stop all the paperwork, all the planning, all the *stuff*. I just stop, put the pens down, the pads away, and focus completely on Olwen moment by moment, to be her physical-energetic container twenty-four hours a day.

It hits me in the face that it is not just Olwen who must let go—our focus these last weeks—but *I* who must let go, *I* who must surrender completely to the process and fully trust it. We are in this together. We will have helpers, but in a deeper sense, there are only the two of us now, as it was in my beginning, as it will be in her ending. The two of us, waiting for Lizzie.

We have a quiet evening—Mother in her chair, flower essences, Reiki, music. She reaches out with her hand, I move my hand to meet hers, we hold hands for a while, she breaks away, rests, and repeats this cycle several times. She embraces the little bear and I am so thankful she is actually taking in the comfort it offers. I say, "I love you." Although it is hard for her to speak, she replies, "I love you, too."

It doesn't matter if the night nurse still cannot venture a time line. Lizzie has spoken the truth. We have moved into the sacred Death Time. These will be the last words Mother speaks.

Thirteen

The Dance of Grace

Only when you drink from the river of silence shall you indeed sing . . . And when the earth shall claim your limbs, then shall you truly dance.
—Kahlil Gibran, The Prophet

The hour between the night nurse's departure and Christine's arrival is intolerably long this Monday morning. I have asked for Dinaz to come, and am anxious to learn her view of the changes in Olwen over the weekend. Olwen is physically responsive, but her eyes are closed, and she is no longer speaking. She is making few large body movements. Her blood pressure is 114/64, and her heart rate is running at 136. Christine is reluctant to get her up.

Dinaz concurs. Raised even to a sitting position, Olwen might have a final event on the spot. Christine ministers to Olwen in her bed, while Dinaz tells me in the living room, "Five to seven days. I doubt she will see the weekend."

Acutely aware of the fragility of Olwen's situation from her first visit, Dinaz now confides that she had thought on first meeting that Mother had only days to live. She has been astonished by her resilience. Today's medical assessment fits with Lizzie's answers and with my long-standing intuition of a significant post-birthday slide. A convergence of three modes of knowing.

No pills; she might choke. No fluids; her swallowing will soon fail. Use ice chips and moisten her mouth with mouth sponges (not too wet) that she can suck on. Toothettes to clear out her mouth and scuzziness. Lip balm, liquid tears, and body lotions for dryness. Ativan for anxiety,

Compazine for nausea, Tylenol suppositories for any signs of fever or pain, and, we agree, hold off on the morphine until her breathing starts to creep up. A low-tech arsenal for her comfort.

I expand my use of caregivers and reconfigure their time. I want someone here every night so I can fall asleep with someone watching over us who can immediately alert me to any changes I need to know about. Rosanna can come tonight and give us daytime hours all week. Sue can stop by in the evenings and do one overnight. A hospice night nurse can come every third or fourth night. Nicole can do one overnight. Dory's granddaughter, an experienced LPN who works in a nursing home, can come this Saturday night because it is her weekend off.

I also need someone here at several points in the day and evening to help me reposition Mother so she doesn't get bedsores. Given her parchment skin and loss of muscle and mass, our biggest concern is where her bones rest against bedclothes. I find positioning the scariest of tasks. What if I do it wrong and break a bone or cut off her circulation? Now it becomes terrifying as her arms and legs start to lose muscular tension, and she might not be able to alert me to a problem.

Because all the people and pieces are in place, I can focus on what is truly important: being with Olwen. I do not have to go out for any reason. Knowing I will be unable to eat solid food, I enlist Becky to bring in more bananas, berries, and yogurt. Now that Mother is not trying to get out of bed and be at risk for hitting the nightstand, I bring it back. I move the beds together and put the nightstand on the outer side of her bed, next to the window and her low chair. Now we have a place right next to her to put flowers, Mama's picture, and water supplies, a drawer for lots of little comfort things to be handy but out of sight, and a shelf for the Kleenex tissues on which I have just stocked up. Flowers are on each of the dressers all the time now. As always, medical supplies are stashed inside the closet door except when we are using them. I get rid of the barely-used commode. Two nightlights with a seashell over them offer subtle lighting as the room darkens. Mother's bedroom is the very antithesis of a bright, noisy, equipment-centered, hospital room.

After Christine leaves, I settle in with Mother, always in contact with her. I affirm what we've done and orient her to where she is. I assure her she will never again have to go to any hospital, and won't be going to any nursing home. I remind her we got her back here, "because we are a team. You did your part and I did mine." I describe things we are doing to make her more comfortable and our physical space even more special. I remind her yet again how brave, courageous, resilient, gallant, and gracious she has been through all of this.

She can no longer speak, but she sometimes makes sounds that do not seem to be random. They occur after I have said something that would be significant, and are positive and affirming in tone and cadence.

"I want to tell you again: you are not going to be alone. I will be right here in this room, okay? I will be sleeping right here in the other bed. I am not going to leave you. I'll be right here with you." She makes an affirmative, responsive sound. Every time I leave her room, even if only for two minutes, I tell her where I am going and how soon I will be back.

"I'm here and we have lots of helpers. Our helpers will be taking turns. Christine, Rosanna, Sue . . . You've always got someone attending to you, making sure you are comfortable, in no pain, and that you feel loved and cared for. When I am sleeping, someone else will be watching over you, and they will wake me up if they need to." Again, she makes an affirming sound, whose closest translation might be "aahh-hmmh."

While Sue is here during the dinner hour, I go up to the roofdeck with my cell phone because I can feel myself coming apart. The exhaustion and tension of holding everything together while living in a state of dread that has built up these last years, months, weeks, and days can now let go. The endlessness and vast range of unknowns have become finite and therefore manageable, and with that shift comes whole body release in uncontrollable sobbing. Now that I know we are "safe" and that I will be with her until the end, I am free to finally feel my feelings, and they rush in a flood of gratitude, love, loss, and grief.

With finitude comes perspective. She has gone downhill today even from last night. Saturday night was the beginning of the end, not a pulling back or plateauing. "Lizzie, I think you're right. 'Hang in there. A couple of days,' you said. Thank you! Please come to her, please, please come! She *needs* to see you. Maybe it's not time yet, but she needs to see you! You need to let her know it wasn't her fault. I've told her over and over, but it was too little, too late."

Downstairs, I sit with Mother, holding her hand, listening to her breath. "We've been going through a long, difficult, complicated, beautiful process these last weeks. You were worried you didn't know how to do it, how to let go, but you did! It got harder and harder for you. It got harder and harder and for me. But we both kept going, we both stayed with it, and that's been true our whole lives. We've never given up on each other. We have never quit on each other. That's the thing about you and me. We've always kept working at it." She makes affirming sounds.

"I want you to know I am going to be okay. I have a lot of support here and back home. Everything is working in my life. I am so very sorry I couldn't make it happen in time for you to see some of the payoff from all you've believed in and supported. You never gave up, you've been my biggest champion all these years, you've been there for me through thick and thin. You know it's going to happen for me, you've always known. But since it's taken this long and I couldn't get my work out in time for you, it can wait a while longer. What's been more important is to do healing work with you and keep you here in your apartment, keep you out of hospitals, out of nursing homes, and out of unnecessary rounds of failing health. And together, we've done that."

She pats my hand reassuringly in the way she always has. "That way you pat my hand—it's so you! I shall be forever grateful I had this chance to be with you in this way, to work with you in this way, to heal with you in this way. I will have that for the rest of my life and you can carry it with you on your journey Home."

"Many times you have asked, why are you still hanging around when all your friends have gone? Maybe now we know something about that. You found your own way that's right for you and right for us. Because of the way your dying process has unfolded, we got to go through all the phases together. We've done a lot of healing and lot of loving with each other. I am so thankful for that. Thank you, thank you! Even though it was physically so hard on you, I hope it was as healing and rewarding for you as it was for me."

She responds, "uhhhuh."

"I hope so, honey."

"huhhmm."

"Yeah. Thank you."

She tries to speak several times over the next few minutes, but she cannot produce more than some version of "uhh-huuhh" each time. I listen to her breathing. It is not heavy, but her exhale is audible. "I'm right here, and I'm not going anywhere. I'll be sleeping right next to you all night."

Mother has a good night with Rosanna watching over us, repositioning her, and doing comfort care. I manage to sleep quite well on the spare bed while keeping in contact with her. However, even with the bars down, reaching across the hospital bed makes my neck and shoulder pain even worse, but it's worth it.

Olwen is resting comfortably Tuesday morning. Her pulse has slowed to 112 and is less irregular than yesterday. Her blood pressure has dropped to 110/56. After Christine leaves, I settle in with tapes, including one by Marina Raye—which is how I began making tapes for her.

A couple of years ago, I had been playing a Raye tape, "Heart of the Mother," during a visit and Olwen started dancing to it. Her responsiveness to this music was delightful to behold. Raye combines native flute, percussion instruments, keyboards, and nature sounds to evoke harmonious sounds and rhythms of nature, and dedicates her compositions to the healing of Mother Earth and All Our Relations. Olwen was eager to know more about this music. Her body and facial expression perked up even more when I told her the title. When I explained that the "Mother" here was Mother Earth, she took it in, thoughtfully savoring this new idea and obviously experiencing it as a big "yes." I could literally see an expansion in her awareness.

I decided to leave the boombox with Olwen, and when I got home, started making tapes for her momentary enjoyment, to help her to relax when she was anxious, or energize herself when she was down. Because I knew that hearing is the last sense to go when someone is dying, I anticipated using this by-then-familiar music when that time came.

Although Olwen was less responsive to Christine's voice or queries this morning, she is extremely responsive—and actively expressive—with me. We play and connect with our hands for hours. Our hand play follows her surges of energy marked by shorter interludes of rest. I am astonished by how powerful her grip still is, and bemused by the fact that she is directing and leading everything we do.

I have an impulse to change the tape so Olwen can hear Welsh being spoken, English spoken with Welsh accent, and traditional Welsh folk music. During a lively Welsh tune, Mother keeps time to the music with her left hand in the air. I watch, spellbound. When a great piece from

Carreg Lafar comes on, I take her hand and keep time to it in the air. Still holding her hand lightly, I rest our hands.

On her own, Olwen begins to keep time to the next Carreg Lafar song. When an exuberant tune by Ar Log comes on, she seeks out my hand and leads an extraordinary dance of our hands.

Mother is completely in charge. Her strength and her ability to find the changing core of the rhythm (syncopated and shifting back and forth between three and four beats) are stunning. It is an amazing, moving, and beautiful moment—her choosing to have this dance with me now that she no longer speaks and her walking days are over. It tells me she is quite conscious, hearing very well, purposeful in what she is doing, still responding viscerally to a Welsh tune, still loves to dance, wants to lead the dance, and to have this last dance with me.

While she rests from dancing and I can be certain she is still hearing well and tuned in, I say a few more things. "There's a very gentle, vulnerable, magnificent being inside of you that got shut away after so many hard things happened to you. I wish I could have seen through your layers more clearly and we could have connected at that level more of the time. But now we are finding ways to connect from our centers. I wish it could have been sooner but what really matters is that we got there." My voice, the tape blessedly reveals, is calm, quiet, loving, and resonant.

A little later, "Let me say this again because it is so important. If you had died suddenly in your sleep like you always wanted to, we would not have had this process, we would not have had this time together, we would not have had this incredible dance that you just led, we would not have reached this place together. Having gotten here, I can't imagine not having had this! So I think we know now why you stayed around so long and chose this hard exit strategy!" A responsive sound from her.

"It is the wisdom of your soul and its hard journey that got us to this place. This is an enormous gift you have given to me, and I hope that I have given to you. Thank you, thank you, thank you, thank you, dear one. We'll always be together. We will always be connected, always." She exhales audibly. "There is no end to us, there is no end to our relationship."

※

When Rosanna comes this afternoon, we reposition Mother, apply lotions to any area of sustained contact vulnerable to bedsores, and apply the treatment patch to the most vulnerable area around her coccyx which is already pinkish. Mother falls into a deep, restful sleep. I take a nap, and feel more rested when I awaken.

Olwen's breathing is a little more labored now, and has crept up to 23-24 respirations per minute. Her pulse is 120, thready, and irregular but her nailbeds are pink. Her body is warm so we give her Tylenol. Dinaz says once she is dehydrated, there can be a little fever or congestion, not to worry. Even pneumonia can develop from being bedbound, but Tylenol is still the preferred treatment. If Olwen develops shortness of breath, then put a nitro under her tongue.

Olwen is able to swallow a few drops of water. We reposition her once again before Rosanna leaves.

I *thought* we had had our last dance this morning. Evening comes softly, ushering in the most extraordinary experience of my life and, I daresay, of hers. No words can capture our final dance because words come from this side of things, whereas this dance was a communion of souls which touched on the infinite, entering the Mystery and becoming one with it.

Olwen directed the entire, silent dance for a couple of hours. No music was playing and I spoke no words. Over and over again, she searched out my right hand with her left hand, holding, touching, dancing, caressing in the most profound way imaginable. She was clear, intentional, strong yet delicate in her grip, completely open, taking enormous risk, fully confident of being fully received, completely trusting, and filling the room with the greatest love imaginable.

Her love was being directed to me, it was about me, her love for me. At the same time, I was her witness, the witness to whom she was showing where she had come to in and for herself—healing the wounds not only in our relationship, but also, I sensed, in all of her life, and an ocean of love poured from and through her, all-loving, all-knowing, all-forgiving, all-encompassing.

Periodically she would gently break off and separate our hands. Perhaps her hand was tired, or perhaps she was signifying our impending separation, or both. Then she would come back and search out my hand again.

If my hand went on top of hers, she quickly asserted herself so *her* hand was *always* on top. This was definitely *her* dance. All fear gone. In its place supreme confidence, knowledge, joy. Anxiety vanished. In its place, utter calmness, serenity.

From the standpoint of her life's paradigm, she was taking a huge risk of putting out that much love, because what if I, in this last fully conscious, fully agentic moment of her life, could not or did not receive it as fully as it was given? What struck me most forcefully was her complete and utter confidence that she *would* be received, that this huge huge huge love was not too much, that it would be received and be held, that it would be met, matched, and given back.

When she went to look for my hand again, it was *always* there. Over and over again, *I* was there. I was *there*. *For* her, *with* her. If her hand had moved further away from mine since our last connection, when she began searching for my hand again, I made sure it wasn't too far away, but I let *her* find it. I also made sure she didn't have to work too hard or search too long.

But such risks no longer mattered because she had shed all that carefulness, measuredness, cautiousness that had marked her search for safety in a world that had delivered such devastating blows. I was experiencing and witnessing the shattering of her low-risk, self-protective paradigm. Even if I hadn't been able to meet her fully, it would no longer have mattered because this was ultimately about her coming back to her whole-self *for herself*.

But I did meet her, and in that moment, she finally knew or remembered who she was, who I was, and who we were. In that moment, I finally knew who she was and why it is I had never given up on her. In that moment, our profound faith in and love for each other was fully realized and shared. In that moment, I knew that each of our lives had been transformed forever.

Somewhere in the middle of our dance, Sue arrived. Speaking no words, she silently took a seat in Olwen's low chair behind me, becoming our witness. About ten days later, we explored some of what we experienced and saw that evening:

Sue: "I think she discovered something that gave her trust, and allowed her to cross over. When she touched your hair, it was like an anointing.

It felt ethereal. It was her spirit touching you, not just her hand. Like a mother touches a much younger child."

Artemis: "I sensed enormous confidence, trust, risk taking, daring finally to let this love, this passion, her real feelings, pour through, confident it would be received, no fear of rejection or abandonment. It felt very personal and interpersonal, expressing love for and to me, and about her relationship to and with me.

"But it was much more than that. It was about her showing me where she had come to about *all* of her life, *all* of the woundings, that she was finally healed, that she was whole, showing me the results of her soul's journey. This was very much a conscious process, she was still here, and in charge."

Sue: "Her life has been so much about loss, but this was not about mourning. It was about rejoicing. It was not a leaving but just getting started."

Artemis: "I was not only to receive it, but also to see it, to know it, to witness it. She was letting me know what had happened for her. Her heart had burst open, like a flower that bursts into fullest bloom or a bird that sings its only song just before it dies.

Sue: "Eclipsing death with life. You witnessed the revitalization of her spirit, the learning of her soul's journey. She was the instructor, transmitting the message. You received it.

Artemis: "She had the will to do it, and I had the ability to receive it."

Sue: "It puts death in its place, it is small. You got as close as you could without dying yourself. She wanted you to—maybe she needed you to—go that far with her. Something happened, you gave her the confidence to let go of you and step forward on her own."

Artemis: "She did it her way. *How* she did it is a mystery. She experienced something magnificent. You and I witnessed her faith being fully realized when she entered into a state of grace while she was still on this side of things and, with her last bit of strength, shared that with me. We cannot do other than rejoice.

"I don't want her service to go backwards into unworthiness and hand-wringing prayers that she *will* get there because we know she already did. It would be like erasing her own hard-won empowerment, her own completion of her soul's work." At her memorial service, my eulogy will lead up to her final dance with me:

"When I attempt words, I can say that Olwen was completely serene and at peace. All fear and uncertainty had vanished. She was utterly confident and intentional in seeking out my hand, directing the movement of our hands, separating and reconnecting, over and over again. She was none of the Olwen personas that we knew, but the quintessence of her whole being, more fully and completely herself than she had ever been, more fully present that she had ever dared to be. She was magnificent and majestic, with oceans of love pouring from her and through her to me. The magnitude, blazing intensity, and profound quality of the love was much more than the far end of earthly love; it belongs to another plane of being. She was glowing and joyous, yet quietly centered around the still point. I knew that all of her wounds were healed, and she was whole and complete. A mother to the end, she was both *giving* this love to me, and *showing* me as her spiritual witness where she had come to: that she got all the way Home while still conscious in this earthly realm and able to communicate nonverbally, and thus able to give herself and me this last incredible gift.

"So Olwen has given us an answer to her question about why she was hanging out on this side of things for almost a century. She had the potential and the desire for completing her soul's work, had been doing her spiritual work and practice all along, and had the stamina and will to stay the course and let the process unfold. Through that process, she achieved a state of grace, becoming one with the Mystery at the same time as she became most fully and completely her unique and magnificent self. She and I came to know the meaning of the words of the poet:

> Only when you drink from the river of silence shall you
>   indeed sing . . .
> And when the earth shall claim your limbs, then shall you
>   truly dance."[1]

I held the silence for a long moment. The soaring space of her gothic church was then filled with the joyous Ar Log piece to which she had lead our dance in that most extraordinary day of our lives.

After Sue leaves that Tuesday evening, I settle back in with Olwen. "Thank you for this extraordinary day. It has been the most extraordinary and important day of my life. I thank you for all the love you have given me through your hands, and all the healing that is taking place.

"This last gift to me is beyond anything I could have imagined. It must have taken all of your strength. Thank you, thank you, thank you. We've come now to this place of total and perfect and eternal love.

"You didn't choose a quick, easy exit, it wouldn't have done anything for you or for me. It would have left things in limbo. You've chosen this really hard way to go, and you did it for us, which is an incredible gift. We got to see each other on the most profound level.

"You see, underneath it all, you knew everything all along. You were always fretting that you didn't know things, but you really did know everything you needed to know, it was all within you all the time. And it brought us out to where we needed to be. And *that* is the mystery.

"A few weeks ago, I said it was about grace, and here's the grace. The Mystery revealed itself, the mystery of how it all comes together, the things that seem so jagged and not together. It all came together through love, an incredible love you showed me through the dance of our hands, which is the dance of our souls that are always together, forever united, can never be separated by mere physical death. So I thank you for this incredible gift, what you have put yourself through, what you have put me through, what I have put me through and put you through. We have been through a lot, but look at where we got to! It is very rare what we did. Very, very rare. And very precious.

"Know that we will always be together, always, always, we never can be separated because our souls are connected forever. We cannot be separated by death. You will live in me always. We are always connected in whatever it is that is way beyond all this. We will always be connected."

I sleep from about 2:00 AM until 5:40. "How is she?" Her caregiver says, "Oh, she is doing fine." But she isn't. Her respirations have increased and she is starting to be short of breath. Yesterday they were 22, 23, 24 per minute, and now they are 26, and within the next hour, they go up to 30. The on-call nurse says go ahead with the Tylenol. We put more stuff on the area around the end of her spine that is more reddish than pinkish now but, thankfully, the skin is not broken. We reposition her.

Dinaz calls by seven. It's time to start the morphine every four hours to ease her breathing and take a load off her heart.

Half an hour later, her breathing is still 30 per minute. I sit with her, counting breaths, waiting, playing the score from "The Hours." It is a very long hour alone before Dinaz and Christine come, confer, and we talk about what is likely to happen. The morphine will probably bring her respirations down but don't be surprised or freak out if they even go up to 40—that does happen. She is having the death rattle at times. It is alarming to hear but is okay. She can't swallow anymore. Her heart is still beating about 120 times a minute, her blood pressure is 100/60.

I make essential phone calls, shower, and dress. Becky arrives with more fruit and yogurt supplies and I make a fruit smoothie. Rosanna is already here for the entire day. I must nap this morning because I am exhausted and my eyes are so puffy from crying. It is a blessing to have Rosanna here not only so I can nap, but also for so many other reasons.

Rosanna is not only gifted with the elderly and dying, but also has fabulous people management skills with the living. She is fielding phone calls and making calls on my behalf. She gives updates with details appropriate to their level of intimacy with me and/or my mother and her sense of what they can handle. She sees what needs doing and takes care of it. Her intuitive gifts are backed up with a broad spectrum of training and experience. She exudes confidence. I feel safe with her here and I am sure that Olwen absorbs that sense of safety as well.

After her second dose of morphine, Olwen's breathing slows to 21. It is quieter, and she is no longer struggling for breath. She is very calm. She knows my hands. I pat her the way she has patted me since I was child. I tell her I will be napping right next to her and that Rosanna is sitting right on the other side of her bed. A friend calls just as I am climbing into bed. She is wonderfully supportive and sings me a lullaby. After I settle in with my iced rag over my eyes, I ask Rosanna to play "She Carries Me," and I fall asleep.

When I wake up, I am thinking about how we struggled through so much for so long to get to last night and yesterday. And now she is letting go. It's all happening in the right order, like the rainbow seemed to foretell—*if only I* could trust the process.

I tell her again things I was saying last night, and pick up a couple of key threads. "I feel sometimes like I spent a lot of my life trying to fix the pain, and I hope, especially in these last weeks, I have been able to help you heal some of those deep wounds from your mother's death and Walter's death and my father's being the way he is, and all the stupid things that I have done that have hurt you and caused you pain. I think we really got there."

"If I have been able to heal some of that wounding, that's always what I wanted to do for you. I always wanted to fix it. Even though I added to the wounding, I also healed some of it. And that's what I wanted to give you. All my life, it's what I wanted to give you. I think in the end, I did. The way your hand sought mine and how we danced together, I think you were telling me that yes, you finally took it in—who you are, the wondrous, magical, magnificent being that you are, that you have had too little affirmation of. I hope you finally feel seen and affirmed. I hope you feel that admiration and love and reverence coming back to you. And that will help you to go in peace and make the journey Home.

"I only wish we could have gotten there sooner. But we both had stuff in the way. The miracle is that we *did* get there. We did get there. I am sorry about how my stuff got in the way. I may be smart in some ways, but I'm dumb in others. But I finally got it. Wouldn't it be nice if we both got a chance to do the whole thing over? We would really get it right this time, wouldn't we? Maybe it's true we come back. It would be nice if we could come back with all the wisdom we gained."

Much of this day I am obsessed with the yearning to push the rewind button so we can do the whole thing over and get it right this time, right from the get-go. My grief for what might have been and wasn't knows no bounds. It is counterbalanced by the great fact that will become my north pole for the rest of my life: we *did* get there. What if we hadn't gotten there at all? Having gone through this enduringly transformative moment, the idea that it might never have happened is completely intolerable. To have missed this is now unthinkable.

"And now that you have gotten to where you needed to go, it is okay for you to let go." On Wednesday afternoon I ask Lizzie, 'When are you going to appear to her? When will she see you? When will she know?"

"Not quite yet."

"But it would be such a comfort to her to experience you at this time."

"Make a ground for whatever unfolds." I haven't a clue about what this means but I write it down.

Midevening, as I am lamenting not seeing Olwen sooner and the pain I have caused her, I sense Lizzie behind my left shoulder. "I know you had great rows, I know you caused her pain, but don't you see how much you gave her?" Sue arrives, and I can't hold onto my sense of Lizzie's presence or what else I might draw out of this liminal space.

In the weeks and months to come, I will brood upon why I couldn't see her sooner, why we couldn't get there sooner, what I could have done differently that might have made a difference.

Sue, as she often does, distills her perception into its essence, "It's hard to see the dimension of somebody who is trying so hard to conceal it."

"Perfectly said. She didn't let people see her. She showed them what she thought they wanted to see."

On another occasion, Sue, with penetrating incisiveness, speaks an even more devastating truth, "she showed so little of herself that you thought she was smaller than she was."

Another friend offers her perspective. "You and your mother were able to experience grace and mystery, but she had to open to it. You can invite, set the stage, but you can't make it happen. When she was able to let go, she was able to feel what she always wanted to, but for which she never had permission. Your gift to her healed her other wounds, the whole lineage.

"She already knew what your mind was capable of. Getting the book published wasn't it for her. It was about you, and *you* did it. The miracle is what happened, and *that* is what needed to happen. She wanted the connection she had with you, that is what she wanted and needed, because she hadn't opened up yet. She got to express her love, and it was completely reciprocal, mutual. The pearl of her heart, the light of her soul coming together with yours."

How would I move through this passage without the wisdom and witnessing of such friends? Much later, my reading will also salve some of my anguish, for such transformative openings, when they do occur, seem to take place only as death draws near.

Mother's respirations have been holding at around 21 since we introduced the morphine yesterday morning. Her breathing is sometimes so quiet I have to check to make sure she is still breathing. Then again, each exhale can be a mild spasm of her whole chest. They said it would be like this. Her heart is racing at 134 beats per minute this morning, Thursday, while her blood pressure has fallen to 82/50. She is, however, as caregivers continue to note, in no pain or respiratory distress.

Christine is off today, and one of her substitutes, Jean is here. Jean and I got off to a shaky start on her first visit, but we both immediately pushed the rewind button and have developed a good working relationship. Jean is very thorough, very systematic, and very careful in her approach, and today, her gentle science becomes a work of art in her repositioning of Olwen. When I come back into the bedroom after she has left, I am moved to tears by the extraordinary care and attentiveness she has given to this dying woman whom she hardly knows and will never see again. In her final act of love, Jean has made highly creative use of pillows, rolled-up towels, and all of the bears to gently hold and support Olwen and take pressure off of any conceivable area of her body that might rub and become painful or produce a bedsore.

Once Jean leaves, Mother and I are alone for the day. I am concerned about repositioning her later on, especially now as she is becoming more limp. Just forty-eight hours ago, she still had a powerful grip and the muscular strength to lead our arms and hands through the air in time to the music.

Yesterday I was grieving her, all that was not and could have been, all that she has lost and I am losing, a grief that has come to focus on her precious hands that I do not want to have to give up. I think of all the things she has done for me with those hands, the last of which are our two extraordinary dances on Tuesday. Those dear little hands, so worn and gnarled, are about to disappear from my life. I am so glad I called Mary yesterday afternoon and asked her to photograph our hands. Mary came over during the magical time between afternoon and evening, the time of day when our final dance and so much else has happened. She took the film to be developed immediately and brought the prints and negatives this morning. They are everything I hoped for.

Today I am saying good-bye by running through Mother's life one more time. I continue to speak of my love, gratitude, and hopes for her.

I tell her again that the dance of our hands was the most important moment of my life, and that it has changed my life forever.

Midafternoon, I call Dinaz because Mother drooled out some stuff, and I can't reposition her alone. Dinaz comes by and stays a while. With all she has to do, Dinaz never appears rushed, and gives each situation the time it needs.

Around five o'clock, Olwen's hands and nailbeds turn a dusky blue. It happens very quickly. Her hands are getting colder. It is terrifying holding her precious hands and watching them turn blue. Her feet are mottled as well.

I tell her I am asking her spirit guardians and Lizzie to help her make this transition and keep her in their care because I won't be able to do that any more beyond the earth. To Lizzie, I say, "it is getting to be time, almost, almost. I've trusted for so long that you'll be here for her. I need a sign. *I* have to know, too. *I* need to know that *she* knows." My impression is that Lizzie says, "very soon now. Your faith will not be in vain."

In a while, Mother's hands become less blue and her nailbeds pink up, although not completely. Sue arrives for the evening and overnight. Will Olwen last the night?

I awaken around six on Friday. Lizzie's response to yesterday's pleas is clear and concise. "Today. You will know." I ask Sue to write this down. Not that I will ever need notes to remember her exact four words.

I need more sleep and I dare not go to sleep with no one sitting next to her bed watching over us. Can Rosanna come earlier than we had planned? She is here by 9:30.

Knowing I have not left the apartment since Monday, she and Christine strongly encourage me to go out for a walk or down the street where an outdoor book and art show is happening. I say, no way. I am not leaving. What I need is a nap.

After Christine leaves, and before my nap, I talk with Olwen. "Okay, honey. It's now the morning of July 11, ten days since your birthday. Another beautiful, sunny day. We gave you a nice bath and got you repositioned so you don't get a bedsore. I know your mouth feels yukky, and we are doing the best we can to help you with that. You'll always be able to breathe okay."

"You are still amazing everybody, because you are such a fighter and you've been so strong and so vigorous. My concern, honey, is that you are still trying to be my mom and take care of me. But I want you to take care of yourself. Do you hear me?

"We had that incredibly beautiful day on Tuesday, where our souls just flowed together in the most healing, loving way through our hands, through our dances together. That was the most important day of my life, and I think of yours. Wednesday, I was grieving the losses so far, the losses to come, and wishing we could have gotten there sooner, but we couldn't. The important thing is that we did, we did.

"Yesterday, Thursday, I thought might be your day of transitioning to another reality we don't understand very well. Maybe you sensed I wasn't quite ready. But, honey, I want you to know that I want you to take care of *you,* I want you to know I will be fine. It will be hard, but I will have all our memories and all we have been doing together for the rest of my life.

"I am concerned about you, how miserable your mouth must feel, and your impending bedsores. We've done what we've needed to do. We got where we needed to go. You got where you needed to be. You entered into the Mystery of Grace.

"I want you to know you are free to go at any time, to go on your journey Home. I do believe—I have *always* believed—that Mama . . . your mother . . . Lizzie . . . will come and she will guide you. I feel the time has now come for the caretaking role to shift from me to your mother and your spirit guardians. They will take care of you in the spirit realm as I have been trying to take care of you in this realm.

"I want you to go in peace. I want you to go knowing how much you are loved. I want you to know how much you have meant to me. I want you to know I never could have done my life work without you. All the ways that you are and that I have become are what have enabled me to persevere in my work all this while that it and I have been invisible to the world. Everyone will come to know this, because I will say it, and I will speak it, and I will write it.

"I don't want you to suffer any more, honey. I don't want you to stay longer for me. I want you to just take care of you. And I hope that soon Mama will come to you, to make you feel safe, so you can let go, and I can hand off your care to your mother."

Periodically, I have to stop and blow my nose. "Look at that jaw line. Whoever saw a jawline like that on a ninety-nine-year old? Look at those little hands . . . so much gentleness. All that gentleness that was always there inside all that strength."

"I love you always, and I have always loved you. And we are forever united. You are never alone. I am always with you, just as your mother is always with you."

In the early afternoon, I am lying next to her, and Rosanna is in the living room. Suddenly I detect an ever-so-subtle shift in her breathing. I climb into her impossible bed so I can cradle her.

Her breaths are gentle and easy but unlike any breaths I have ever heard. Her face is utterly beautiful and peaceful, exquisitely delicate and young. Just beyond my focused line of vision is the artery in her neck, an artery I have checked so many times over the years. It hesitates, slows, beats, but is fluctuating and the strength of its pulsations is growing weaker.

In all her life, I have never seen Mother so serene and trusting. Not an iota of fear. Only complete surrender and beatific delicacy.

Something awesome and indescribable is happening as I feel myself becoming Mama or merging with her or turning Olwen over to her, or all of these things and more all at once. I could say that I, or that Lizzie and myself, are the Mother and Olwen the Child being reborn in another world, but that does not really capture this profound three-way merging.

During our long, eternal moment, we three are completely one. My arms around little Olwen are simultaneously Lizzie's arms—indeed, her entire being—surrounding and permeating her daughter and granddaughter. My containing presence letting Olwen go is completely infused by Lizzie's powerful, all-embracing presence receiving her into the spirit world while merging with and embracing me and letting me know beyond all doubt she is with us.

The pulsing hesitates, weakens, barely beats, and stops. The shining little beam of pure light that was Olwen finally gives out.

Part IV

Dancing with the Ancestors

If you know who you are and you know where you've come from, then you'll know what you must do.

—Ancient Celtic Proverb

Fourteen

Unexpected Gifts

Through mourning we let the dead go and take them in.
—Judith Viorst, *Necessary Losses*

I can be fully with Olwen in the hours after her death because Rosanna is managing the interface with hospice, undertakers, the equipment supply company, and everyone else. Dinaz officially pronounces the death, and repeatedly exclaims, "she is smiling!"

What should Olwen wear for her final outing? I go directly to a cotton dress I have always loved. I had forgotten the little matching scarf she used to tie around her neck and its belt; these I get to keep. We change her into the dress, and I remove the ruby heart necklace from Ginny, the birthstone necklace I had put around her neck on her birthday.

One pragmatic consideration mars the afternoon and cuts short my time with Olwen. I cannot abide the presence of hospital equipment and am compelled to cleanse the room of its existence. The supply people won't come, however, until the undertakers have left. I absolutely must get rid of this stuff, but they will be closing for the weekend. Pushing my time with Olwen to the limit on both accounts, we have some hours together but not enough. With Rosanna's help, I emancipate the bedroom from all foreign equipment.

Weeks later, another option comes to mind: move Olwen to the spare bed, take apart the hospital bed, move the equipment into the hall, call the undertakers when I feel ready, let the supply people come on Monday, and if anyone complains about the stuff in the hall, tough. Then again, given the way things unfold on Friday evening, perhaps I was unknowingly doing exactly what Lizzie had said to do: "Make a ground for whatever unfolds."

When all the intruders are gone, it is a blessing to have Rosanna here, doing laundry and whatever needs doing, and being the all-important presence. I ceremonially rip up the blank Medicaid application and have brief conversations with a couple of friends. And now what? I am rattling around in the living room, wondering how it will be to go back into the bedroom.

After Rosanna leaves, I move the nightstand where Olwen had been, and light the candles in Olwen's crystal candlesticks. I am astounded by how I am welcomed.

The bedroom, so spacious with but a single bed, is massively full of swirling fields of exuberant yet coherent energies, as powerful and intense as on Tuesday but in a different mode. I get out my pendulum and it is whirring around like a helicopter blade and almost flies out of my hands. The personal and transpersonal love and energy emanating from and flowing through Olwen a few days ago is now flooding the entire space.

During our dance of hands, the mode was subtle, gentle, holy, reverent, serene, healing, yet profoundly joyous in a powerfully quiet and concentrated way, a meeting of souls in perfect love, knowing, and forgiveness. It was about Olwen's coming into wholeness, entering into grace, and participating in the Mystery.

Tonight, the bursting energy is vibrant, robust, welcoming, warm, joyous, wild, and deliriously happy. Our dance of healing and grace has flowed into a dance of reunion and ecstasy. Lizzie and Olwen together at last! They are sharing it with me because this moment is for and about the three of us. A lifetime of hope and faith in their being reunited has been realized.

The Knowing of it envelops me in a blanket of peace, serenity, and completion unlike anything I have ever known. I am finally done! We did it! The three of us! I am not feeling alone and devastated as I thought I would, but encircled and infused by their love.

"You will know," Lizzie promised a mere thirteen hours ago, an aeon it now seems. Yes, I do indeed now know. Our merging during Olwen's transition was exquisitely subtle and at the same time, monumentally powerful and awesome. If Lizzie's active presence so permeated *my* being, then surely she must have permeated Olwen's more expansive, transitioning consciousness and dying body. Perhaps feeling Mama's arms embracing and welcoming her explains why Olwen became so delicate, trusting, and young.

Now, in this moment, it is unmistakable that Olwen is free and joyous, *and* that she and her mother are together. How do I *know* it is both of them and not just Olwen's liberated spirit? I simply Know. It is the most self-evident, powerful, and transparent gnostic experience of my life. It is beyond all doubt.

"Make a ground for whatever unfolds." Certainly this room could not have been the magical space it became with that dreadful bed in here. Olwen's spirit did not need two or three days (as mystics often say) to escape from her body. She was more than ready to leave it behind. Having her body here longer wasn't something *she* needed, it would only have been for my own process of letting go.

Yet by my giving up her body sooner than I would have liked, I received a gift beyond anything I could have imagined. Such is the mysterious nature of the sacrifice. But who would have ever thought it would unfold like this? Lizzie has kept her promise in ways I could never have anticipated.

I sleep in the spare bed in Olwen's bedroom tonight and the rest of the time I am here as well as on my two trips to plan and hold the memorial service and close out the apartment. The energy will never again be as powerful as this evening, but it continues to be palpably present. So much so that I will find it unbearably difficult to leave each time to return to my own home.

※

The dance of grace and healing continues the next morning when I call my father. He is alone—unusual on a Saturday morning in summer. We have the most extraordinary conversation we have ever had.

He asks, in tones respectful and deferential, would I think it "unwelcome" or "inappropriate" or "intrusive" if he were to come to her service? I say it would be absolutely magnificent, altogether welcome. Michael would think it was great and would love to see him. Mac would sit with us. His coming would continue the healing process in which so much has happened, and help him bring some closure and resolution to his relationship with Olwen and with me and with himself. That is so important, especially as his own health gets ever more precarious. Yes, yes, by all means, do come.

What about flowers, he asks. He would like to send some, but would it be "appropriate" or "acceptable"? He doesn't know what she would like or what I am planning. I tell him his offer is absolutely lovely, and that Olwen, too, would have been pleased by it and by his desire to come. I tell him my plans for the gorgeous arrangement of red roses I saw at Hugh's calling hours and my hope the florist can do something with lilies similar to what hospice had done on her birthday. I invite him to be part of that in any way he likes, or choose something else if he prefers. We talk of related matters. I will come down after I finish with the funeral director.

At the end of my afternoon visit, my father escorts me to the door and comes outside, leaning on his cane and against the cottage, shifting from one position to another. We have the second extraordinary conversation of the day, one which he manages, despite his physical discomfort, for a good 25-30 minutes.

I sense something has changed since this morning. Mac says he doesn't know if he can come. He is clearly shocked and dazed by the uproar his intentions generated among "the family," which he self-corrects with perfect grammar to, "the part of the family with whom I live and on whom I depend"—his wife and his daughter. And how exactly did they react? They said things like, "No way! What will people think? People will say, 'What's *he* doing here?'"

What he is visibly still reeling from, however, is the intensity of his wife's reactions. He acknowledges he has "never seen her like that." It is a stunning revelation that the "winning" wife and her first-born are apparently still threatened by the first wife and her daughter half a century later. More startling is the fact that he has actually admitted their reactions to me. It adds a new angle through which to refract the many facets of this old and painful story.

I go first to the substance of their concerns. "Virtually everybody who ever cared about all this is dead. You and Olwen outlived them all. Would anyone else care after all this time? Besides, most people wouldn't know who you are. If they did, they would think it was absolutely fabulous you were there, a great tribute to Olwen and a great tribute to you. If someone nudged them and said, 'That's her former husband,' then great for you and great for her!"

In phone conversations that follow this visit, I will bring feedback from Michael, from Ginny's son, from others who knew him, and from my friends who know the story. I will point out that every one of them thinks it would be the absolutely right thing for him to come, right for him and right for Olwen. I will tell him he has a whole cheering section *in absentia* that is applauding and supporting this authentic impulse that has come up from some deep part of him, this impulse that wants to heal the bitterness as he himself gets ever closer to death.

Standing there that afternoon of the Day After, I address the deeper issue, "This bitter divorce has caused so much pain for so many people for so long. It has to stop!"

He emphatically agrees. "Yes, it must stop! It's way past time."

"Your coming would be a big step in bringing that bitterness to an end and letting the healing continue. Your time is getting short, and it is important for you to experience as much healing and resolution as possible." Although he says "yes" when I ask if his coming might still be an open question, I suspect we have already lost this last great opportunity for his healing the central rupture of his life, a rupture that replicates the bitter schism between his parents.

I refocus on the present moment, the only one we have, and perhaps the only one we will ever have. "I love you."

"And I love you." We hold each other a long time. The primary glimpses of truth between us are those moments when I am taking my leave and we hug good-bye. Those embraces carry the pain, the woundings, and the reservoirs of feeling that have no place in his chosen world, and yet I know he carries them silently, as do I.

I inquire about the old days. He recounts ancient office stories with amazing detail. I dare to ask, "What do you think drew you to Olwen?" Yet even at this moment of his maximal opening, he cannot acknowledge himself as the subject of his own desires, the protagonist in his own story. He reverts in the telling to his having been such a young lad, susceptible to this older, powerful woman.

Somewhere in our conversation he refers to Walter dismissively as "that farmboy." Has he really forgotten Walter's name while remembering all those office people? Is there still a shadow of resentment of Walter that can be activated after all this time?

If only he could see what his being "so young" really meant. That he hardly knew who he was or what his needs were. That he projected his domineering mother onto the strong women to whom he was drawn. That Olwen was ultimately not right for him and he was not right for her. That he and Olwen were both disconnected from themselves. That she needed and he wanted what the other couldn't give: someone who could help her reconnect with herself, and someone who was willing and able to make connections on his behalf. If only he could begin to forgive himself for not knowing, begin to forgive her for being who she was and not his fantasy, and finally allow some movement in what has been stuck and frozen in him all these years.

I am not surprised he cannot sustain his openness or suddenly show evidence of insight into himself. It's sad but I let it go by because of all we *have* been able to say and be today. I again affirm and reinforce his impulse to come to her service and send flowers, tell him how healthy it is, how important for him, and that I hope we can find a way for it to happen. Even if it does not, the most important thing is that he had this authentic impulse and shared it with me.

In subsequent calls, his coming to the service is still on the table but I can tell it is not likely. When I need to order the flowers, I again call my father. His response comes from his old standard position and erases the original authentic impulse. It is not that he would like to come but can't—whether because of his health, or because they won't let him. Now *he* has disowned his own best impulse toward resolving a half-century of bitterness. He is back in the cocoon as if he had never stepped out of it.

I will always hold my father's impulse that morning of the Day After as his best self reaching toward a moment of healing and closure. With his waning strength, he rose to the occasion, and stretched as far as he could. It was, in my entire life's experience of him, his finest moment.

That moment was opened by Olwen's death, the relief it afforded him, his own impending death, and my healing journey with Olwen, for such energies flow in mysterious ways among those who have been connected and made part of the journey together. It is the best he can do.

Even as he confronts his own death, he is not able to cross the fragile bridge he dared to imagine.

I come away from our conversations with a new clarity. The self-protective mythology he built so long ago has become his family's cocoon as well as his. It may be even more rigid for them. Whereas he is still inside of his myth and knows that not everything fits, they meet the myth from outside, and the next generation seems unaware of things that do not fit the picture they have constructed. Although Mac's defense structure began as a way to take care of himself, it now entraps him. He cannot break out—except in extraordinary moments—*and* his supportive co-inhabitants have unknowingly become invested in making sure he does not.

My moments with Olwen and with Mac during this week, following a lifetime of struggling with each of them, make it so painfully clear what it is we *all* do: build fences to protect ourselves from what we can't cope with at the time. But the fences become a wall, and eventually can become a heavily guarded fortress. Everything that comes in or goes out must struggle to pass through its walls. Our real job in life—our soul's journey—becomes one of understanding the fortress and why we built it, dismantling all that no longer serves us, journeying back/forward to our wholeness, and living a life that unfolds our evolving whole.

As the power of Mac's cocoon becomes more evident in the wake of Olwen's death and his own death soon after, I see more clearly than I ever have how perfect my parents' ill-fated union has been, not only for my emotional, intellectual, and ultimately spiritual growth, but also for doing the work I am here to do. Had I lived in a cozy cocoon with no contradictory, non-integratable pieces, I would never have stretched in the monumental ways I have. I would not have become a questioner of claims and surfaces, always probing deeper. Without my parents' conflicting constructions of reality, I doubt I would ever have become so fascinated by the monopolistic nature of a reality, nor been compelled to create new lenses through which to tell more encompassing stories than can hold apparent oppositions and contradictions.

My parents' imperfect marriage, divorce, and aftermath was the shattering gift that set me on my long, difficult journey to wholeness and gave birth to a way of seeing that would allow me to complete the journey for all of us.

∽

The crematory is a blessedly old, small, country place, set in an old cemetery. After following the beautiful white hearse at a funereal pace along an old and familiar road for many miles, I am able to have a long and final farewell with Olwen. Just this morning I was able to think of exactly the right things to bring for this nearly final step of our journey together. When I leave the little building, I wander around the cemetery for a while, a cemetery with hip-high headstones. After a while I come to a stop, leaning back on one, watching smoke curl out of the chimney into the cloudless July sky, making my mind a kind of blank at the appalling nature of the smoke.

I am interrupted by hearing Olwen's voice in the full, authoritative tone of her prime. I sense her leaning back on the neighboring headstone to my left. "You don't think I'm still in that old body, do you? Don't waste your time here, dear. Get along with all you have to do."

I am startled by the unexpectedness of her voice, its clarity, its being full strength, and the use of exact phrases she used to say to me. It's her all right! Still trying to run my schedule! I have to chuckle.

"I'm not wasting my time. That body was the vehicle for your being, it served you well, it was a remarkable body."

"I'm already gone, I'm free, you know that. I'm with Mama now. I'm very happy, dear. Thank you for doing all this for me."

In deference to her stated wishes, I will—this time, this day—do as she says.

∽

In the weeks following my mother's death, the stepdaughter of one of Olwen's oldest friends decides for no particular reason to finally tackle her stepmother's boxes that have been sitting in her attic for a decade. She finds a letter which she knows must come back to me.

Olwen had written on initialed stationery to her friend Charlotte in New York the day after I was born. The letter begins, "I am so happy I can hardly contain myself." Olwen's happiness radiates throughout the entire letter. After my immersion in her last hard years and this grueling exit strategy, it is such a gift to hear her be so thrilled and joyous. It is also gratifying that I am the source of this happiness. My mother had always told me she wanted a girl but the intensity of that desire (and her attempt to contain her disappointment if it were not fulfilled) is brought home by the letter:

> "She was born 7:24 AM & it was after 11 before I woke up & Mac was standing right side of my bed. He told me I was fine & so was the baby & I couldn't believe it was over. I had to feel my stomach to make sure. And then when he didn't say right away the baby was a girl, I thought sure it was a boy so I said, "Is it a boy?" and he smiled all over & said it was a girl. I said, "you are not kidding me, are you?"

Her desire for a daughter comes through even more vividly as she describes Mac's reactions outside the delivery room where he waited with one of her friends, Carrie:

> Then the nurse came out and said, "It's a boy" & Mac said, "What a blow for Olwen after going thru all this." Then the nurse said, "But *he's* not *yours*." Carrie said his face was a study. And finally when she came out & said ours was a girl, you can imagine.

The letter also reveals a glimpse of my father and their marriage very different from the one seen through the lens of his After. His concern for and attentiveness to Olwen and her situation is striking. Despite his later distancing and rewriting of history, he was at this moment completely involved in Olwen's well-being and the safe arrival of their child. As recapped by Olwen:

> "Mac was going to call you as soon as he got home last nite. He had such a hectic day—no sleep Wed. nite—here until after 2 on Thurs.—then a bearer at his grandmother's funeral & a department dinner & open forum last nite & here in between—left the dinner as soon as the discussions were over to get back here. He sure looked all in. Even the nurses tell me that he was the perfect worried movie father—his ear glued to the delivery room door. Carrie was with him & I guess it was a good thing. She said he was a wreck . . . Love, Olwen"

I read the letter to my father on my next visit, but nothing registers. I ask him if he has any idea what he meant by "what a blow for Olwen after going thru all this," but he has none.

※

Just as Charlotte's letter found its way to me after Olwen's death, so, after his death, I will receive pictures of a pre-teen me along with cards and postcards I had sent my father during the post-divorce era. His wife will write that he had carried them in his wallet or kept them in his drawer, and perhaps I would like to have them.

This little package will startle me on two accounts: *that* he had carried these ancient artifacts around with him or kept them close, and that *these* were the fragments or crumbs he held onto—or thought were all he could have. They will trigger a memory of one of our brief visits to his dark continent when I had pressed him as to why he had not built more of a relationship with me. Although he at first insisted that he had had no choice because Olwen had called the shots, it finally came out that he had felt he had no right to "come between you and your mother. You're all she had."

The little package cracks an old lens. In the either/or world he inhabited—perhaps inherited from the chasm between his own parents—leaving his wife and building another life for himself apparently meant giving up a real relationship with his daughter. What had long appeared to me as evasion of his responsibility can be seen through his lens as the only honorable course of action. Out of respect for Olwen and recognition of her needs, he abdicated his position with me. To have sought more would have risked breeching the right he felt Olwen had to my allegiances, and he chose not to do anything that might dilute that bond. By stepping back, he was, in his own way, I now see, trying to accept the consequences of his decision to leave the marriage, a decision he took many years to make.

※

Although I had thought I would go directly into my book and its proposal after my mother died, I instead find my energy being pulled to gathering photographs, sorting them by decade and era, and preparing them for a collage that in one visual sweep spans the century from stone cottage to grand hotel. The letter to Charlotte dovetails with what I am seeing in pictures I am cropping and enlarging, important things that did not jump out from small Kodak Brownie prints crowded with background clutter.

Olwen's body language holding her infant daughter and being with her young daughter is that of pure joy, deep pride, and profound satisfaction. I see that I brought back the joy that died with Walter. I see how Olwen contracted during her marriage and began to expand afterwards.

My experience with the photographs mirrors my work on her eulogy. I find myself drawn to constructing the story of her formative years, her resilience, her capacity for picking up the pieces of her life and resurrecting herself each time it was shredded, and creating a rich tapestry in which she thrived for decades. Is it any surprise that I became a sociologist or that my thinking focuses on the fabric of relationships rather than on separate entities? My eulogy leads up to her living legacy in me and in how she chose to make her transition from this world:

"Although I found my soul's path quite early, staying on it for the last thirty years has required my drawing on all the qualities that were Olwen's signature. It has demanded overwhelming commitment to my project, infinite perseverance and resilience, not giving up no matter how hard it gets, hanging in during the times when nothing is working and there is no end in sight. It demands being a self-starter who is self-structuring and does things her way, irrespective of what others are doing. Because of Olwen, I have had the stuff to see it through because like her, I'm a long-haul kind of person. The dedication to my book (which I framed and gave her at Christmas several years ago) begins:

> for Olwen, the Weaver, who gave me the gifts of this life and the most profound and steadfast love, the value of life-long friendships among women, her in-the-bones knowledge of weaving and reweaving the fabric of community, her faith that I would weave a tapestry of my own, and her Welsh resilience and tenacity for staying the course and completing the impossible.

I develop her eulogy and service the way I do everything: gathering elements together, following my intuition, letting the organic order unfold, and progressively clarifying the rhythm and story. During one of her incarcerations, I had found a scrap of paper—her propensity for scraps of paper drove me crazy—which listed three pieces of music, her lot and plot numbers at the cemetery, and the funeral director's phone number. No mistaking her intention here. I write them in my datebook lest *I* misplace this precious scrap of paper. One of her friends points me to the magnificent soloist I engage. When I hear her singing the *Ave Maria, Abide with Me,* and *I Know that My Redeemer Liveth* during rehearsal, I collapse weeping in a pew and wonder if I can hold it together in real time.

I also know I want the Ar Log piece, Welsh hymns, the sound of the Welsh language and bagpipes. I know nothing about polyphonic Welsh hymns but the couple who plays a leading role locally in such matters offers to play some on the piano and sing them for me. During rehearsal, I am bowled over by their power and beauty on the organ, and it becomes easy to make a final selection. I track down a master piper to set the context, lead us in, and lead us out.

Sue and Olwen sometimes read the Lord's prayer together, and I would like Sue to read it in English (as well as to speak for herself) but who will read it in Welsh? Likewise, I ask our friend and neighbor Sharon (who writes a poem about Olwen for part of her remembrances) to read the passage about "a time to live, and a time to die..." that I want us to hear also in Welsh. I am led to such a woman, herself now in her nineties, who can read Welsh scripture.

Ar Log is my biggest challenge. I knew nothing of Welsh folk music until host Gail Gilmour played some pieces on her Celtic music program on a day when she featured triple harpist Robin Huw Bowen during his tour of "A Welsh Christmas." I had taped for Olwen their conversation, his music, Welsh poetry, and pieces by Carreg Lafar and Ar Log—the music that would lead Olwen to dance on her deathbed.

When Gail returns my call, I tell her about the Ar Log dance of hands and we have a lovely connection about our mothers. On her own time, she generously researches the piece until she finds it. With difficulty, I locate Ar Log's tapes and CDs and begin exploring Welsh folk music and the musicians who are serious about keeping it alive. I have finally found *my* music, the music of my bones, the music that belongs to me and to which I belong. The Ar Log dance led by Olwen has opened to the music I most need for my healing and nourishing my roots.

After a hiatus of several months, Lizzie's picture begins turning again toward her three daughters. Two shelves down, a picture of Olwen holding her infant daughter has also begun to turn. Holding the angle of their original position on the intermediate shelf is Elizabeth as a child with her doll carriage.

On Olwen's 100th birthday, Sue, Mary, and I sit down to dinner at Mary's. We have set a fourth place for Olwen. Just as we raise our glasses to Olwen, a tremendous crack of thunder is followed by the lights going out for a couple of hours. We cannot listen to Ar Log but we can speak of Olwen and feel her presence.

Back home a few days later, I madly clean the house for another celebration honoring her birth, the first anniversary of her death, and friends who supported me during the end of Olwen's journey.

> [T]he attempt to reconstruct a world of meaning is the central process in the experience of grieving.
> —Robert A. Neimeyer, PhD

The culmination of allowing this year to unfold organically is a journey to Wales, which will unfold into a second journey the following year. I am compelled by an overwhelming sense that my future and my roots are inseparable.

Where is this powerful urge coming from? Apparently, it is not enough for me to have come to peace with each of my parents in very different ways, to see why they were so "perfect" for my growth and the work I am here to do, and thereby make more complete sense and meaning of my own life. There is something more I must do. I long to recover more of Lizzie's world and perhaps a deeper understanding of Lizzie herself, and to understand more about what the American branch carried from the old country. I am compelled to reconfigure my story within a larger familial context, and to complete my work with my lineage.

My journey and the story I must tell are no longer only about recovering and completing Olwen's story, but also about reconstituting my own. The story and the journey into the unknown now shifts.

Family Tree of People Named in Book

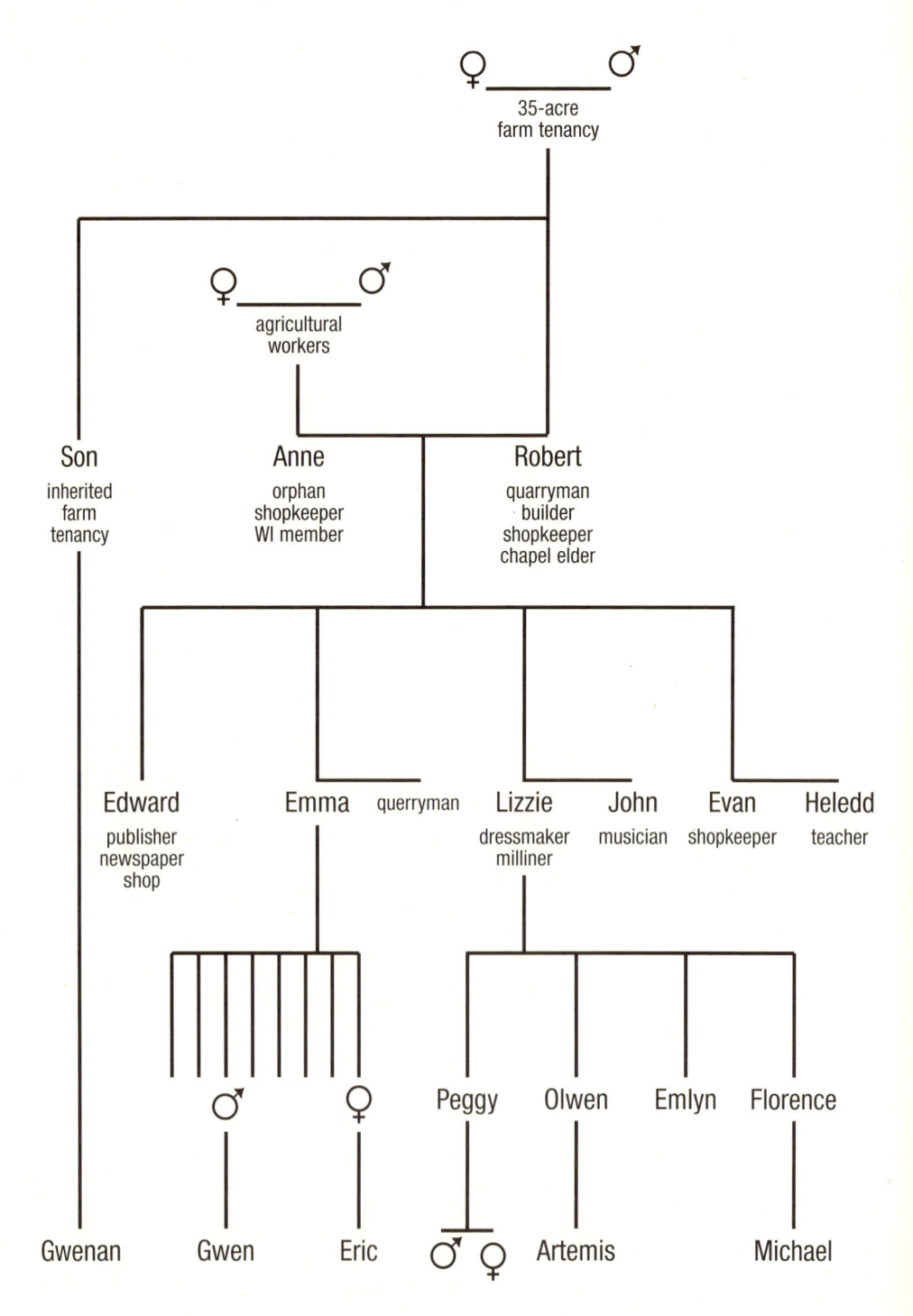

♀_____♂
35-acre farm tenancy

♀_____♂
agricultural workers

Son — inherited farm tenancy

Anne — orphan, shopkeeper, WI member

Robert — quarryman, builder, shopkeeper, chapel elder

Edward — publisher, newspaper shop

Emma — querryman

Lizzie — dressmaker, milliner

John — musician

Evan — shopkeeper

Heledd — teacher

♂ Gwen

♀ Eric

Peggy

Olwen

Emlyn

Florence

Gwenan

♂ ♀ Artemis

Michael

Fifteen

The Houses Speak

To be rooted is perhaps the most important and least recognized need of the human soul.

—Simone Weil, *The Need for Roots*

How do I recover Lizzie's world and my roots? No one is left in Pen-y-Dyffryn. Computer searches and centralized UK repositories have produced no records. Few family stories have been handed down on either side of the Atlantic, and those that have are rarely grounded in dates or specifics; they are more like legends or myths. How does the mythic reality relate to historical reality? Can I reconstruct a larger story that holds them both?

To begin, I have two letters, some pictures, Lizzie's marriage certificate, her mother's obituary, and the address of the "family compound" in Pen-y-Dyffryn. Several cousins have similar scraps. My new tools will include birth and death certificates, census data, wills, maps, and tax books.

My primary artifacts, however, are the houses Lizzie and her family rented, owned, built, lived in, were promised, or inherited. Their history gives structure to the family story, grounding it in time and place. Even this spine, and certainly fleshing it out, will take leg work, conversations with local people, helpful clerks at local records offices and registries, historians of slate willing to answer my questions, and my experience of towns, villages, hills, mountains, rivers, and quarries.

My organic research process of pulling threads and following leads will run into frustrating dead-ends, but also to moments of elation and discovery. By allowing my discoveries to inform and query one another, my open-ended journey into the unknown will take me much further than I ever expected.

Central Story. The central family story handed down from Lizzie's sister Emma alleges that despite disapproving three of his children's mates (or perhaps because of it?), their father endowed each of them with a house. They could live in it, rent it, or sell it as they chose. Robert was a contractor who built these houses, each of which had three stories, on Llyn *(thlinn)* Road, a few blocks from the family compound. Compelling tale, but is it true?

Lizzie told a similar story because Olwen wrote on an old envelope: "Gwen [Emma's granddaughter] corroborates my memory of all my mother told me about Mama's father Robert Morgan. He was a contractor and built homes, including one for each of his children." A 1916 letter to Lizzie from her younger brother Evan supports the story: "As you know, mother owns two houses on Llyn Road and three on Carreg Mawr. I have heard Mother mention several times that the lower house in the middle will be yours."

Clearly, Robert left behind at least five houses. Yet it is obvious from Evan's letter that as of 1916, Lizzie had not yet inherited "her" house and neither had her siblings, now in their forties, inherited theirs, even though their father had been gone for years. I will discover Robert left no will. The houses and "effects" valued at over £400 (twice the "rateable value" of the houses at the time) were transferred administratively to his wife, Anne.

Why did a man apparently so committed to endowing his children not leave a will? I suspect he believed his intent was so well understood that nothing more needed to be said. Yet, what exactly *was* his intent in building each of them a house? To give them an inheritance when they needed it? When he died? When Anne died? The story is silent on this critical point.

It is equally silent about the particulars of another part of the story that I first heard from Emma's grandson Eric: "Lizzie turned down her share." What? I never heard that one before. Was there in fact an offer she turned down? If so, exactly what was she offered, by whom, and when? And, if she did turn down an offer, what could have been so powerful to motivate her gesture?

These questions about Robert and Lizzie will inform my search, especially during my first trip. They give me something to work against as I try to sort out and connect the disparate pieces I unearth.

> *We write about what we don't know about what we know.*
> —Grace Paley

Family Compound. On my first day at the records office, I find my family was established in Pen-y-Dyffryn by 1881 at 13 Carreg Mawr. In that moment, they materialize from the mists of the "old country" and touch the ground. Not only did they live here, but they already owned this corner house heading a row ("terrace") of two-and-a-half-story, stone houses.

Most quarrymen—as I soon discover Robert to have been—rented their cottages.[1] Slate mines, according to slate historian Griff Richard Jones, "depended on the expertise of rockmen," the skilled artisans such as Robert who decided how to set the explosives and remove the easily shattered slate. "Rockmen could make or break the quarry, but they were not rewarded for it."[2]

How then could a rockman with four children have scraped together enough money to buy his first house? Most likely, by borrowing money from a building society, many of which were organized around chapels. Quarrymen sometimes built their own houses, or co-developed a row of cottages with other quarrymen. By the 1870s, however, there was an influx of professional house-builders in slate towns.[3]

Could Robert have been involved in constructing the house on the corner? Not likely. He was living elsewhere when Carreg Mawr's infrastructure and terraced cottages were being developed. The homogeneity of the terraces speaks to well-capitalized, professional development. Pen-y-Dyffryn was acquiring sanitation and gas lighting during the 1870s, and the estate on whose land Carreg Mawr houses were built had adopted a policy of "controlled leasing," according to slate archaeologist-historian David Gwyn. "They stipulated the quality of houses that were to be built, and, by the early 1870s, they seem to have been insisting on proper privies attached to sewers."[4]

Yet there is family lore that Robert brought produce over to sell in this boom town prior to moving there by 1881. Could he have had his eye on the choice corner lot near the High Street and town center—

much like Olwen had her eye on another lot seventy-five years later? Did he check on its construction, even if not on a daily basis as Olwen could? I would not be surprised.

Twenty years later, Emma was settled next door at 15 Carreg Mawr with her quarryman husband and their growing family, while Lizzie's two brothers, neither of them yet married, still lived at number 13. Gwen says our great-grandparents did not want Emma to marry a quarryman, but the reasons are unclear. Perhaps it was the desire for mobility out of the quarry and into the shop, perhaps it was concern about risks to health and longevity, or both. Emma continued to live next door to her parents, and then to her widowed mother, until after the Great War when she and her family moved to Liverpool where there was more work.

With a shop in 13's front parlor, two grown sons at home, Emma married and beginning a family, and Lizzie and John returning from London, practical needs would explain why Robert acquired number 15 and, based on structural evidence and local hearsay, promptly enlarged the two houses as a joint project.

Lizzie's House. Evan's reference to Lizzie's "lower house in the middle" would be an odd designation for a terrace house, and I cannot find any record our family was associated with 17. Nesta, a long-time neighbor, demystifies the "lower house in the middle" as a free-standing house built *behind* 13 and 15 at the end of their lengthy "long gardens" which slope gently downhill, forming a second corner to the joint property.

It is evident from Evan's letter that Lizzie was familiar with this third house in the family compound and knew the intention behind it. Was it Robert's way of giving Lizzie an economic base, a choice he might have felt necessitated by John's difficulties in making a living? Was John already talking about America, and was this an inducement to stay? Questionable, as there is no family story or documentary evidence they ever lived in the lower house in the middle. Rather, given the birth of their first child at 13, it appears the young couple lived temporarily with Lizzie's parents after they returned from London, and then moved directly to a rental cottage five minutes away—the cottage where Olwen was born, and from which they would emigrate to America.

Was Lizzie's and John's living situation a contentious issue? Would Lizzie have preferred to remain closer to her family? Or, did she want more distance? I suspect John was comfortable with being a little further away from her family, a feeling that might have been mutual. Or, was "Lizzie's house" never actually offered as a living situation, but as a legacy for her future? Just when and under what conditions Lizzie was to inherit her house are not clear.

What I will eventually affirm is that Lizzie's house was the first legacy house to be built, the only free-standing house, and the only one that was part of the family compound.

Robert and Anne. In the margin of Anne's obituary, a year is noted in Olwen's writing, followed by a question mark. I picture Olwen coming across the obituary in a drawer years after the fact, and marking it with her best but uncertain recall. Using this date, the name of the cemetery, and the known gap between Robert's and Anne's deaths, I sift through microfiche of grave data for hours and find nothing about either of them.

My difficulties are serendipitously resolved when a local official tells me his sister has made a record of every gravestone inscription in that cemetery. Within an hour, his sister gives me their dates and inscriptions. Now I can get their death certificates.

It is then I discovered that Lizzie left for America *after* her father died, and that he had been a slate rockman who, I will later reconstruct, was associated with quarries not just in Pen-y-Dyffryn, but also for much of his life. This is a surprise because his quarry work has been given only passing reference in family accounts—such as Olwen's undated note about his work as a builder, which she follows with: "He worked in a quarry early on."

Was this emphasis part of the desire for mobility out of the quarries? Or, did it reflect Robert's central project and identity as a builder during the third act of his life—or possibly even earlier? Or, was this emphasis an inadvertent effect of how parts of stories get lost and other parts embellished (by the speaker or the listener) as they are handed down?

Whereas Robert's age is consistent from one record to the next, Anne's fluctuates. Even though census data variably identify the shire or towns where they were born, I cannot find records of their births in any of the potentially correct records offices or registries.[5] I do find her baptism, however. A family tree sent by her great-nieces to my mother makes it easy to know when I have found the right family with an Anne of the right age in the 1851 census, which states that both of her parents were agricultural laborers. After 1851, I find no trace of them. This is consistent with a brief letter Evan's wife wrote Olwen just before the war in response to her queries about her grandparents:

> We don't know where nain was born. She lost her father when she was nine years old, and she lost her mother soon after, so she had to go to service when she was twelve years old. I heard her say many a time that she had to work hard when very young. Taid was home from work for ten years without going to the quarry where he worked, and then nain was a widow for twenty years.

Curious that even Evan doesn't know where his mother was born. As hard as she worked in other people's houses and as lonely and precarious as it was to be an orphaned girlchild, Anne apparently gained exposure to the quality of life and the quality of furnishings she and Robert would pull themselves toward and gradually acquire through decades of hard work. Even in her seventies as a house-poor widow with bills to juggle, my great-grandmother was, according to a local informant, well dressed, active in civic and chapel life, and good friends with the mother of a quarry owner. Her obituary describes her as intelligent, well-read, knowledgeable, and kind. She had come a long way from her orphan days and the humble cottages in which, I will ascertain, her children were born.

Curious phrasing about Robert: not that he had retired, or quit, or been injured, or become sick, but was dwelling in a seemingly openended situation to which he might return. I have no account of why he was home from the quarry for the last ten years of his life. He did not die of any of the lung or miners' diseases that were so common, but of "apoplexy" or what we now call a stroke. He lived well into his sixties, way beyond the average rockman.

The one picture I have of Robert is in a family portrait with his wife and four adult children when he was about sixty. His deep-set eyes, expansive forehead, and broad-boned face are handsome and remarkably young in appearance. His hands, on the other hand, appear damaged. It would not surprise me, given the nature of his work and the kinds of hand tools (like "jumpers" and crowbars) used for pounding and digging into rock. Or, it may just be the way he was holding them or the way the shadows fell on them. But if they were damaged, how could he build houses? Perhaps because he was acting, as the family story suggests, more as contractor and overseer.

It is no accident, I think, that Evan's wife makes no mention of Robert's building houses for his children while running a shop with his wife. She says nothing that would acknowledge his intended legacy. From her phrasing, you might think he had idled under foot around the house.

About the shop itself I know only that Robert identified his work as "grocer" in the 1901 census, and that they sold provisions such as flour. Robert's gravestone reads, "Siop Carreg Mawr," a device which would differentiate him from others bearing the same name. Since numerous houses on Carreg Mawr also had shops in their parlors, was there also something distinctive about the Morgans' shop that caused it to be known by its street name only? Or would it have been colloquially known, as most shops were, by the wife's name—in this case as "Mrs. Morgan's shop"?

Anne's Standing. On my second visit to Pen-y-Dyffryn, Nesta takes me to visit Mrs. Parry who, at age 102, is sprightly, mentally sharp, and moves with the spryness and ease Olwen had until those last few weeks. I have brought a picture of Anne when she was about eighty. Her life is etched in her lined face, now a tad mellowed with just a hint of sweetness—much the way Olwen mellowed in her early nineties and with a remarkably similar expression. Will Mrs. Parry remember my great-grandmother?

Oh, yes! She smiles, and speaks energetically in Welsh with Nesta and in English with me. Mrs. Morgan, as she refers to her, was a member of the Women's Institute (WI), and attended Carreg Ddu *(thee)* Chapel. Mrs. Morgan was well-dressed in dark clothes, smart jewelry, and had her hats—black hats—made in the millinery shop where Mrs. Parry worked when she was young, a shop she and her husband would later acquire. Nesta recognizes its name as having been a fine shop.

In those days, Mrs. Parry continues, "we never went out without a hat," and a customer came into the shop and described what she was looking for. "We fixed a shape to suit her and try on." Measurements were made, fabrics picked out or ordered. When one of Mrs. Morgan's hats was ready, it was delivered to her at home. "The fact that her hats were delivered is an indication that Anne was a person of some standing and a valued customer," Nesta explains.

Mrs. Morgan was friendly with the widowed mother of a quarry owner who lived with her family in "the big house." She and her friend attended WI meetings together and often came into the hat shop together. Edward's wife (whom Mrs. Parry calls "the young Mrs. Morgan") also came shopping with her mother-in-law. It is clear from Mrs. Parry's tone that she liked and approved of all three of these women and is enjoying the fact that a young person like myself is interested in her memories and finds them valuable.

Mrs. Parry warmly remembers how she was invited by the young Mrs. Morgan for tea at her house during the break between afternoon and evening sessions of the all-chapel Gymanfa Ganu. It would have been difficult, if not impossible, for Mrs. Parry to get all the way home and back again. The young Mrs. Morgan extended this courtesy to her—apparently over a period of years—because, in Mrs. Parry's view, "I gave personal service from the shop." All in all, she said, "the family was [what Nesta translates as] 'true blue.'" Nesta elaborates, "'True blue' might be said of an upstanding person, someone you looked up to."

True blue—except for Evan's wife. It is stunning how eighty years later, Mrs. Parry remembers these details about Anne and her older son's wife with such fondness and admiration, and how her voice and expression change when she remembers that the "other" Mrs. Morgan—Evan's wife—occasionally accompanied her mother-in-law. I am impressed not only with Mrs. Parry's memory for salient details, but also her keen judgment of character and its having stayed with her all these years.

The "Other" Mrs. Morgan. Evan's wife, Heledd *(helleth)*, was the third of the spouses of whom Robert and Anne disapproved. Their uneasiness about Heledd might have been more difficult to put their fingers on than with Emma's quarryman and Lizzie's musician. If they had, they might have said she did not have a generous or open nature and, try as they might, they just didn't trust her.

When Olwen journeyed to Wales in 1965, she and one of Emma's daughters visited Aunty Heledd, now a childless widow living at 15 Carreg Mawr where she and Evan had moved during the 1940s. Olwen, who rarely had a bad word to say about anyone and tended not to be suspicious of people's motives, described a significant moment when the widow claimed as hers things that Olwen and her cousin, exchanging glances, were certain belonged to their grandmother.

Nesta describes incidents and patterns that show her neighbor Heledd to have been oddly reclusive, excessively religious, and mean. She knows a few particulars about what I have always heard: the avaricious Heledd dispersed our family's material legacy to her own family in South Wales. I am finally able to document that story after I track down Heledd's will.

Astonishing in its detailed instructions for distributing tons of furniture crowded into number 15, her will also leaves a tidy sum of £7700, most of it derived from Robert's, Anne's, and Evan's estates. I think of how Anne survived being an orphan and those hard years of domestic service, followed by birthing and raising her children in rugged conditions, and how she and Robert scrimped and saved to get a real foothold in life, to own houses with real furniture and real china, to earn respectable and honored places in their community, and secure a modest level of comfort and solvency, and then poof! it's all erased into the netherlands of people for whom their struggles and stories mean nothing.

Anne's Will. Eighteen months after Lizzie died, Anne made a new will. It is short and simple. She leaves the house named Ty Gelyn (tee gellinn) to Emma, and all three houses in the family compound and their furnishings to Evan. Edward is a witness, so either he had already cashed in his share, or, his business was sufficiently successful that he turned it down. There is no mention in the will of Lizzie's children in America.

Thus, although long promised to the adult children, most or all of the parental endowment was not realized until my great-grandmother's death when *she* still owned the remaining four houses, her children were in their fifties, and Lizzie had already died. Although Robert seems to have had a generous and open mind about how his legacy would be used to benefit his children, he was committed to equal shares. I doubt he would have approved Anne's skewed distribution, which set up Heledd's thievery.

When I track down Anne's will, I have a moment of anger. "Why did you forget us!? This is *not* what Robert would have wanted!" It passes. I can imagine how Evan and Heledd insinuated themselves in her life, how much she may have come to depend on them in her late years after

Emma moved to Liverpool. The slyness, secrecy, and manipulativeness I pick up from Evan's 1916 letter was amplified by a more than willing and stronger partner who had no conscience about appropriating his parents' entire estate.

Llyn Road Houses. Although I was able to sort out the family compound on Carreg Mawr during my first trip, I could not reconcile the account of Robert's building three, three-story houses on Llyn Road with what I saw when walking up and down the street: only one three-story house, and, it was not named Ty Gelyn. I suspected that Emma, known to be pretentious, had inflated her family history after she moved to the big city.

When I return to Pen-y-Dyffryn, however, Nesta points out a cluster of three attached houses further down Llyn Road—around the corner and out of sight. This set of houses *does* have three stories, but you wouldn't know it from the street; the third story drops down into the valley terrain in back. The end house is named Ty Gelyn, the house Anne left Emma in her will.

The family's association with Ty Gelyn comes into Mrs. Parry's account as well. The house where she was invited for tea during the break between Gymanfa Ganu sessions was Ty Gelyn. Thus Edward and the "young Mrs. Morgan" must have lived at Ty Gelyn during some part of the 1920s.

The houses are undergoing renovation and a local official informs me of a discovery. Each of the two purlins is a single great timber that runs across all three houses. The houses were all, therefore, "fixed together," as she puts it, and built at one time. (Purlins, or side timbers, are a structural component for supporting the roof. They are continuous, horizontal timbers running parallel to the ridge or apex of the roof.)

These bits of evidence all support the story that Robert *did* build these three houses on Llyn Road, bringing to six the number of family houses. Did he leave all six? Without a probated will, there is no enumeration of the houses at his death.

Did Lizzie Turn Down her Share? Given that Anne owned "only" five houses in 1916, she may have had to sell one of the Llyn Road houses to pay her own bills sometime before that. Given that only Ty Gelyn was left by the time she died, another Llyn Road house was sold during the following decade. That Anne was house-poor, short of working capital, owed money, and was owed money is suggested not only by the sale of two of the houses, but also by Evan's 1916 letter to Lizzie, which opens with the news that Aunty Jane (Anne's sister) has just died.

> Aunty Jane was worth about £150 including the furniture. They had to deduct bills and costs, and then divide the rest into five shares. Mother's share was used to pay taxes, and the balance was used to buy flour. Mother was deceived by several people in the past two or three years . . . Honestly, mother has nothing to buy goods for the shop, all she has are the houses she owns, and the rents are not enough to pay ground rents, taxes, and repair. I am enclosing the bank receipts. She had borrowed about £20 to pay for various items; she managed to pay part of the loan, she now has a balance of £8. I made the payments as they became due. Remember to return the bank receipts and make sure you send them to me at the shop; nobody will know then that I am telling you a few secrets.

Knowing of Anne's hard childhood and orphan history, and seeing her formidable presence in the family portrait when she was in her fifties, I have a strong sense that Anne in her prime was shrewd and clever about survival and financial issues, and developed a flinty cast to her persona. The mellowing visible in her later photograph, together with Mrs. Parry's account and Anne's obituary, suggest her imposing exterior was tempered, especially in her later years, by a kindness of which others may have taken advantage. Without Robert, it must have become harder to supply her shop, while local and larger market forces were no doubt eroding the viability of parlor shops. I suspect Anne sold the sixth house and later the fifth to pay off debts, keep her head and shop above water, maintain her standing, and indulge her small luxuries such as new black hats.

Evan is also apparently not making ends meet—and on a grander scale—because, "I had to find somebody to lend me £100 to pay my debt to Aunty Jane to settle her estate which was quite an undertaking." His sense of secrecy continues, "Remember Lizzie, all I have said is a secret between you and me. If Mother found out she would be very offended with us, but it's only fair that you get all the news. Remember this is all a secret."

Why would Anne be offended about what Evan conveyed to Lizzie? Pride? False pride? Did she not want to worry Lizzie? And what is his motivation in telling Lizzie "all the news"?

Evan proposes to Lizzie that they sell her house for her benefit, while conveying that their mother might herself need the proceeds from the houses. Knowing how concerned Lizzie would be about Anne while being unable to do much from so far away, was Evan actually trying to get Lizzie to do the one thing she could do: say no, at least for now, to cashing in her share? Was *this* the offer that has been interpreted as Lizzie's "turning down her share"?

> Although you are in the United States, if something should happen to mother before me, you can rest assured that everything will be taken care of, just as if you were here. As you know, mother owns two houses on Llyn Road and three in Carreg Mawr. I have heard Mother mention several times that the lower house in the middle will be yours. I have said in front of Edward several times that I'm sure you would prefer to get the money because what would the house be worth to you when you are so far away. The rest would have to be used to pay ground and rent taxes. The way to get the money would be for me to sell the three Carreg Mawr houses in order that you can get the money, the balance to pay any bills, costs, and debts. Mother and Edward could see my point in selling the houses. Remember now, Lizzie, don't mention any of this in your letters. When you write, send the letter to me at [he refers to his own shop], then nobody will see it. I will try and persuade mother to carry out your wishes. My belief is that around £350 would be a thousand times better than the house. I regret that I myself bought a house.

Interestingly, Evan assumes that the proceeds from selling "Lizzie's house" would go to Lizzie, and not to Anne, as I conjecture the proceeds from the first two houses did.

I have to wonder if these ideas percolating in little brother's mind were just his flights of fancy. Did they ever turn into a family discussion of selling one or more of the houses, including Lizzie's, while her mother was still living? Was it in response to such a conversation—if it ever happened—that Lizzie may have "turned down her share"? Or been (mis)interpreted as doing so? Was her turning it down (*if* she did) only for the duration of her mother's life?

Yet if Evan had really been having all these conversations with his mother and older brother, why was Lizzie admonished not to reference their conversations and become a part of them? Why was there no mention of Emma in the house conversation? Was she left out?

It is through Emma's descendants that we hear Lizzie turned down her share. On what was Emma's story based? Emma, her grandchildren say, wasn't much of a letter writer. Lizzie, on the other hand, as Olwen told me long ago, corresponded weekly with her mother and regularly with Evan. Emma, therefore, must have received most of her information about Lizzie second-hand through her mother or brother. Did Evan lead Emma to believe that Lizzie had permanently turned down her share?

What if Lizzie had felt freer to tell her mother about her own financial uncertainties and John's shortcomings? Would the outcome have been, "I told you so"? I do have a sense—from my experience of Olwen, from working with this material, and from conversations with Emma's grandson—that Lizzie continued to feel she had to prove her choice of a mate, and/or that false pride, whether on her part or Anne's or both, was operating. If Lizzie had broken through that, might her mother have made Lizzie's children beneficiaries of Lizzie's house and their share of her things? If so, might they have then felt less orphaned, less abandoned, and more like they were part of a family, more like they had a place in the world, even if it was far away?

Or would Lizzie's little brother and his wife have manipulated the situation to his advantage in any event? Having insinuated himself in his mother's life more fully after Emma moved away, he became executor of his mother's estate. We know that he was already skilled at getting poor widows to take care of him because he owed his aunt two-thirds of the value of her small estate.

To Olwen's losses in the wake of Lizzie's death we can add her grandmother who was her strongest link to Wales, the matriarch of Olwen's disappearing family. To Olwen's shadowy might-have-been's we can add whatever Lizzie had told her about her share and the expectation or trust that it would be honored.

Lizzie certainly did discuss this with Olwen because Olwen spoke to me about it long ago before I could appreciate its significance or ask the right questions, and she took it up with our cousin Gwen. The fact that Lizzie or Lizzie's children did not get her share was an ongoing issue for Olwen. I can still hear her saying, "I just can't understand why Mama [or did she say 'we'?] did not get her share." Olwen clearly believed an injustice had been done, one that was hurtful. For her to have felt that way:

- Lizzie *had* to have conveyed to Olwen the understanding that when Anne died, Lizzie would still receive her share even though she was in America.

- Lizzie, therefore, cannot have believed anyone in her family thought she had turned down her share—at least not permanently.

But Lizzie died first and Anne made a new will, one that made no provision for Lizzie's children. Olwen understood the intention behind her grandfather's building the houses for his children well enough to know he would have wanted Lizzie's children to receive her share.

My best guess is that Lizzie opted to postpone her own interests temporarily in favor of her mother's needs which were so skillfully presented by Evan. Although appearing solicitous of Lizzie and as if they were conspiring together to take care of Anne, Evan may have been setting Lizzie up to do just that. As the years went by, he may have conveniently forgotten that Lizzie never gave up her share permanently, or been helped to revise his memory by the avaricious Heledd. In Heledd's 1938 portrayal of Robert being home from the quarry, she shrewdly omits his "retirement project" of building the houses for each of his children.

Who *would* benefit from the story that Lizzie turned down her share? Not Emma, who still got one and only one house. Not Edward who had either already cashed in or turned down his share. Only Evan, who got Lizzie's house plus two others, and the furniture and household items.

Olwen, Gwen tells me, thought her uncles were involved in cheating Lizzie's children of their share, and that rings a bell in my own memory of the concerns she shared with me long ago. Olwen was probably right on target as usual. Anne's will bears both the marks of both brothers, one as witness, one as executor. Did they work together to prevail upon Anne to forget Lizzie's children? Did one or both persuade her that Lizzie really had turned down her share? Was Evan lying to himself as well as to their mother when he persuaded her to leave the entire family compound, including Lizzie's house, to himself?

The betrayal and abandonment of Lizzie's children and the subversion of Robert's intentions by her brothers amplified her children's betrayal and abandonment by her husband.

It is clear that Robert did indeed own, build, and/or expand six houses with the goal of providing legacies for his children. The house project suggests Robert had a strong sense of equity and of his responsibilities as a father, and the character to hold to those principles despite his disapproving three of their marital choices, and despite concerns or disappointments he may have had with some of his offspring.

The question will always remain, however: Why did he not set down his precise intentions in a will? Since Robert's house project and life trajectory indicate someone who thinks and plans for the long term, it seems not in character. As I sorted through this material, the most likely explanation still seems to be that he assumed his intentions were so clearly understood that it simply wasn't necessary. He may have trusted that his heirs would be as honorable as he was.

Robert appears to have personified the upright, nonconformist, Calvinistic Methodist quarryman with a firm sense of equity and justice. Doing the right thing and doing things right were apparently not just part of Olwen's response to Lizzie's death, but a legacy informing a deeper strain of her character.

Yet beneath that Calvinistic structure organizing both of their characters was something larger, more open, more forgiving, more generous. The man who emerges from the houses seems marked by generosity of spirit as well as strong practicality. Ultimately, it was Robert's integrity, his way of being in the world, not the houses, that form the enduring legacy from the man who built them. His gift of place was an inner rudder for navigating life.

I see now where Olwen and I formed our backbones and resilience: from the ancient, rugged Welsh landscape by way of our ancestors who worked its less than bountiful land and unforgiving rock, and did things for the long haul.

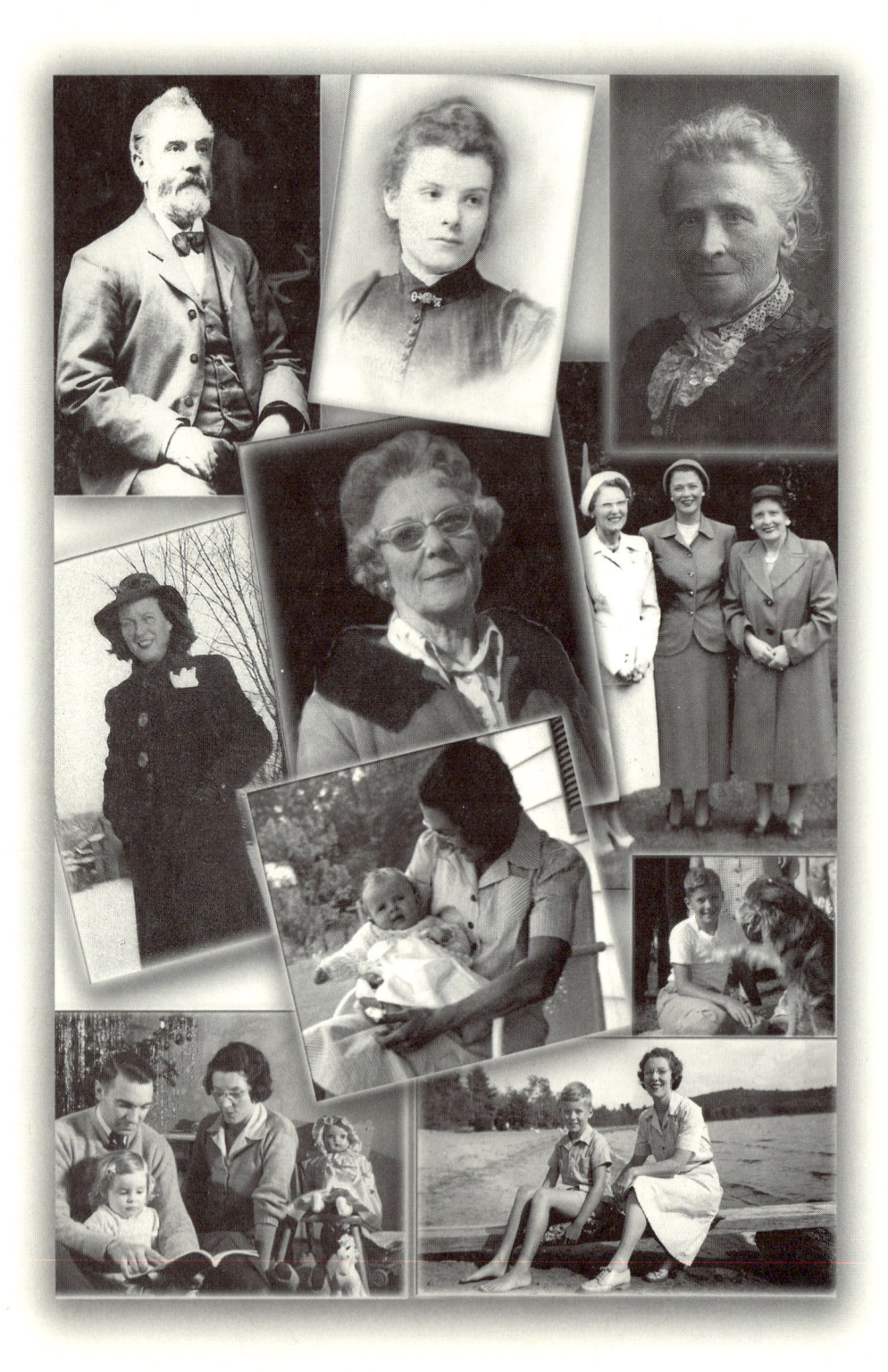

Sixteen

Roots and Completion

> *The longing to tell one's story and the process of telling is symbolically a gesture of longing to recover the past in such a way that one experiences both a sense of reunion and a sense of release.*
>
> —bell hooks

Following the threads of the house stories grounded Lizzie's family in time and place, revealed something of Robert's character, Anne's struggles as a widow, Evan's manipulations, the historical truth of the central family myth, and the falsehood of the claim that Lizzie turned down her share. Pursuing two discoveries—the words "rockman" and "wharf houses" on death and birth certificates—will lead me deeper into their story, and retracing Lizzie's footsteps leads to a new lens through which to see her life.

Through my journey with the ancestors, I will find my roots and gain a sense of lineage forged out of the wild and demanding Welsh earthscape. Robert, Anne, Lizzie, Olwen, and even John have shaped my consciousness, my character, my holding to my dream, and given me the stuff to do what I am here to do. My journey and this book find their own natural completion.

Rockman. Once I learned that my great-grandfather had been a slate rockman, I became fascinated with slate, his work, and what it revealed about Robert.

The veins of slate running through northwest Wales were compressed at various angles between layers of granite 400-500 million years ago. Slate can be extracted and split, but it takes great knowledge of the rock to do either. Indeed, the art form of splitting became an arena of competition at the National Eisteddfod.

Quarrymen were skilled artisans who self-organized into teams typically consisting of two rockmen, a splitter and a dresser. Each team made its own monthly "bargain" with management, often working in a particular "chamber" for a year or more. Settling up monthly, they could actually lose money in this entrepreneurial arrangement if they had encountered bad rock or other problems. The quarrymen had to buy their own explosives, tools, candles, ropes, and chains, and pay for repairs and tool sharpening out of their twenty-five shillings (or less) per week.[1]

Quarrymen did not earn much more than those who cleaned up, transported rock, and engaged in sundry support tasks but they were held in great respect. To be able to look at the rock (in dark, underground chambers by candlelight) and know how it would respond to one's action was an ability that took years to acquire, and some men never could. Most quarrymen started in the mines or quarries as lads, growing up with the rock and learning in their bones the demanding and unforgiving nature of slate. The mystique of slate built camaraderie among quarrymen and contempt for managers who knew so little about the living rock.[2]

The rockman decided how to place black powder so its blast loosened rather than shattered the next slab of rock he wanted to extract. He also had to know how the slab would fall to the chamber floor below when, using a crowbar, he levered free a huge, now-loosened slab. To drill holes, set the powder, and lever the rocks, rockmen hung over the precipice—sometimes forty or fifty feet up from the floor of the chamber—and worked at an angle almost perpendicular to the rockface with their feet propped against it and a rope or chain wound loosely around one thigh. Huge slabs were reduced on the spot to a manageable size for transport to the surface where teammates milled, split, and dressed the slates.[3]

What kind of a man can become skilled at such work? Someone who inhabits his own body, trusts his own judgment, and has an affinity with living, natural processes and geostructures, especially the ancient formative processes now held in strong, yet easily shattered slate. Through his ongoing dialogue with the rock, his confidence in his judgement would deepen.

Quarrymen were also legendary for prizing their independence and having some control over their work and working conditions. One form this took was being extremely protective of the entrepreneurial nature of the bargain, even when most of the bargaining power was on the other side.[4] In conversation with me, slate historian-archaeologist David Gwyn gave even greater scope to their independence than did Merfyn *(mair-vinn)* Jones' now-classic study of North Wales quarrymen:

> A surprising amount of quarrying was done part-time or by subcontracting to others. Some men took up bargains in separate quarries and turned up to work whichever one they felt like. Clashes between managers and quarrymen may at times be better understood as clashes between two sets of people, each of whom saw themselves as managers. It sounds very much as if your ancestor was one of those chaps who envisioned his own future and did not see himself in any way, shape, or form as an employee, but as an independent businessman.[5]

Wharf Houses in Glyndwr. Although Olwen had told me the name of the village where Lizzie was born—Glyndwr *(glinn-dooer)*—it was not until I returned home that all my phone calls and visits to records offices paid off. Her birth certificate reads, "Wharf Houses."

The image of proximity to commercial activity on the water is quickly dispelled during my second trip. With the help of farmers whose families have owned their farms for over two hundred years, I locate the foundations of the wharf houses and learn some of their backstory.

The houses were connected with a slate quarry. The "wharf" was a loading area where slates were stacked onto railway cars and sent to ports for shipping all over the world. The "wharf houses" picked up the designation from their proximity to this wharf.

Near the bottom of the mountain quarry in Glyndwr, the ground had been leveled in the 1820s to build the Old Coach Road from London to Holyhead (from which the ferry leaves for Dublin). The wharf cottages took advantage of this. Their foundations abutted the road embankment. A few yards beyond where the front door must have been, the mountain continues to drop down to the railroad below, a flood plain, and the river. A railway link to one of the west coast port towns was completed in 1868, just as the quarry was opening.

I am struck by the juxtapositions between the spectacular, peaceful, lushly green setting of the Glyndwr area, the grittiness of slate carts going up and down tramways, the smoke and sounds of railroad engines below, and the cosmopolitan aura of this superhighway connecting the great political and cultural centers of London and Dublin. I picture the challenges of raising four small children here. However Anne managed it, I am impressed. None of her children were run down by coaches or horses, nor killed themselves on the sharp slopes, nor drowned in the river, nor let their curiosity lead to a lethal run-in with the tramway, slate carts, or trains.

In those days, I am told, the cottages were not as isolated as they now seem. In addition to deliveries from afar via the Coach Road, there were shops close by in an easterly direction and a significant market town two miles west, and people sold things from their wagons. A Calvinistic Methodist chapel was built in the village, about a mile away if one walked along the river, longer by wagon or carriage. The village had recently been connected by rail to the east, and wealthy people from London were already building second homes there.

How did all of this impress itself on Lizzie's young sensibilities? Did London's being at the end of the Old Coach Road and of the railroad bring it closer or make it more real than it might otherwise be? Did it lodge in her subconscious such that her elopement to London was less of a leap than it might have seemed? What did this proximity to the Old Coach Road mean for Robert's and Anne's access to political and other news? For their sense of the larger world in which their lives were unfolding?

Torn down 30-40 years ago, the two or three wharf houses had been built by quarry managers who, in the view of my informant whose farm is part way up the mountain under the quarry, "looked after their most important people." Since all four of Anne and Robert's children were born in the wharf houses during the 1870s, I now know that Robert must have been working in this quarry for all or most of that decade, and that he was one of the quarry's most skilled and valued workers. Gwyn conjectures more specifically:

> The fact that he was living on the wharf and was provided with company housing suggests that he was very much a trusted employee, a skilled quarrymen who had made the

grade in the quarry itself, a reliable man of steady habits who had been promoted to be an inspector at the wharf. If so, he would have been responsible for making up the loads from the quarry, which means he was basically in a managerial position. He was somebody who commanded respect from his employers and probably from the men as well.[6]

This possibility would allow the documentary evidence for Robert's quarry work to converge with the sense I get from family lore that he was not "just" a quarryman but played some kind of managerial or quasi-managerial role. When he moved to Pen-y-Dyffryn and worked in its much larger quarries, perhaps he again became a rockman. Or, for whatever reason, Edward distilled his father's quarry work and work identities into "rockman" on his death certificate.

Farm Connection. Eight miles from the wharf cottages, Robert's family lived on a farm where his older brother assumed tenancy after their father died just as Robert and Anne were starting a family. His brother's great-granddaughter has found a document which shows that our great-great-grandfather began living and working at Tyddyn (*tuthinn*) around 1850 and that Robert's brother was a tenant there until he died several years after Robert. Thus, Robert moved to Tyddyn as a boy, and presumably had a connection to this 35-acre farm throughout his life.

Was Tyddyn a source of produce for the shop in Carreg Mawr? It is possible, especially given that railway links to Pen-y-Dyffryn were in place by the time Robert and Anne were settled there in 1881.[7] The attraction of Pen-Dyffryn may have been not only the quarries, but also that people there had money to spend.

Despite decades of association with quarries, Robert lived sixteen years longer than the average rockman. I suspect this was partly constitutional, partly better diet, partly that he was doing things other than quarrying, possibly spending some of his quarry years outdoors on the wharf, and partly his living in a house with his family, not a barracks where men slept in airless, often disease-spreading conditions. I would guess he had access to more vegetables and dairy products than most quarrymen whose notoriously bad diet of bread and tea did little to fortify them against the cold and damp and the many diseases to which miners were vulnerable.

Robert, the Builder. Everywhere I have tracked Robert—the area of his birth, the farm tenancy at Tyddyn, the wharf house in Glyndwr, the houses in Pen-y-Dyffryn—there was proximity to slate quarries *and* a connection to raising and/or selling produce. While many quarrymen had no connection with the land, many others had small holdings or gardens. Some thought of themselves as using quarry wages to remain on the land or supplement farm work, while others thought of their holdings as supplementing their quarry work.[8] I suspect Robert began in the first category, migrated to the second, and moved beyond it. He is likely to have begun working in the quarries when still a boy. As he developed a real affinity for the rock and skill as a rockman, the slate became his primary work. Yet he may never have fully identified with his "day job" as a quarryman, or even as a semi-managerial inspector.

Robert's self-concept is likely to have been more complex than any combination of farmer, quarryman, grocer, and shopkeeper. He had an eye for slate and a head for business. He was active as a chapel elder, building houses as his legacy to his children, and may well have been engaged in other building projects. He was, as Gwyn suggests, transforming himself into a small-scale businessman with diverse interests. In the broadest, archetypal sense, not only the house project but the whole of Robert's life reveals him to have been a Builder.

Slate was a much bigger part of his life than family stories had ever indicated, but his slate story was more complex than the "rockman" designation Edward put on his father's death certificate. "Rockman" simultaneously divulged what had been glossed over in family accounts, and obscured a more encompassing and quintessential truth of their storied image of Robert as entrepreneurial builder.

A common thread in all of his work is that it was independent, entrepreneurial, self-structuring, creative, risky, and relied on his deeply trusting himself—no doubt why I find myself developing a strong affinity with my great-grandfather.

Father and Daughter. I have gradually formed an impression that Lizzie was particularly close to her father, and/or that Lizzie was his favorite. It emerges from my sense of who each of his children was, of who he was, and how, beneath his rectitude and even-handedness about their legacies, Robert may have responded to each despite himself.

Emma's grandchildren say Lizzie had a generosity of spirit missing in their self-centered grandmother. I suspect Lizzie and her father recognized that generosity in each other, resonating at a deep level and forming a silent bond. Whereas Lizzie—like her parents—took pride in her work, Emma was a princess who expected to be waited on, demanded butter and cream for her scones, and her doting husband obliged.

Emma seems to have personified the stereotype of the idle and extravagant quarryman's wife—a sour stereotype historian R. Merfyn Jones has questioned as overblown. Yet Jones also recognizes that women denied their traditionally important role in production quite expectably developed "an interest in appearances, both of themselves and of their houses," resulting in "tiny parlors filled to overflowing with gleaming possessions, pieces to look at, not to sit in."[9] Jones' statement seems to fit Emma, and speaks to my puzzlement about how there could have been so much furniture stuffed into 15 Carreg Mawr (as indicated by Heledd's will).

Evan seems to have been weak and wanting in many departments, and to have gotten by with secrecy and manipulation. Edward, on the other hand, was an entrepreneur who put pieces together to build a vertically integrated business platform—printing, publishing, newspaper, and a shop that sold newspapers, magazines, books, hymnals, music, and stationery. He became a player in the community, a recorder and shaper of its political conversations, and, like his father, a chapel elder who put a protective roof over the head of his blood and business families. Robert was likely to have been proud of his reliable eldest, and somewhat disappointed in Emma and Evan.

Yet I cannot find a spark in Edward, a spark I have come to sense in Lizzie, the sort of spark that can endear daughters to fathers even if that spark also tries a father's patience. It is that spark, that sense of adventurousness and independence in Lizzie that I tap into during my journeys to the old country, and that forms a new lens through which to see her life.

> *Like billowing clouds, like the incessant gurgling of the brook, the longing of the soul can never be stilled.*
>
> —Hildegard of Bingen

Lizzie's Independence. Despite the bleakness of its weather, terraces of light gray, stone cottages, and mounds of gray-black, slate waste, I can imagine the vigor of Pen-y-Dyffryn when it was thriving. Even as a shell of its former glory, it exerts magnetic force due to its magical earthscape. Situated in a spectacular valley, it is nestled within mysterious, brooding, powerful yet intimate mountains whose richly textured surfaces turn every shade of green, gold-brown, and gray according to the light and season. Mountain streams generate cascades of waterfalls after a rain, and heather clings to the rocks, casting a rosy-purple hue during late summer and fall. It is an earthscape that inhabits and haunts the soul, and to which one belongs. How did this rugged valley and the embrace of its mountains shape Lizzie?

In slate towns, employment opportunities for women were very limited. Yet even by age sixteen, Lizzie identified herself as a milliner and dressmaker at a time and place when five out of six women aged fourteen and older did not engage in paid work.[10] Her skills—perhaps honed in a dressmaking or millinery shop—and her time in London may account for the fineness of her clothes and her sense of classic style, passed down to Olwen.

Lizzie stands out not only by her having acquired and used marketable skills and having had a work identity, but also by what that identity was. She did not identify herself as "merely" a seamstress—one who sews. Rather, she was, and saw herself as, a milliner *and* a dressmaker: one who designs hats and clothes, makes patterns, guides the process of choosing fabrics that suit the design and the customer, cuts the fabric—and, also sews.

Her self-designation suggests a creative inclination, an entrepreneurial orientation, and self-confidence with giving definition and form to the vagueness and fantasies put forward by clients. Not only is Lizzie her father's daughter, but she also prefigures my intellectual and work life of bringing form and visibility out of amorphousness and silence.

Independence, self-confidence, and willingness to take risks were also manifested by following her heart to London despite parental disapproval of John (at least as a mate) and the stir it likely caused in her chapel community. Such a step could not have been taken lightly or without due consideration.

Lizzie also broke tradition with her living situations. She may have lived in London for all or part of two years when she and John were most in love and just married. When they moved into their own place in Pen-y-Dyffryn, they rented a two-story cottage on the other side of the High Street. On both accounts, she was the first to leave the "family compound."

In addition to her sojourn in London, Lizzie lived in three other vital, thriving places—a village, a town, and a small city—each during their prime time, and each directly connected (by coach and/or by rail) to the wider world. The earthscapes surrounding her Welsh homes were stunningly beautiful, character-forming, and soul-nourishing. Her eminently respectable family was well connected with chapel and civic communities. Perhaps a secure sense of place in her family, community, and earthscape underpinned Lizzie's predilection for taking risks and pushing some of the boundaries that circumscribed the life of her siblings and peers.

Working as a dressmaker and milliner, having a work identity, choosing a musician and eloping to London, leaving the family compound—these things point to young Lizzie as having a mind of her own and the confidence to act on it, behaving in ways that would become part of the signature of the "modern woman." While keeping one foot in the Victorian/Calvinistic Methodist world, Lizzie pushed the envelope of certain of their constraints, venturing ahead of her time. Like her father—and like me—she trusted herself, and, like Olwen as well, set her own path.

Lizzie, the FormBreaker. Whereas Robert, being a man, was free to pursue and assemble his multiple interests, Lizzie had to create space to breathe and be herself. Archetypally, we could say Lizzie was a FormBreaker who simply would not be contained by all the conventions limiting women's choices and lives. Her form-breaking adventurousness variably informed Peggy and Olwen, and most of all, myself.

Peggy, careless of her reputation and lacking discretion in what she said to whom, paid a price for her impetuous behaviors. Olwen, carefully attuned to social conventions, was better able to make her own way in the world with, she felt, no one to really guide her after Lizzie died. She carefully crafted a life as an independent woman in ways that drew admiration and support.

My own life and work have been self-structuring and groundbreaking, with no guides or mentors, no maps or language for my journey into the unknown. Like Robert, I worked in the deep, dark, underground with only a candle and trust in my own radar and judgment that I would find a way to demystify the origins and structure of the deadly Story in which we all caught.

But when Lizzie was cut off from her roots, her family, and her history, I sense that her adventurous self became a wanderer, displaced in her new world, and her life became more form-bound. Despite the liveliness of her new city, Lizzie could not transport the history and context which underpinned her life and had no doubt mitigated John's shortcomings—shortcomings which I suspect became more pronounced as he got older. Alone in a new country across the ocean, Lizzie would have become more dependent on the quality of the relationship with the only person who knew her story, but he was unable to see who she was or support any dream but his own. Without the recognition so essential to nourishing her soul, Lizzie no doubt lost some of her confidence and high-spiritedness.

Somewhere along the way, migraines set in—a not uncommon symptom of women's constricted lives in the Victorian and Edwardian eras.[11] Olwen spoke of her mother's loneliness in the new world, and her not having the same quality of friendship and community she had always known. Olwen was attuned to her mother's sadness which she did not fully understand or know how to fix, and that sadness, as well as the trauma around her death, haunted Olwen all her life.

Lizzie's life was not fully realized because it was cut short, her husband was preoccupied with his own dream and incapable of seeing her in her own right, and society did not support the longing of women's souls to realize themselves. For John, someone existed only to the extent that they fed him and his music—as perhaps his mother had done, as Irma would do, and as perhaps Lizzie grew tired of doing, becoming restive, and longing for something she could not name and for which there was no language, and yet could not be stilled. What might it have been if she had had a partner who could see her in her own right, if she had been validated and supported by her society, if she had lived in a culture that allowed her to give voice to her soul?

Just as Lizzie exuded confidence and adventurousness before her marriage and during its early years, Olwen was more confident before and after an asymmetrical marriage than within it. Although not conscious of it, neither mother nor daughter was able to adjust fully to cultural or husbandly expectations of being a mirror reflecting him, let alone, as Virginia Woolf sardonically reflected, at twice his size.

John's Dream. During the years following his London studies, John became active and prominent musically in Gwynedd. Press clippings from his aunt's scrapbook say he trained some of the best voices in North Wales and adjudicated at scores of eisteddfodau which flourished at the local, provincial, and national levels. If recognition and prestige were what John needed, it would appear he was getting his needs met.

But were all his musical activities adding up to financial viability? The town which had boomed for decades was starting to shrink. Throughout his time in Pen-y-Dyffryn, John identified himself in records by his day job as a tailor's cutter, sometimes adding "music teacher." Apparently he was not making ends meet as a musician. Lizzie continued to identify herself as a dressmaker which suggests they drew on three streams of income.

Still, "to get more work" seems oversimplified as an explanation for John's uprooting his growing family and sailing to America. Why were his sights so set on crossing the ocean? John must have been engaging in local travel for his adjudicating and been known by many people who mattered in music. One would think there were plenty of opportunities in music in other areas of Wales, or even England. Or did the grass look greener from afar? Did John think he might he become a bigger fish on the other side of the big pond? What part of his dream could he not fulfill at home? Something seems to have been driving him as well as pulling him.

I puzzled over this. Did he choose never to see his mother or father again? There must have been adjudicating possibilities in Wales that would have paid his way. Then my cousin Robin found a newspaper clipping in his great-aunt's scrapbook that revealed John's mother had already died before he emigrated.

When a records office clerk graciously takes on the task of finding her death certificate, a new hypothesis emerges. John sailed for America one year to the day after she died. I cannot imagine his leaving on the first anniversary of his mother's death was incidental or accidental. If he had been thinking about America for some time, he may well have been postponing it during his mother's decline. His beautiful mother, of whom I have but one picture courtesy of her nephew Emrys, suffered from "dilatation of the heart" (congestive heart failure) for five years and from "dropsy" (edema) for two years according to John, the informant on her death certificate.

Perhaps his mother's death freed him to pursue his dream in America. Or, was it part of what was driving him far away?

I now suspect that rather than being indifferent to his parents, John was deeply affected by his mother's death. She was perhaps his first music teacher, and their bond through music and voice is likely to have been strong. Since, as I will come to postulate and have confirmed by members of his second family, John did not know how to express feelings except through music, getting as far away as possible may have been a deeper motivation driving him to America.

I cannot help but wonder if the lure of the anything-but-beautiful Irma, with her powerful solo voice and willingness to idolize and revolve around him, was that it resonated the bond he had once had and forever lost with his mother. I cannot help but wonder if his inability to "grieve in place" and his need to flee on the first anniversary of his mother's death was a forerunner of his inability to deal with Lizzie's fateful illness and his once again fleeing, this time to his studio.

What of the father John never saw again? I know only that he subsequently returned to his natal village where he died a decade after John emigrated. Did his father represent the world John thought he would never escape—his day job of tailoring—if he stayed in Pen-y-Dyffryn? Did he feel his dream could never be realized in a slate town that was already past peak?

Like my grandfather, I have held to my dream, distanced from my day jobs, and never settled for less. Like him, I have been preoccupied all my life with voice—metaphorically, socially, and politically. Like him, I have followed my gifts, and there are always very high costs to be paid for that.

Just before heading to the airport for my second journey to Wales, I remembered to take a picture of a cup and saucer that was Lizzie's, a small treasure Florence had given me years ago. I had seen some of this distinctive china the previous year, and wanted to find out more about it. To take the picture, I removed the pack of "angel cards" I keep in the cup.

Slightly apprehensive about what my subconscious would lead me to in my harried state, I chose three cards. In order, I drew "gratitude," "release," and "grace." I was astonished and relieved, yet at the same time I thought, "of course. That *is* what this second trip is about. This will be my intention."

Retracing the footsteps of my ancestors, I was flooded with gratitude and with awe for all they have done, all they endured, all that has made it possible for me to be me. I absorbed the earthscapes to which I already belonged and which had formed me just as they formed Olwen, Lizzie, Anne, and Robert. I, the ParadigmBreaker and ParadigmMaker, have unknowingly built upon them all, trusting that through the work I am bringing into the world, I will recover the sense of place we lost a century ago.

Following my second trip, Lizzie's picture stopped turning. I dearly miss that connection we had for several years, and part of me keeps hoping she will start to move again. A deeper part of me knows better. I have done what she needed me to do, and she is at peace. I have done what I needed to do, and I have been released.

My sense of what it means that "it all comes down to me" has expanded. Yes, I am the holder of the pictures and the memories, the names and the stories, the rugs and the crystal, the flatware and the furniture, but there's much more. I, the Storyteller, am the one who not only had to retrieve Olwen's story and work with her and Lizzie to heal our lineage, but also must take our story forward and complete it.

My Dance of Death with Olwen and the mystery of grace which infused our lives have forever transformed me and our relationship, and prepared me to fulfill the legacy of my lineage by completing the work I am here to do. My long journey recovering Olwen's story and finding my roots is, I now see, one and the same as my long journey giving voice to the social Structures of Silence and has perfectly prepared me for telling their much larger Story while completing us.

Part V

Giving Cultural Form and Visibility to the Dance

*Wisdom, then, is born of the overlapping of lives,
the resonance between stories.*
—Mary Catherine Bateson

Seventeen

The Caregiver's Story

> *Our experience and research tell us that family caregivers are the backbone of the long-term care system, they are not doing well, and current public policy does little to support them.*
>
> —Susan Reinhard, RN, PhD, innovator and policy-maker in aging services and long-term care

The Caregiver's Story is my distillation of what we, as family caregivers, are dealing with and trying to manage, especially during the last phases of caregiving. It is a model of the inherent structure underlying all our unique stories—thus its capitalization.

This Story plays out in hundreds of ways through millions of stories. Each caregiver's story is unique, yet many, perhaps most, also "belong" to this Caregiver's Story. My map allows the caregiver to experience and the observer to see the underlying coherence in what appears to be a highly unstructured situation. Rather than feeling overwhelmed by our situation, we can see it from the outside even when we are living inside of it.

The Caregiver's Story is an orienting device for those going through the process and validation for those who have completed the journey. It helps the caregiver get her bearings in a situation of extraordinary importance that may be invisible to those around her, and certainly has little visibility or value in the dominant culture.

Unlike most models, the Caregiver's Story is not a set of generalizations told from an expert point of view positioned comfortably after the fact. Instead, it is situated in the present moment from the perspective of the caregiver who is composing a duet with her dying partner.[1]

Intersecting Axes

The Caregiver's Story pivots around four intersecting axes: the course of decline, disease, and dying; the consequences for the health and life of the caregiver; the relationship between the caregiver and her dying elder; and the uncertainties and dilemmas about which she must make decisions. The pushes, pulls, tensions, demands, and requirements within and between these four axes and their eight poles underlie, organize, and shape each dying/caregiving story.

> *Not long ago, people generally "got sick and died"—all in one sentence and all in a few days or weeks . . . Now most Americans will grow old and accumulate diseases for a long time before dying . . . Many elderly people are inching toward oblivion with small losses every few weeks or months.*
>
> —Joanne Lynn, MD, physician-champion for improved end-of-live care

Course of Disease and Dying Axis. The first axis in the Caregiver's Story revolves around the course taken by disease and failing health over weeks, months, and years, and the impact it has on the physical and mental abilities—and thus the functional needs—of the elder. At one pole is the ability to function with only the support any adult needs (e.g., transportation, social networks); at the other end is complete dependence. In between lies every form and degree of functional impairment. Depending on the disease course and how slowly or rapidly it unfolds, the needs of the elder differ.

If we plot this course on a graph, we see the shape and speed of decline in functionality over time. According to geriatrician Joanne Lynn, three major trajectories occur.[2] The person functions quite well, even very well, until there is sharp drop-off in the final months or weeks, as exemplified by fatal cancer; this is the path of about 20 percent of Americans, and these deaths peak during the mid-sixties. A second trajectory is marked by slow decline in physical abilities punctuated by health events, typified by congestive heart failure; this affects about 25 percent of Americans, and deaths peak a decade later. A third trajectory is marked by gradual deterioration to low levels of functioning, requiring years of care. About 40 percent, mostly in their mid-eighties and older, dwindle toward frailty; roughly half develop dementia.

Although it is difficult to sort out changes from fluctuations as they occurring, it is important to catch inflection points where the angle of decline turns downward. There may be several, subtle inflection points, but eventually, decline inflects toward dying.

During the decline process, we try to reduce the speed and angle of the trajectory. Caregiving is geared to preserving her safety and maintaining her quality of life at the highest level possible. That usually means helping her stay in her own home or apartment. It means studying her home environment and finding ways to reduce safety hazards embedded in its design. It may include proactive investments in alterations with regard to bathrooms, stairs, and ramps. It may call for hiring part-time caregivers to help her manage her own life and help us assess her situation, particularly if we live at a distance. Finding part-time caregivers whom she likes in advance of a crisis may prove to be a wise investment.

During her decline, we try to sustain her autonomy and pride and the self with whom she identifies. We do not do for her what she can do for itself, yet are ready to close the gap as she is able to do less. If your parent, like Olwen, has been super-independent, she may need to learn that it is okay to depend on others and receive what they want to give her.

> [T]he worst kind of solitude when you are dying is not being able to say to the people you love that you're going to die.
> —Marie de Hennezel, PhD, palliative care psychologist

When the downward curve bends toward dying and an irremediably downhill quality of life, we need to look right at it, and not be in denial. We redirect our support to removing artificial barriers so that she may complete her journey in the best way possible.

These artificial barriers are deeply rooted in our death-denying culture and the philosophy, practice, and reimbursement incentives of a mechanistic medicine which tries to keep body parts that are wearing out going forever, irrespective of the consequences for the dignity and wishes of the whole human being and the burdens this generates for the family. The party line has been absorbed by many families, impeding their ability to let go of their dying members, and often generating painful family conflicts. When we do not know how or when to let go, we fall behind the curve, and impose our own agenda on the dying. In the end, everyone loses.

> *Caring for a person who will not recover is one of the most stressful of human experiences.*
> —Stephen Connor, PhD, and Jocelia Adams, RN,
> National Hospice and Palliative Care Organization
> & Center for Caregiver Training

Caregiver Consequences Axis. The second axis in the Caregiver's Story pivots around the physical, emotional, and financial consequences of the disease course for caregivers. At one pole is bodymind exhaustion, immune system depletion, financial hardship, and even bankruptcy. At the other pole are caregivers whose life and health are still intact, have not lost their homes, and are financially solvent—due to greater wealth and incomes, but also in part due to achieving balance through self-care.

Even when the principal family caregiver does not give hands-on care, she makes it possible for direct care to be provided and does not escape sustained, high levels of stress. Caregiving is often initiated by our noticing something that gives us a queasy feeling of alarm in the pit of our stomach, ever after which we are on alert, waiting, wondering, anticipating. As tension builds over what is often many years, some part of us is always waiting for a shoe to drop. Whether managing from a distance, nearby, on the spot, or by commuting, the family caregiver has no limits on her unpaid time or the scope of her activities, responsibilities, and decisionmaking. Suddenly or gradually, she takes on primary responsibility for the life and welfare of another human being who is no longer able to care for herself completely, if at all, and is becoming less and less able to negotiate with the rest of the world on her own behalf—although she may still think she can, which loads more stress onto the caregiver.

Although family caregivers provide 80 percent of long-term care in the United States,[3] they are not paid. Their contribution to the invisible "gift economy"—which underlies and enables the monetized economy—is equivalent to one-fifth of the healthcare bill. It dwarfs spending for nursing homes and professional home care combined. It is roughly equivalent to Medicare spending, and exceeds Medicaid spending.[4]

Not only are family caregivers not paid or supported, but they themselves pay a steep price for the impact of caregiving on their own lives and health. They rearrange work schedules, miss work, come in late, leave early, take leaves, pass up promotions and transfers. They quit jobs and draw down their savings. One-third experience severe financial setbacks such as losing their home or going bankrupt.[5] Back injuries are common. The stresses of caregiving and of death can compromise their immune systems and general health, and make it more likely that they themselves will die in the near term.[6] Most of the increased mortality risk for survivors is associated with caring for someone who is mentally and/or physically disabled, presumably because of the unrelenting and repetitious demands their conditions make on caregivers.[7]

> *Almost all family caregivers, especially those providing the most intense levels of care, report significant physical and emotional stress. Many encounter serious loss of income and job opportunities . . . [T]he high economic toll that caring for terminally ill patients can take adds to their emotional as well as their physical stress. Their grief and loss absorb immense energy.*
>
> —Rosalynn Carter, Rosalynn Carter Institute (for caregivers)

Who bears a disproportionate share of these costs? Women. Caregiving is a gendered issue in which, overall, women give more than they get. One study describes this asymmetry: "Three out of four [family] caregivers are women, who themselves are less likely to be cared for by a family member than their male counterparts."[8] Women's caregiving may be "rewarded" by ending their own days in a facility. A Hastings Center report observes, "Many former caregivers, mainly wives and mothers, with no family left to care for them, will themselves die in nursing homes."[9] Long-term care (LTC) in such facilities is summarized by LTC innovator Jude Rabig as, "poor women taking care of poor women."[10]

Many caregivers who provide hands-on care are the primary or sole provider of care. The sleep deprivation and the physical and emotional toll this can take is beyond words, especially when care extends over many years and/or during the last phases of care. Gerontologist Andrea Sankar describes the latter:

> There is a period before death, lasting as much as several months or as little as a week, when the body begins to break down . . . Several problems characterize it: the extreme fragility of the dying person, the often intense intimacy of the caregiving process, the significant levels of responsibility the caregiver must assume, the physical and emotional stamina

required of the caregiver because of the unremitting nature of the task, and the cost.[11]

Because we have been segregated from the intimacy of dying by its medicalization and institutionalization, the fragility of the dying is often a surprise for family caregivers, as are the physical demands on the caregiver.[12] Transferring adult bodies that are becoming dead weight, repositioning rigid or fragile bodies, preventing bedsores, keeping the dying person clean and dry, helping them to drink water or take a pill—such projects consume unbelievable amounts of time, can damage our own bodies, and are profoundly devastating. A being our child-self once installed on Mount Olympus is now crumbling before our eyes.

> *We send people home who are very sick and do not make the correlation that an untrained person or family will have to do the work of an entire hospital staff.*
> —Stephen Connor and Jocelia Adams

The demands on family caregivers differ and change. Over what period of time must you compensate for which losses in functionality? Are there programs available to supplement those losses, or are you thrown back on your personal resources? Can you leave your elder alone and get out of the house? How long can you be gone? Can you still carry on your own life? What physical and emotional demands are being made on you? Is it your back that is breaking? Or are you ready to explode from the hundredth time she said that today? How early in her trajectory, and over what period of time, is your sleep routinely interrupted, often several times a night, and inadequate to support your own well-being?

Caregivers' own most vital need, whether acknowledged or not, is for self-care. This can be the hardest thing for caregivers—especially women—to justify to themselves and the easiest to let go of. Yet self-care is an absolute necessity. We need a full night's, uninterrupted sleep. We need quiet space, alone or with good friends, counselors, or support groups and away from the caregiving scene. We need to share our experiences, feel that we are seen and witnessed, recenter in ourselves, and feel like "me" again. For those of us in long-term caregiving situations, it is essential that we sustain our own lives and move forward. Otherwise, we can be ground to a pulp, which undermines the quality and consistency of our caregiving as well as our own health.

Some parents may have made a career of neediness and dependency which, as they move into their declining years, can burn out their caregiver(s) years before the end-game occurs. In that case, we should resist—and sometimes that means strongly resisting despite what may be heaped on us—regressive pulls toward premature dependence. We need to support every bit of autonomy and self-pride that we can for as long as possible. Olwen was still taking the keys and returning them to their box and pushing her own elevator buttons on her very last outing six days before she died.

> T]he healing of a broken relationship in the last hours, or even minutes before death, can reframe the history of the relationship and the biographies of everyone involved.
> —Ira Byock, MD, palliative care physician-champion

Relationship Axis. When a parent is dying, it is the last chance to realize the hope, fantasy, and yearning to meet in love, understanding, and healing. The love and history we share makes it possible *despite* our past struggles and woundings. The push-pull between our history and our hopes forms the relationship axis which is the wellspring of motivation that feeds the caregiving process and informs the dying process.

Parent-child relationships are complex and often difficult. The mother-daughter bond is arguably the deepest and most complex bond we ever experience. Our natural bond is bombarded, however, by cultural meanings which sentimentalize motherhood while devaluing real mothers and women, pull mothers and daughters apart, and pit women against each other. Many of us in the current caregiving generation came of age when, for the first time, we began to have language for understanding the socio-cultural processes dividing us from our mothers. Often we could not bring our mothers fully, if at all, into the liberating perspectives we had struggled to achieve. Our intergenerational struggles can be seen as expressions of frustrated desires to share, connect, and feel on the same side.[13]

We may have longed for and tried to have The Conversation which we fantasize will bridge whatever has separated us, heal old wounds, and magically usher in a new level of connection, understanding, peace, and healing. As our mother's caregiving needs escalate, we are getting down to the wire. We don't know how long she will be conscious, able to talk, or be sufficiently lucid for the conversation we imagined. As death draws closer, The Conversation may take physical-energetic rather than verbal form. Indeed, physical-energetic forms may be the deepest way to connect.

Our fantasy of The Conversation may merge with the emotional and spiritual needs of our dying parent. Whether or not those needs are conscious or articulated, they are as important for dying well as freedom from pain and unwanted interventions, and not being left to die alone in some hospital byway. Although not everyone chooses to deal with their "unfinished business," most dying people do long for peace of mind, and that is said to derive primarily from finding meaning in and of one's life, and mending and completing important relationships.[14]

Approaching the end of life presents opportunities that go beyond "getting to say good-bye" or even reaching a sense of completion about relationships. As those nearing death shed what no longer serves them, their hearts may open and invite the living to meet and match them. When a parent and adult child are fully present and open to the moment and each other, old sticking points and defenses may vanish. They may find themselves flowing together in new territory where growth and healing and all that had seemed impossible are suddenly possible.

Reality Axis. Most realities are socially constructed, but some realities are existential: built into the human condition in a world delimited by time and space. The fourth axis organizing the Caregiver's Story revolves around the existential uncertainties and dilemmas in the face of which we must decide and act.

- Uncertainties are rooted in the fact that we simply cannot know the answers to critically important questions.
- Dilemmas are rooted in the existential fact that two or more lives, two or more centers of subjectivity are engaged in this process.
- Nonetheless, we must place our bets and make decisions, some of them only once (e.g., where she will reside), and some over and over (e.g., when we will come and go).

Heading the list of uncertainties is the timetable of our dying parent. Without a timetable, all planning is difficult. Although some decline/disease courses are more predictable than others, we do not know at the beginning (and often until near the end) just how long this overall process will take, let alone its phases. We do not know the end-game scenario, or whether we will be able to handle all of it at home.

Therefore, unless we are wealthy, we don't know much money our parent has for her care because we don't know how long we have to make money stretch, nor how the needs of our parent may escalate and when, and thus how long each phase of care may need to be sustained. We don't know how much money we can spend on outside help this week (if we can spend any at all) because we do not know how many weeks, months, or even years are ahead of us.

Because we don't know the overall timetable, its major events, and phases, we also don't know how to pace ourselves. We don't know if this is the time to quit or take a leave from our job or start phasing down clients and new work, or whether we should postpone such decisions for the "real crunch" that may come. Postponing carries the assumption that we will see the signs in time or get a "heads-up" to make those changes later when, we imagine, it will "really" matter. To avoid burn-out and often to sustain our own lives, we may start identifying other caregivers whom she will accept and whom we can trust, and begin to phase them into her life.

Uncertainties are built into the situation because we cannot know the answers about her unfolding situation in advance. The uncertainties associated with a parent's decline constrict our breath as we wait and watch and hope; they can overwhelm us at times. Yet we do place our bets, whether consciously or through our trail of decisions.

> *Decisionmaking is the most extensive area of responsibility, followed by actual hands-on care . . . Speaking on behalf of the dying person [when there is cognitive impairment] becomes much more difficult because the caregiver not only has to interpret what the patient cannot say but also has to assess whether what is said is actually meant.*
> —Andrea Sankar, PhD, gerontologist and medical anthropologist

It is not only what we don't know that gnaws at our innards, but also inherent, existential dilemmas generated by the fact that two or more lives, two or more centers of subjectivity are involved in the caregiving story. Needs of the frail and dying are sometimes pitted against the needs of our own lives and the lives of our chosen family. Many dilemmas confronted by the primary family caregiver are tensions between "her life or mine." We can't be in two places at once, and there is only so much of us to go around.

The intensity of our dilemmas and the consequences of our decisions shift to another level if we live outside commuting distance. We have to decide how we are going to manage being a long-distance caregiver, and whether, and at what point(s) in our parent's decline or dying we are going to uproot our lives and be with her. If we are going to come and go episodically so we can keep our own ship afloat, how do we choose times to be with her so that it will matter the most and/or we can do the most good? During acute episodes and/or their aftermath? To set up the next level/round of support? When she is more herself and more good stuff can (so we think) flow between us, or when she is failing and frightened, or getting close to death, or at the moment of death itself? Or do we simply come and go on a fairly regular commuting schedule shaped by our jobs and other commitments? However we arrange our comings and goings, we are going to need another relative or private caregiver(s) to be our eyes and ears on the spot.

One way to resolve the long-distance and/or work-versus-caregiving dilemmas is to temporarily uproot our lives, often with no guarantee we can pick up where we left off. Those who quit their jobs, draw down their savings, and put the rest of their life on hold to undertake this journey may jeopardize their own financial viability, job and/or career, other relationships, and even their own health. If and when we decide to become a virtually full-time caregiver, we are unlikely to secure an open-ended leave of absence from our job (let alone a paid leave), and even if we do, our organization may have moved on without us by the time we return. If we quit our jobs, are self-employed, or are not working, then becoming a hands-on caregiver depletes our savings (if we have any) which can raise scary spectres about our own future. Nothing is coming in, yet our expenses don't stop, and our savings are flowing out. The move may turn out to be the best choice we ever made, but we don't know that until after we have risked it.

The uncertainties about our parent's situation and the dilemmas between attending to her and to the rest of our lives do force us to make decisions, however, whether consciously or by default. Our trail of implicit and explicit choices gives us *de facto* answers to our caregiving uncertainties and dilemmas.

In the moment, it is often difficult to know the best or optimal choice to make, and most of our choices have risks—often very high risks—attached. Buffeted by capricious winds and perilous currents, we sometimes feel like our little boat will be pulled to pieces and sink from the relentless demands and the juggling of so many unknowns.

Caregiving decisions have a crossroads quality because each decision needs to be informed by the emotional history and hopes of our relationship, *and* by the harsh realities with which we have to deal, by our assessment of the course of dying, and by its impact on us. *It is the crossroads quality that makes coming to any decision so exhausting, frightening, and stressful.* Figure 17-1 locates the caregiver at the intersection of these axes.

Many of our decisions are indeed momentous: any decision we make may be a point of no return. The stakes are very high, and we get to visit each decision point only once. There is no rewind button.

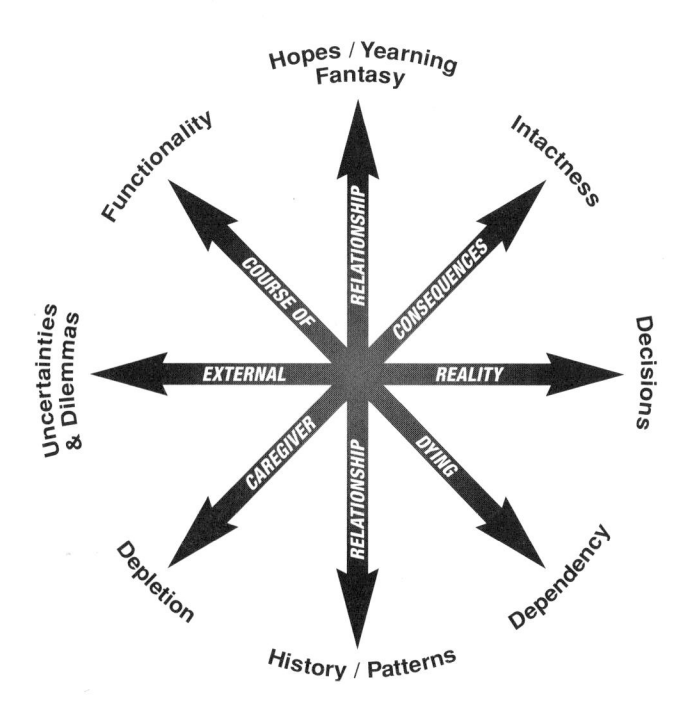

Figure 17-1. Axes and Poles of the Caregiver's Story

Constraining/Enabling Context

The Caregiver's Story operates within a larger context that is predominantly constraining because the caregiver deals with a host of outside decision-makers who must abide by and enforce rules and regulations. Yet that same context is potentially enabling because some professionals may become resources and allies.

Professionals and administrators have the power to decide: whether one's mother can stay in her residence; how her medical conditions are to be treated and where; whether she will be accepted into their program or facility; what services they can provide; whether particular services will be paid for by their program; when she can leave their facility; and where she can go next. These players include doctors, social workers, government representatives, program directors, facility directors, administrators, insurers, home health care agencies, and hospice staff. We must work within or around rules made by the state, the medical profession, the hospital, the rehabilitation facility, the assisted living facility, the skilled nursing facility, the home health care agency, the hospice, Medicare, Medicaid, and healthcare insurers.

To counteract the constraints and turn the challenging environment into a more enabling and supportive one demands persistent, proactive involvement by family caregiver(s), and that requires time and energy we may not have. As best we can, we try to gather information about her disease, her options, and the resources available to us, and try to bring attention and interest to her case. If we are lucky, some of the people we encounter or seek out will be experienced, reliable, and even wise sources from whom we can gather information, explore options, and make informed decisions that enhance the quality of our parent's living and dying.

More likely, many of our forays and encounters yield information that is incomplete, not fully accurate, biased, or contradicts other things we have been told or read. We are left to work our way down multiple learning curves, digging further to make some sense of inconsistent bits, and pull things together as best we can, often in acutely time-constrained situations. Whatever we can learn in advance and inventory for future reference will pay off later. Even when we can do some homework in a timely way, a good deal of what we will need to know about will be specific to the unfolding of her dynamic situation, and we do the best we can with learning on the fly.

Nationally and regionally—but not always locally—many trained and experienced people are available, and the array of innovative services and modes of delivering them is expanding. Yet identifying resources and assessing which are most appropriate for us is a project in itself, while gaining access can mean yet another set of time-consuming projects. In my experience, finding a match is difficult. Publicly-funded resources require our needs to fit into reimbursable categories, while better-fitting alternatives may be too expensive or not available locally.

When we know the direction in which we want to head, we try and get the evolving cast of players on the same page and work with them to make our care as seamless as possible. We try to screen out those who cannot fully face and honor the process of illness and dying, and screen in those who can, and who are highly attentive, observant, compassionate, and proactive. We try to turn potential adversaries and overworked professionals and para-professionals into interested allies working on her behalf. Building good working relationships with them benefits our parent and ourselves. Some of them, especially hands-on caregivers, may become our biggest supporters. The bonds I built with those who actually knew my mother and attended her in her dying process are not like any other.

So, we must expand our diagram of the Caregiver's Story as I have in Figure 17-2. Our history and hopes, her functionality and the impact on us, and the uncertainties and dilemmas rooted in our situation all play out in the overall context of healthcare organization and funding, with its institutional power, authority, rules, and regulations personified by decision-makers. To get the outcomes that you want, you—as best you can and to the fullest extent possible—must engage and manage these players, and create an *ad hoc* team allied around the purpose of helping your mother and supporting you.

> *The hospital is a place of disconnection.*
> —Sharon R. Kaufman, PhD, medical anthropologist

In dealing with external players and facilities, we also have to be a watchdog and patient advocate. Safety and quality problems in American health care are structural, systemic, and of epidemic proportions because they are embedded in how work is done and how the healthcare environment is organized. It is estimated that up 98,000 people die every year through hospital errors; almost as many die due to the two million infections patients acquire each year while in hospitals.[15] Unless we can afford to hire private nurses around the clock, we lay folk have to be on top of the medical situation as best we can.

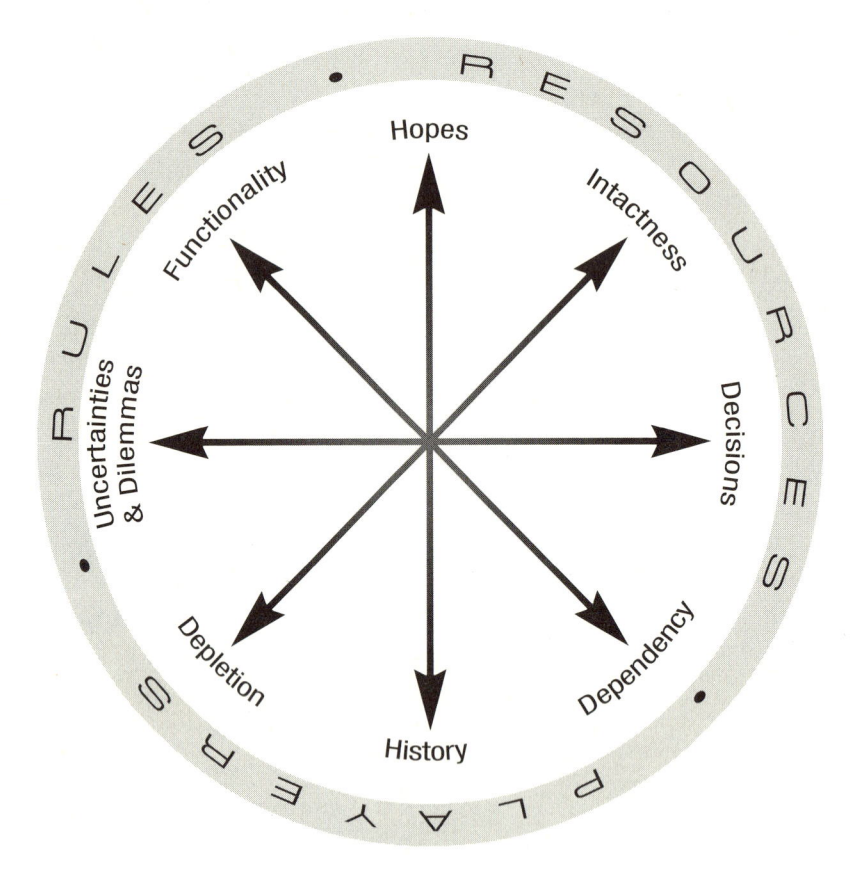

Figure 17-2. Structure and Context of Caregiver's Story

Identifying problems, initiating interventions, thwarting infections, remedying errors, reducing neglect, preventing enforced incontinence—any and all may fall in our lap. If we hope to get back the same (or nearly the same) person who went into the hospital, then it is up to us to prevent our parent from becoming disoriented—a real danger. Although it is an uphill battle, it is a battle with such high stakes that we must do whatever we can to win it. The very fact that we show up, hang out, ask questions, and take action lets staff know our parent is not alone in the world, and may get them more and better attention. Yet we walk a tricky line because we are dependent upon some of the people whose practices we are scrutinizing, and we are not there to watch them all the time.

> *Hospitals are not geared for the intensive, non-invasive nursing care required by dying patients.*
> —Andrea Sankar

Sometimes, you must take power—such as when her physician's behavior runs contrary to the reality of your mother's situation and wishes; and/or providers are unable to treat you as her surrogate decision-maker; and/or their ego, fear, ignorance, empathy deficits, or felt impotence in the face of death are harming or demeaning your parent, making her situation worse, or narrowing her options. Researchers have documented that communication between physicians and patients is far from ideal, and worse with the families of elderly and dying parents. Coordination among specialists, attending physicians, residents, and nurses is rarely seamless and more likely inadequate, while many factors work against continuity of care from one caregiver to the next.[16]

Is it any wonder, then, that we get overwhelmed, exhausted, cranky, or burned out? To add insult to injury, most of what we are doing, feeling, and coping with is often invisible to anyone who isn't inside of it with us. Public policy does not support us; indeed, its absence, deficiencies, and perversities add to our pressures and negative consequences to ourselves from our gift of caregiving.

Cultural and Medical Phobia about Death

> *Too many Americans die unnecessarily bad deaths—deaths with inadequate palliative support, inadequate compassion, and inadequate human presence and witness. Deaths preceded by a dying marked by fear, anxiety, loneliness, and isolation.*
> —Bruce Jennings, True Ryndes,
> Carol D'Onofrio, and Mary Ann Baily,
> Hastings Center and National Hospice Work Center

The Caregiver's Story is permeated by cultural and medical phobia about death that makes the caregiving role difficult and lonely, and escalates the chances of our parent's dying badly. This phobia keeps us from getting up close and personal with death as an integral and natural part of our life cycle. Most of us cannot tap the accumulated wisdom of our elders because society does not support gathering and informally transmitting experiential knowledge from one generation to the next. Few of us receive honest, reliable, concrete information about the dying and the death process even if we ask for it, and most of us don't have independent, informed sources to ask.[17] As a result, we treat the dying from a place of ignorance, and the dying process is often so much less than it can be for the dying and ourselves.

Our difficulties in getting forthright statements from medical professionals are compounded by confusing messages sent by physicians who continue to treat the dying. As young doctors told Sharon Kaufman, "Dying is not billable. You can't treat it."[18] Whereas people used to be allowed to die on their own time, Medicare's "Diagnostic Related Group" or DRG reimbursement system changed "the financing of hospital care, and thus the organization of death" in 1983. By putting a price tag on each diagnosis, and linking reimbursement to treatment, the DRG system disallows *"waiting* [for death] without specific, listed diagnoses and treatments." Kaufman connects the dots: "Medicare's reimbursement methods dominate what happens to the majority of hospital patients at the end of life," which may include unwanted interventions and treatments.[19] Reimbursement practices, a healthcare system geared to acute-care interventions rather than chronic or preventive care, and the fix-and-cure medical paradigm together lead to a predictable outcome: "[A]lthough most people die in hospitals, hospitals are not structured for the kinds of deaths that people claim to want."

As the caregiver for our dying elder, we have to work in and against cultural ignorance about death and dying. Cultural reality and the organization of medical care infect the way healthcare providers practice, the way they talk to us, what they will and won't say, and their lack of forthrightness. Because of our societal and medical cultures, we may find ourselves rushing to catch up and fill in some of the gigantic holes in our education about what is really important to know. We may feel angry and frustrated at what we don't know and can't seem to find out. We may feel we have no one to talk to about the most important questions we have ever asked.

Because our death-denying culture surrounds and pervades everything in the Caregiver's Story, Figure 17-2 is incomplete. Think of this diagram as representing a sphere whose entire space is suffused by the denial of death and thus ignorance of the process of dying. Color it murky gray, cloudy, opaque. Our cultural phobia about death leads some friends to back away, pits family members against each other, and aggravates our stress levels and the impact of caregiving on our health. Worst of all, because we can't get the right information and don't have the experience of dealing with dying, we may cheat the dying and ourselves of the most powerful, meaningful, and transformative experience of their or our lives.

Summary

The Caregiver's Story situates us, the caregivers, at the center of things, trying to navigate a path through multi-faceted, multi-leveled pushes and pulls, hopes and history, uncertainties and dilemmas, constraints and opportunities, rules and regulations. Its structure helps us to see where we are by laying out all we are dealing with and by revealing an inherent order in the seeming chaos.

This structural map organizes and normalizes an often overwhelming situation in which most of us have had little or no experience. It validates the scope and complexity and devastatingly powerful nature of caregiving our dying parent. It gives visibility, shape, structure, and dignity to the experiences, processes, roles, stresses, conflicts, and triumphs of caregiving, and to the love through which the lonely act of dying may be transformed into an intimate dance.

Navigating the Caregiver's Story

The path we navigate is easiest to see in retrospect. Like the wake behind a ship, it is the trail we leave behind by our choices as we try to match our mother's unfolding situation to the space we create for her journey to complete itself.

But how do we navigate in real time? The Caregiver's Story lays out the territory and locates us in it, but it doesn't tell us much about moving through its territories. It doesn't tell us about the paradoxical Dance at the heart of this Story, nor help us to dance from moment to moment.

By reflecting more deeply on what I was doing intuitively in my dances with Olwen and with Pandora, I have articulated my intuitive mode of operating, identifying four basic dance steps as well as our more comprehensive role, and elaborating guiding principles that helped me to dance. These principles help us not only with the intimate Dance itself, but also with navigating through the caregiving territories in which the Dance takes place.

Eighteen

The Dance of Death: What do We need to Know and Do?

> *[H]ealing and wholeness are always possible. Even after years of alienation, of harsh criticism, rejection, or frustration, . . . Even as people confront death (their own or others'), they can reach out to express love, gratitude, and forgiveness. When they do, they consistently find that they, and everyone involved, are transformed—for the rest of their lives, whether those lives last for decades or just days.*
>
> —Ira Byock, MD, palliative care physician-champion

Although my experience with my mother compelled me to write this book, the metaphor of the "Dance of Death" had been turning around in my mind for several years. It first came to me during Pandora's days of dying.

We had been given a prognosis of 6-24 months. Nowadays there are web sites devoted to the memory of cats who have died of chronic renal failure, and most still die within a couple of years of being diagnosed. Pandora was thirteen-and-a-half years old when diagnosed, and she graced my life with another eight years and seven months. During those years, we were already living the principles I would later follow during her days of dying and Olwen's months of dying. Some friends characterized our healing dance as simply "love." But how was love enacted?

I never looked away or procrastinated. Our healing journey was initiated the moment I saw her hanging over her water bowl. When, following a two-day kidney diuresis, the vet was casual about the future ("check back in a month or two"), and I discovered he had never told me her kidneys had been shrinking for some time, I immediately changed vets.

During the few days before our appointment with Dr. Wiesman, chief of medicine at a veterinary teaching hospital, Pandora got alarmingly weaker. Her creatinine had shot way up. Wiesman was thorough in his exam, and cautiously optimistic about the near term. Another round of diuresis and ICU was indicated. I visited twice a day for five days, and her creatinine level dropped by half.

The central questions with which I was wrestling during Pandora's ICU days were: Is it her time? Does she want to be here? I was clear that these were her calls, not mine. I promised her and myself, "We are doing this heroic thing once, but I will never put you through this or anything like this again. It doesn't feel to me like it's your time to go, but it is your choice. I will bring you supportive therapies, and, if you so choose, you can use them to heal yourself."

To find those supportive therapies, I instinctively initiated a dial-a-thon, calling everyone I knew who might have ideas or leads about alternative and complementary medicines, energetic modes of healing, and working with animals. Intuitively following the paths those conversations opened not only enabled me to bring Pandora what she needed, but also led to networks of people who became important in the next stage of my life, and to my making breakthroughs that would transform my life's work. Those breakthroughs allowed me to see where my underground journey had been heading all these years; my trust in myself and my path thereby settled into my bones.

I kept my promise and Pandora did choose to heal herself. Dietary changes, supplements, subcutaneous fluids, herbs, homeopathy, and energy healing were our tools. Because Pandora was imbued with exquisitely subtle energy, I took my cues from her and studied Reiki to channel healing energy more effectively in my hands-on work with her. Virtually no one was doing Reiki with animals in 1990. I chose Reiki because it is gentle, does no harm, and the body wisdom of the recipient chooses how to use it. Pandora was in charge, and use it she did.

Following her ICU ordeals, we did Reiki daily for months. During our sessions, she sat in my lap without purring until we were well into the second side of my favorite Enya tape before she jumped down (thereby relieving me of the responsibility for knowing when we were done!). By contrast, when she came for a snuggle, she purred but rarely stayed more than five minutes. Pandora always knew the difference between healing work and snuggles.[1]

When Pandora's days of dying came, we walked every step together. When she gave me the soul-piercing Look, our eyes locked for a very long time. She knew that I knew, that I would do all that I could to support her, but that I would not try to keep her past her time. I began thinking about the terrible and beautiful dance in which we were entwined as the Dance of Death.

The Dance of Death

I experienced her dying as a dance between two subjects, one of whom anticipates the moves of the other. The caregiving partner stays ahead of the dying partner's curve. We are not in denial, or stuck in the past, or lagging behind, or imposing our needs on her.

Being proactive and staying ahead of the curve were not new ideas for me. I had absorbed them from Olwen since childhood. If she heard a not-right noise in her car, she got it checked out immediately. She kept her cars running well and rust-free for up to eighteen years. It was the same with her furnace, her roof, her shrubbery. She never smoked and was opposed to sugars and fats decades before the rest of the world. Giving up her driver's license on her ninety-fourth birthday was one of her most difficult decisions. Much as it compromised her independence and quality of life, Olwen did it because she knew it was the right and wise thing to do.

Mother also stayed ahead of the curve with dying. Throughout her life and throughout her dying process, she was never in denial about her own death. She saw it as a real event that would in fact happen. She talked about wanting to make things easy for me "after I'm gone." Every so often, she insisted that we go through her accounts and papers; she kept meticulous records that often carried explanatory notes intended for me. She made out advance directives and we discussed them. From time to time we visited the funeral home so she could revisit her choices. Since childhood, I had gone with her to visit her mother's grave. As a child and teenager, I remember Olwen's taking the big clippers and a stepladder to trim the bushes she had planted for my grandmother long before I was born. Olwen took comfort not only from visiting Lizzie's grave but also from being on intimate terms with her own final resting place.

My mother was unknowingly teaching me what to do during Pandora's years of healing and days of dying and later her own days of dying, as well as how to live: look at life and death squarely in the face, stay ahead of the curve, and get on with it.

Core Idea. The Dance of Death is an intimate duet of movement composed by the dying partner and her caregiving partner(s). We, the caregivers, cannot control the Dance. The beloved who is dying is the lead, and we must take our cues from her. We must follow, and yet paradoxically, in other respects, we must lead, anticipatorily staying ahead of her curve, even though we cannot know just where she will go next, or when.

So we must shadow her, yet be simultaneously translating what we see into anticipatory action that keeps us slightly ahead of her. Our role in the Dance is a paradoxical one of "anticipatorily shadowing our beloved dying."

Our primary guide is deeply attuned intuition informed by a lifetime's knowledge and full, bodymind listening. The overarching principles for dancing the Dance are to be deeply attuned to her and our own intuition while staying ahead of the curve.

Core Question. Embedded in the idea of *her* curve is the single most important question we have to ask throughout each phase of her decline and dying: What does she want? Her subjectivity is the centerpost around which the dance pivots. The Dance of Death is a relational model in which she who is dying is an active subject and partner.

Answering this question becomes more challenging as she gets closer to death and/or her mental faculties erode. The question may morph into: What *would* she want? Answering well requires deeply attuned listening.

In my mother's case, she had always been clear about what she wanted: to live independently and never end up in a nursing home. Her dread became concrete when she went into rehab. Olwen's dread and determination were so powerful that she, who had rallied so many times over the years, harnessed her anger and her indomitable will for one last big rally to get herself home again.

Her visceral reactions to rehab together with oft-repeated statements about not wanting to live forever and not wanting to go on and on gave me a clear, overarching goal and directive for navigating my path and creating a safe space for her: get her home, keep her out of a nursing home, get her off the medical treadmill, and let things unfold on her own timetable and in her own way. Having such a clear and unambiguous North Star by which to orient my caregiving was a gift by which not all caregivers are blessed.

Elaborating the Core. I have translated into words the intuitions that guided me during my Dances with Pandora and Olwen. Although they may seem obvious, the pain, guilt, and regrets I have heard from others who have not intuitively followed them (as well as my own failure to follow my intuition about the timetable for Elizabeth's death) tell me that they are, in fact, not obvious, nor easy to sort out and act upon in real time. The awe many friends have expressed about these Dances tell me they are well worth sharing.

I begin by elaborating my overarching principles into what we need to *know* and what we need to *do* in order to stay ahead of the curve. Four key questions that we need to keep asking are matched with four key steps in the Dance that help us answer them.

What We Need to Know

> *The caregiver with privileged access to the details of the person's daily condition may be the best judge of the cause of a change in a condition. This level of responsibility is a significant and singular aspect of the home care of the terminally ill.*
>
> —Andrea Sankar, PhD, gerontologist and medical anthropologist

The Dance of Death pivots around answers to four key questions that define her situation and the viability of our responses:

- What does she really want?
- Where is she now on her multi-dimensional journey?
- What does (and will) she need?
- Does the response (still) match the situation?

We are dancing the Dance of Death because we need to keep asking and rechecking our answers to these questions about her dynamic, unfolding, often volatile situation. We stay ahead of the curve when we intuit valid and viable answers and responses.

What does she really want? This question is first among equals because her subjectivity is the centerpost around which everything else should pivot. The other three questions come into play as she begins to lose—whether gradually, quickly, or intermittently—her full adult, mental and/or physical capacities.

What she wants can be on many scales, from a glass of ice cold water immediately to hearing a favorite story again, to not feeling abandoned, to going Home soon. As faculties and systems fail, her ability to translate her needs and wishes into words may also be failing. Nonetheless, her insights and utterances may sometimes surprise us by their clarity and profundity. She may communicate her needs in physical or novel ways. The more open we are to how she communicates and the multiple scales or planes on which she may be communicating, the better the quality of the flow between us, the more effective we can be on her behalf, and the better we will feel about ourselves both in the moment and in the forever that follows her death.

Where is she? Her journey is emotional and spiritual, supported by her body systems, her mobility, her mind/brain, and the all-important intangibles of drive and strength of will. We have to assess, as best we can, all of these aspects of herself while they are in motion, changing, fluctuating, and interacting. There is no room for denial, only for clear-eyed attending and assessing that is at once compassionate and dispassionate. What is very tricky is trying to distinguish between fluctuations in her strength and abilities, temporary changes (due to hospitalization, drugs, or outside events), and permanent changes that are part of a downward trajectory. Trajectories never follow a smooth, even course, so we can easily be fooled, especially if we are in denial or not paying close enough attention, or paying attention to indicators that turn out to be misleading.

What does/will she need? Our answers to the questions of what she wants and where she is are the basis for answering the third: What does/will she need? Sometimes it is obvious, like the right support pillow, knowing where her glasses are, or being in charge of the keys, but often we have to figure it out by tapping a lifetime's knowledge without letting old stuff get in the way. Many anticipatory actions relate to her physical and financial needs or to the rules of the players, organizations, programs, and institutions that shape and constrain our action arena. Many others try to affirm her life, her value, and her meaning, and address anxieties that arise from "unfinished business."

Do our actions match her situation? Her dynamic, fluctuating-yet-ultimately-deteriorating situation is composed of what she wants, where she is, and what she needs. As caregivers, we are trying to translate our understanding of her situation into responsive and anticipatory actions. We continue to check on their viability: do they meet and match her needs? "Responsive actions" respond to immediate or manifest needs. "Anticipatory actions" are geared to where her curve is headed as well as to her deepest needs, which may be unspoken.

The Four A's: What We Need to Do

How do we go about answering these questions about what she wants and where she now is? What do we need to be doing? What *is* the Dance? Are there steps, or is it just free-form?

I have decomposed the Dance into four steps: attending/attuning; assessing; anticipating; and acting/advocating. These steps are fluid; in the real world, they flow into and out of each other. The "Four A's" are also iterative: we keep going through cycle after cycle of testing, recalibrating, and revising our observations, assessments, and actions. Through iterative cycles of the Four A's, we try our best to understand what she wants and where she is, and we invent anticipatory actions that meet her as she moves further into her journey.

Attending/Attuning to the dying means hanging out, staying open, seeing what is present and what is absent, where holes and gaps exist, what isn't there to hold, meet, or support her, and responding appropriately. It is not about filling silences with chatter; it is about listening with one's whole being and becoming attuned to hers.

Attunement is at the very heart of the broader process of attending. As her mode of communication changes, our mode of listening has to shift. We take our cues from what we observe and what she says—especially about her impending death—treating her utterances with respect, not dismissing them, or denying them, or changing the subject. When she begins to let go, we are a presence and bear witness. We do not cling to her because we haven't done our own homework. She is doing the hardest work of her life, and we should be doing no less.

Assessing the dying is enabled by immersing ourselves in the daily process while maintaining enough distance to pick up cues, notice changes, make comparisons and assessments, and hypothesize about what is going on. It is often difficult to distinguish fluctuations from changes. It is also often difficult to assess the source of observed changes, especially as multiple body and/or cognitive systems become compromised.

The clinicians involved in overseeing her clinical care may be helpful and able to answer some questions that help us with our broader assessments, but they come and go, have a segmented acquaintance, and may have met her but recently. Hands-on caregivers who spend time with her (such as hospice nurses or privately hired caregivers), like family caregivers, make micro-observations on a daily basis that are essential to assessing the situation near the end of life. Those who are drawn to this book are likely to know her better than anyone else, or at least have lifelong knowledge. Our challenge is to gather all the micro-observations and professional experience together with our knowledge of our parent to assess the situation.

Anticipating is the basis for preparatory actions in the inner and outer worlds that surrounds our dying partner, and for changes in our own psyches and readiness for what lies ahead. It requires detaching from old patterns and assumptions, and giving up what worked yesterday, but not today. Anticipating assumes that we are not in denial and are willing to walk each step as it comes. It asks us to discern the trajectory, as best we can, through the confusing veils of fluctuations, episodes, and discontinuities, and the ups and downs among the multiple variables we are tracking. It requires that we stay open to upticks and surprises, make the most of them, but not be drawn into false hopes. It means enlisting resources when and where they can be of the greatest help.

Acting/advocating refers to the responsive and anticipatory actions we need to take to address her situation, current and future. We try to respond to needs that are manifest and latent, spoken and unspoken, physical-financial and emotional-spiritual. We assess how well our current actions match her situation, and make adjustments. Many of our actions require assertiveness, others require receptivity and presence, and some require balancing both.

Cycles

As with any dance, the steps keep repeating in regular ways. As we trace those cycles, we try to pick up downward inflections in the rate of decline.

Figure 18-1 depicts the four major steps in the Dance of Death as they iteratively feed and flow into each other. They help us to understand her situation—most critically, what she wants and where she is—and take actions that are not only responsive, but that also anticipate where and how she may next need to be met and held. We are trying to match her unfolding situation to the space we create for her journey to complete itself. We keep reassessing the match: what is still working and what needs to be added or changed or revisited?

Intuitively staying ahead of the curve thus entails cycles of attending and attuning; noticing cues; listening in new languages; making comparisons; forming hypotheses, yet staying open and flexible; taking anticipatory actions, and testing their continued appropriateness; acknowledging and letting go of what has been lost or is being lost; and repeating cycles while moving on in the journey with open hearts and minds.

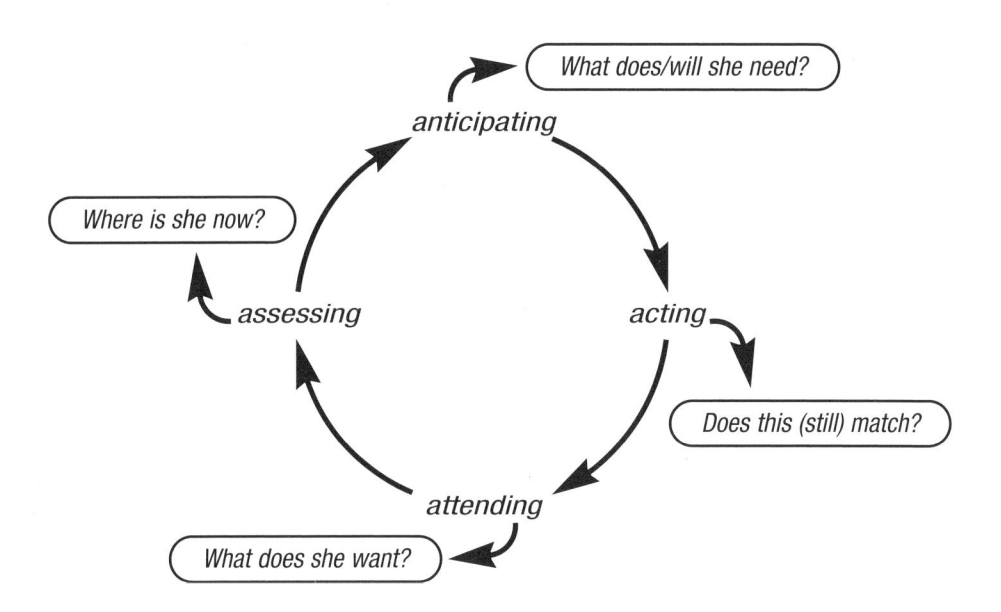

Figure 18-1. Intuitively Staying Ahead of the Curve: Steps in the Dance

The Three P's: Building a Containing Space for Our Dance

The Four A's do not take place in a vacuum. Our ability to pay attention to the Four A's is interdependent with the quality of the space in which we are dancing. Does that environment undermine what we are trying to do and make us dance uphill? Or does it enable and support our intimate Dance so that it can unfold as fully as possible?

In an ideal world, a supportive ecology for the Dance would already be in place, and we would have grown up learning in our bones how to be in that space. In the world as it is, we do our best to reshape the environment of dying by building a "container" of alignment, safety, responsiveness, presence, and engagement which befits the completion of a life and our relationship.

Building a container is our most comprehensive role in dancing. Being conscious of it gives coherence and meaning to all of the things—many seemingly small, mundane, and unrelated—that we and many others may be doing to enhance the dying process.

Our container has three levels—the Three P's: a palliative paradigm of care; a physical-energetic ecology of comfort, respect, and privacy; and our evolving quality of presence.

Palliative Paradigm. We should not have to be struggling with an uncoordinated, fix-and-cure, DRG-driven bevy of medical professionals and institutions when our parent's body insists on moving toward death. The foundations for dying well begin by aligning the medical paradigm, the clinicians involved in her care, and their integrated care plan with what she needs: freedom from pain, management of symptoms, responsiveness, and authentic engagement.

Hospice can help us to shape the caregiving environment by shifting the paradigm to palliative care, providing medical expertise and backup, supporting us as well as our parent, and giving us the courage and confidence to oversee her care. Its staff embody the respectful comfort with the dying that we want in our caregiving family. Innovative palliative care units are also shifting the paradigm and trying to provide a physical environment more attuned to the dying and their families.

Physical-Sensory-Energetic Ecology. The standard hospital environment—with its dreadful and disrespectful blend of intrusiveness and abandonment, cheeriness and denial, fluorescence and chemical air—is the very antithesis of what a dying person (or a recovering sick person) needs. Although it is often not possible to keep an elder at home throughout their decline and dying, it is the ideal that most Americans say they want. The familiarity of home is comforting, orienting, and, we hope, provides privacy and emotional as well as physical safety.

The physical-sensory-energetic ecology we create or modify and how we use it are of enormous importance. When we are able to offer home care, we try not to turn a living room or bedroom into a hospital room. We rearrange furniture to facilitate contact and connection, and we keep medical equipment and supplies out of sight as much as possible. We can respond immediately to her physical needs—for ice water, getting to the bathroom, being too hot or too cold. To set the tone, we can use warm, subdued lighting; flowers; and create a sound environment that is not harsh or intrusive, and uses appropriate music, silence, and comforting sounds. We can control air quality, temperature, who comes and goes, and when.

My transformative journey with Olwen could only have happened at home. Her body knew she was in her safe, familiar place even if her mind could no longer name it. We had complete privacy, which allowed her to express herself according to her own needs and rhythms, out of which extraordinary intimacy and moments of healing and transformation emerged. Such moments were not interrupted by institutional schedules or the intrusions of roommates' families. In my experience, *knowing* that they will not be interrupted is part of what allows them to happen in the first place.

> *Those, like myself, who accompany the dying know just how much we receive as a gift simply by accepting the commitment to embark on this ultimate experience in a human relationship that is proffered to us by the dying patient . . . The gamble of this ultimate relationship seems to reside in the attempt to reveal oneself as one really is, or, to use Michel de M'Uzan's expression, to "give birth to oneself in the world before leaving it."*
> —Marie de Hennezal, PhD, palliative care psychologist

Presence. Psychologically and interpersonally, we create a container through the evolving nature of our containing presence. We evolve in relation to her eroding abilities and emerging needs.

Just as a "good-enough mother" provides a psychological "holding environment" in which an infant becomes a person,[2] so does the mature adult child provide a holding environment in which their failing parent moves through decline toward death. But rather than progressively pulling ourselves back in response to the child's increasing abilities, we progressively move into our parent's personal and decision-making space, filling in gaps and losses, substituting our judgment for hers, and propping up her life and, sooner or later, her body. Through intimate knowledge of a parent, we create a supportive context that holds and tries to meet her fears, needs, and hopes. We fill in blanks, unstated references, and use that knowledge to follow the shifting currents of her mind.

Just as good-enough mothering allows the child to keep expanding their limits, so also does good-enough dancing meet and hold her without supplanting her own initiatives, movements, and modes of conversation. Over the course of decline and dying, we create a series of spaces in which, through our containing presence, she can be all that she can be at that time or in that moment.

If she becomes disoriented by hospitalizations and eventually by the failure of bodily systems, we need to be aware that we ourselves constitute her primary context. The more a disoriented or dying person loses

> Creating a "container" has parallels with being a "good-enough mother," but it is not a role reversal. The notion that we reverse roles with our failing parents is misguided. The parent is always the parent and the child is always the child. That biological and psychological fact, our generational difference, and our long relationship history do not change or reverse themselves. However, becoming the *mature* adult child for a declining or dying parent represents a dramatic shift from earlier phases of parent-child relationships, and it does have parallels with effective parenting.

their bearings in relation to their surroundings, the more dependent they become on their caregivers to provide a feeling of safety, familiarity, self, and connection.

Our presence evolves from deep listening and authentic engagement to being an often silent witness whose presence is communicated energetically and through physical contact. Ultimately, the greatest gift we can give her is to ourselves embody a safe physical-energetic-emotional-spiritual container for the awesome mystery of letting go of her life.

Summary

The Dance of Death is an indivisible whole in motion. Dying becomes a duet of movement co-composed by the dying partner and her caregiver who is anticipatorily shadowing her. The overarching principles for dancing the Dance are to be deeply attuned to our dying partner and our own intuition while staying ahead of the curve.

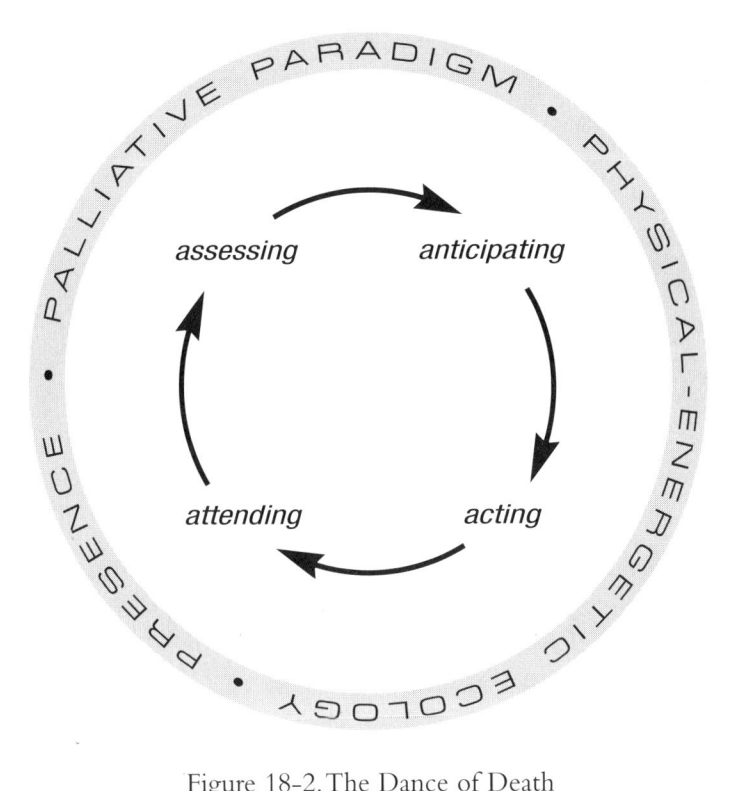

Figure 18-2. The Dance of Death

I have elaborated these ideas by asking four basic questions and answering them through the Four A's which describe what the caregiver does. The movement of the Dance is expressed in these four iterative steps that flow into and out of each other and allow us to stay ahead of the curve.

We find the coherence in all that we (and others) are doing when we see ourselves as creating a safe, respectful, responsive, intimate, and ultimately sacred container that is physical, sensory, psychological, interpersonal and energetic, and that is clinically and culturally supported by a palliative care philosophy. Because each of the Three P's is a holistic quality organizing and permeating the dance space as a totality, I have drawn them as an embracing circle around the Four A's in Figure 18-2.

Nineteen

Dancing the Dance of Death

> *At the moment of utter solitude, when the body breaks down on the edge of infinity, a separate time begins to run that cannot be measured in any normal way . . . [W]ith the help of another presence that allows despair and pain to declare themselves, the dying seize hold of their lives, take possession of them, unlock their truth. They discover the freedom of being true to themselves. It is as if, at the very culmination, everything managed to come free of the jumble of inner pains and illusions that prevent us from belonging to ourselves.*
>
> —François Mitterand, former President of France
> and quiet champion of compassionate dying

The Four A's tell us about the dance steps, while the Three P's direct our attention to building a container of alignment, safety, responsiveness, presence, and engagement for dancing and letting go of a life. They make conscious important things we need to be doing. What we still have not addressed is *how* to dance the Dance of Death. What principles can guide our empathically attuning, attending, and anticipating? How do we become a containing presence?

Guiding Principles

My principles for guiding our dancing direct our attention to the one thing over which we have some control: ourselves. We cannot control the Dance, but we *can* dance with intention. The guiding principles orient us and give us a way of dancing that improves the chances that the Dance will go well, or as well as it can, given the situation. They help us come back to what is really important. They bring us back to our deepest and best selves when the situation is chewing us up and we feel like we are disappearing.

These guiding principles, like the dance steps and the three P's, are not intended to add more layers to the burden of caregiving, or ratchet up the standard so we feel we have never done enough—as has happened with parents who turn themselves into pretzels around their kids. Rather, they are directed to our internally reconfiguring our intention and our priorities—and, when necessary, jolting our mental and emotional default settings—so that the urgent does not crowd out the important. These steps and principles are not about spending *more* time and energy, but paying conscious attention to what we are doing with the time and energy available to us, so that we are doing what truly matters.

Being Fully Present. How do we stay ahead of the curve, develop our intuition as a trustworthy guide, and enable ourselves to become a containing presence? By being fully present to ourselves, our beloved dying, and the situation.

Making decisions based on one's intuition requires trusting yourself; no one can confirm your intuitions, and others' well-intended recommendations may ran counter to them. I found that whenever I trusted my intuition, my choices were virtually always right. What enables intuition to become a reliable guide? *The interaction between our deep knowledge of our beloved dying, and an unblinkered attunement to the present. The past informs, but does not blind us.*

That same presence and attunement to your partner and her rhythms is the key to the paradox of leading what we must follow. Our focus shifts from the interaction between past (knowledge) and present (attunement/attending/assessing) to the interaction between present and future (anticipating and preparing for what is to come). What enables us to work ahead is being fully present to her and her current situation—i.e., being *on* her curve. The clearer we can be about the present, the more effective we can be in working ahead.

We anticipatorily shadow our dying person or animal companion not only so that material stuff, other players, and the next arrangements are ready, but also so that we can catch ourselves up psychologically and emotionally with where she now is and where she is heading. We shadow her so that we are ready to meet, hold, and support her in the next moment. There are many facets of being fully in the moment with our dying parent. For example:

- We look disease, decline, and death squarely in the face. We don't look away, or pretend this is not happening. We don't procrastinate. We walk every step of the process, step by step.

- We offer, but do not force, a spectrum of support and healing modalities for sustaining the quality of life. For as long as is appropriate, we support the physical maintenance of life. We do not, however, forcefeed a body whose failing systems can handle food less and less and, eventually, not at all.

- We meet her where she is, take our cues from her, peg our activities to her rhythms, energy level, and lucidity.

- We use our voice and words to convey important things (including leaving and returning to the room), but do not chatter to fill the silences, or avoid being present, or make ourselves comfortable.

- We try not to allow the urgent to crowd out the important. When you find yourself swimming in the urgent, pull yourself back, take stock, and refocus on the truly important.

    > Much of what you have to manage is time-critical and urgent—e.g., the immediate needs of the dying, communications with other players, scheduling caregivers, getting people on the same page, meeting deadlines imposed by rules and regulations. Caregiving time requires "doing" activities, whether with her, on the phone, or out in the world. Yet, this can crowd out what is truly important: being-with your dying parent in the moment.

    > In my experience, temporal separations are the key to finding a balance between doing stuff and being-with, between outer activities and inner presence. Being fully present-and-with is *part* of your day, but not the whole day. Neither she nor you can sustain the prolonged

intensity of being-fully-with around the clock. She must rest and do end-of-life work, and you must recenter and do stuff.

- Being-with is not hovering-over or intruding-upon. Being-with requires you to be as centered and relaxed and open as possible so that you can be available to her without intruding on her space.
- We form an intention (such as gratitude, if you do in fact feel it) to guide our important time with her. While she is still conscious and cognizant, you may want to create an honoring ceremony, or informally lace your time together with remembering and honoring.

  This may not be possible in relationships that have been abusive or neglectful, but you may still find ways to be open to surprises and moments of connection or healing.

- We tune into our intuition, respect it, and, after due consideration, are not afraid to act on it—especially if we know her more deeply and more fully than anyone else.

  Intuition needs to be grounded in empathy and supported by the capacity to tune into what *she* wants. It is not about projecting our will on her and everyone else.

  Remember, no matter how well we dance, we cannot act on our attunement and intuitions perfectly because there are far too many unknowns. We cannot control these unknowns, and we must trade them off against competing demands in our lives. Do not expect perfection from yourself. You do the best you can at the time and try to optimize among competing and conflicting demands.

- We trust the process. Trust her timing.

While the principles of staying ahead of the curve and looking at death and dying squarely in the face were instilled in me through my mother since childhood, following intuition, being in the moment, trusting the process, and trusting the timing were things that Mother had been cut off from long ago, and from which I became cut off in childhood. (She did trust her Lord, however, and so she carried a sense that there was a reason she was still here, and that there was some kind of higher, unknowable logic that had a hand in such things.) Over decades, I regained these abilities, in part through trusting my healing and dying Dance with Pandora and having them borne out.

Trusting Mother's process and timing was the most challenging of all of the principles for me. The times I didn't follow my intuition made things less than they could have been, but fortunately, on really critical decisions—especially continually saying no to respite care—I did stay in the moment and with my intuition. It made all the difference.

> *Most people who are dying still have the capacity to change in ways that are important to them. Their transformation can also make an enormous, and lasting, difference to the people around them.*
>
> —Ira Byock, MD, palliative care physician-champion

Letting Go and Staying Open. What helps us to be fully present? In my experience, the more we can let go and open our own mental space, the more present we can be, and the more we can create space with our dying partner for something new and unexpected to happen. Letting go is a mutual, two-way street. She is doing the hardest thing in her life. Why should it be easy for you?

Although it appears as if your dying partner is the one who has to let go and surrender, *you,* too must let go—not only of her, but also of your assumptions; habitual patterns in your relationship; projections; what you thought was true a day or minute ago; your sense of right timing; and your inner timetable for your own life and moving it forward. Giving up my strong, inner timetable and surrendering to the situation and her inner timetable was the hardest and scariest thing I had to do.

- Catch and challenge yourself when you see yourself doing old stuff. Try to let go of old patterns, assumptions, and defenses that may not be serving you well. Try not to project them onto her.

- Even though you may know her better than anyone, do not assume you know all about who she is. She may reveal or express parts of herself that were there all along, but you never saw or noticed. Don't block them out now.

- Let go of forms in which you may hold your hopes. The Conversation may turn out to be much less verbal than you fantasized and may happen in scattered odd moments.

- Don't tell her how she *should* react or respond to her decline, to a hospitalization, or, most of all, being put in a nursing home. She needs validation, and the freedom to find her own way through such ruptures to her sense of self, independence, and security.

One moment can retroactively flood an entire lifetime with meaning.
—Sandra Bertman, PhD, death-and-dying educator

The most important and transformative moments during my mother's journey all had the element of surprise. Only by my staying open and receptive did we have those profound and healing moments together.

- Stay open to what she says or does, to moments that may happen between you, and to the form in which they occur.

- If they come "out of the blue," do not continue on the track you were on, but stop, tune in, and let her know you heard her and you get what she is saying. *If she is (finally) pitching, you had best be catching.*

- When she tells you (in whatever way) it is her time or gives you The Look (as animals often do), immediately stop anything else you may be doing or saying and meet her where she is. Acknowledge that you know, and that you know she knows.

- Hold her gaze, do not joke, discount, or invalidate those profound moments of her acknowledging her impending death and your impending separation.

Olwen sometimes responded tomorrow to yesterday's question, which suggests a different, slower, and perhaps, deeper way of processing. Yet, she captured the heart of the matter over and over again, grasping the meaning or the gist of what was going on, despite the fact that she could not do rapid-fire, question-and-answer sessions. Many of her utterances were holographic and multi-scaled in nature. They raise intriguing questions about the substructure of consciousness beneath society's artificial rules of thought which become irrelevant when we are engaged in the great project of bringing life on earth to a close.

- Do not map the artificial rules of our constructed reality onto the one who is dying. Let go of the judgments and categories enforced by these rules.

- Do your utmost to respect rather than dismiss or judge unfamiliar states of consciousness or unconventional modes of speech. Listen carefully and take notes. You may be surprised later by their insights and wisdom.

Our three-dimensional, time-ordered, linear reality has been constructed and superimposed upon a vast reality that may have eleven or more dimensions, some curled up inside our accepted dimensions, and operating on nonlocal or quantum principles about which we know next to nothing. Yet our waking consciousness has been molded by the same mechanistic principles that have organized science and society since the seventeenth century. When we use those antiquated standards to enforce conventions of linear thought and speech, we can easily dismiss thought patterns of the very ill and the dying as "confused" and derogate their visual impressions which we cannot see as "hallucinations." We thereby potentially harm the dying and cheat both them and ourselves.

What if some of their non-linear, verbal expressions or visual impressions are not products of delirium, disorientation, dementia, drugs, infection, or a failing bodymind? What if, as the conventions of speaking loosen their hold and drift away, a dying person's consciousness begins to function in other modes—modes not easily represented by linear language, modes more suited to the end of life than conducting daily business? What if the dying process tears down the three-dimensional fences and allows the journeyer to move far more fluidly through her expanding consciousness and begin merging with a greater Consciousness? What if the dying have things to teach us about consciousness?

Stay open to extraordinary experiences which may or may not be in accordance with your belief system. By allowing extraordinary experiences to flow through us without resistance and without trying to map interpretations on them, we can open to something larger and potentially transformative.

- Do not discount these experiences as unreal or label them dismissively. Do not overlay them with religious beliefs that constrict and foreclose on their meaning. Materialist scientism and conventional religion can both close down that which most needs to be open.
- Simply stay open and let those moments flow through you. *They don't need a name or a label.*
- If you stay open, such extraordinary moments can profoundly alter your consciousness and transform your relationship—permanently.

Why is it important for us as caregivers to be at ease with extraordinary experiences? As their mental structures for living in this world fall away, the dying seem to flow in and out of other dimensions and forms of consciousness, and become receptive to what may lie beyond this world. When we enter deeply into their dying process *with* them, suspend our own mental furniture, and allow ourselves to become open and receptive, we are less likely to squash, dismiss, or mislabel their expanding consciousness, and cheat them—and ourselves—of their dying's being all that it can be. We can go much more deeply with them on their journey, and their journey may complete itself in a fuller way that has powerful and permanent effects on everyone who is intimately involved.

Summary

What enables us to dance well is being fully present to the moment. Our ability to be present is enhanced by letting go of all that no longer serves us or her while staying open and receptive to the moment and surprises. What binds everything together is the understanding that our role as a mature adult child is shifting: we are becoming a containing presence for our parent's decline and dying, the bookend to her having created a holding environment for us in our infancy. As she moves closer to death, the space we create for her to let go of her life becomes sacred space.

Dance and Story

The Dance of Death is both the heart of the Caregiver's Story and its containing context. By integrating all the models in Figure 19-1, we see why the process is so all-consuming, exhausting, and uniquely rewarding.

- You are trying to understand what she wants, assess where she is, anticipate her needs, and navigate a path through your choices, which create space for her life to complete itself in the fullest way it can.

- Dancing well is enhanced by: being fully present and open to the moment; letting go of anything blocking that; attending and listening; following attuned intuition; and recognizing your most comprehensive roles as containing presence and shaper of the space in which the Dance unfolds.

- Your Dance plays out within the context of the hopes and history of your relationship, the shape and speed of her trajectory of diminishing functionality, the impact and consequences of the demands of caregiving on your health and life, and your coping with uncertainties and dilemmas that can rip you apart while managing an often considerable cast of players and decision-makers within the constraints of many sets of rules—all within a death-phobic culture that does not validate or honor your process and makes it much harder and lonelier than it needs to be.

Figure 19-1 gives coherence to the Dance and Story so we can get our arms around them. It is a tool for orienting ourselves to all we are doing or did, and perhaps for communicating with others who do not yet know what we are talking about. It situates us at the center of it all, with a grasp of what we have to manage. Yet even with a map and conscious knowledge of steps and dance principles, it is overwhelming. How on earth do we manage it all?

The Heart of the Dance. Ultimately, we meet the demands of this profound process by digging way down into our love, experiencing at the deepest level what it means for love to "crucify" as it "crowns" us.[1] Thus it is that those who have midwifed the journey Home for some-

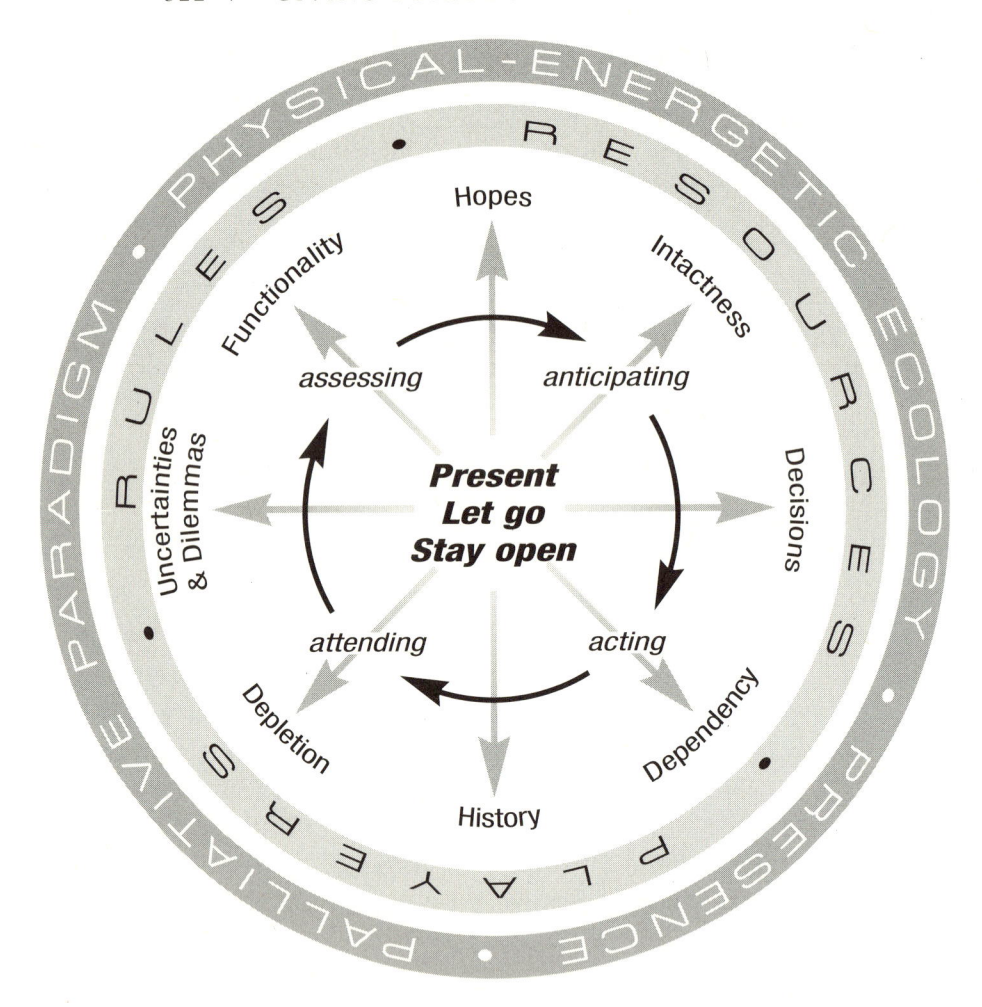

Figure 19-1. Dance of Death: Heart and Container of the Caregiver's Story

one they love often believe, as Andrea Sankar tells us, that it was their finest hour, the greatest accomplishment of their lives.

Love is the living, transformative force that makes sense of this daunting process and charts a path through the maze. Without a deep reservoir of love to tap, into the Dance will not go well or even be danced.

The Limits of the Dance. Despite our best efforts, our Dance may be very far from perfect. We will screw up and the doctors will screw up and the nurses will screw up and even hospice will screw up. Sooner or later, everybody will screw up. If we're lucky, the screw-ups and their consequences will be reversible and we will learn from them and make course corrections.

Some screw-ups happen because our structurally fragmented healthcare system is organized around insurers rather than the patient, and routinely produces and condones an unsafe, inefficient delivery system. Some screw-ups are products of a society that dumps onto individuals the responsibilities of the local and larger communities and does not support family caregivers. To achieve consistent, high-quality, end-of-life care at drastically lower costs, we must:

- fundamentally reorganize healthcare delivery and shift to a single-payer system;
- de-institutionalize long-term care and end-of-life care, and create home-like alternatives (e.g., Green Houses) to the 17,000 fossils—nursing homes—now warehousing many elders who cannot stay in their own homes;
- change perverse financial incentives and financial misalignments which, among other things, force unwanted treatments on the dying, and make family members feel guilty if they don't "choose" to do "everything possible";
- make attentive and respectful palliative care standard for end-of-life care in any setting;
- adopt, implement, and institutionalize public policies that support family caregivers, home care, as well as the de-institutionalization of long-term care.

Sometimes, what feel like screw-ups are simply by-products of being human with limited knowledge. We are not omniscient; we cannot control the dying process; and we have our own needs. We will make choices that in hindsight, we will wish we could rewind and do over. Even though we do the best we can with what we have at the moment, we will later see how we could have done something better or another way, or that we had more options than we realized at the time, or that there were other things we could have been doing that we never thought of. We try to dissuade our friends from beating themselves up on such accounts, and we have to find the same compassion for ourselves.

The most overwhelming and pervasive emotion that surrounds the caregiving of failing and dying parents is guilt—guilt that we did not do enough, whether in prime time, the declining years, or in the dying process; guilt that we did things to take care of ourselves when we "should" have been with her; guilt that "if only" we had done thus and so, something would have turned out differently; guilt that we got frustrated and angry when we should have been patient and calm.

When guilt and our imperfections overwhelm us, we need to remember the forest and not the trees. The container is built from all you did do, not all the other little things you didn't think of. Ultimately, what matters is your containing presence which registers at such a profound level that your dying parent can trust she will not be abandoned.

There is no "perfect" here. *Caregiving is about doing the best we can with what we have and where we are at the time.* In telling my story and sketching out my suggestions for dancing the Dance of Death, my intent is to help you shed guilt and the sense of powerlessness. Given that our culture does not teach us how to bring closure and resolution to the most important and powerful relationships in our lives, nor how to facilitate dying well, this book is intended to help you gather more awareness, knowledge, and wisdom for dancing as well as possible.

As Gerda Lerner has written, to be the person whom the beloved dying needs for their dying is a heavy and blessed experience. My intent is to help you have a blessed experience as you navigate your journey by providing a few maps, more awareness of what you may encounter, more compassion and validation for yourself, and guiding principles to orient and direct the only thing over which you have control—how you choose to dance your half of the Dance.

A Relational Paradigm for Dying Well

A mutual relationship is a relationship where neither person is at the center. Relationship *is."*
—Judith V. Jordan, PhD, Jean Baker Miller Training Center

The Caregiver's Story and its heart and soul, the Dance of Death, are relational models about interacting, interconnected subjects—models which I drew out of my journey with Olwen. I did not set out to create a "relational paradigm for dying well," but early readers recognized such a paradigm in our dance.

By "relational," they and I reference the model of human development co-created by Jean Baker Miller, Irene Stiver, Judith V. Jordan, Janet Surrey, Alexandra Kaplan and an ever-expanding network of relational psychology colleagues whose hub is the Stone Center and Jean Baker Miller Training Institute at Wellesley College; and by Carol Gilligan, Mary Belenky and colleagues rooted at the Harvard School of Education.[2]

Launched by Miller in 1976 as a "new psychology of women," this body of work is now understood as a model of *human* development based on a natural path of connection and empathy that boys and men are routinely pushed out of by the construction and demands of a disconnected masculinity.

Over the past three decades, relational psychologists have built a powerful and persuasive body of work demonstrating that we can only grow into emotionally mature, authentically individuated adults *through* caring, empathic relationship and connection. They began their paradigm-shattering work by exploring in great depth the neglected subject of empathy, recognizing that it is the key to movement and growth in relationships.

Empathy is emotional attunement to the other that allows one to be with them in their experience while inflecting that experience from a different center. When both parties are open to being affected by the other, the combination of emotional responsiveness and difference generates movement in each person and in their relationship. "Empathy is the sense of connection and the connector."[3]

Mutual empathy is thus the pivotal dynamic nurturing growth. Self and relationship are inseparable, interdependent partners in human growth—like twin strands of DNA. In relational psychology, one's expanding capacity for authentic, empathic relationships is the key barometer of maturation.

This work fundamentally challenges traditional psychologies which insist we can only become persons (and boys become "masculine" men) by disconnecting and separating from relationship (and from women). These psychologies thereby make self and relationship antagonistic opposites, especially for men, and disparage women as lesser beings ("dependent," "enmeshed," "weak") because of their propensity for relating to others.

This disparaging of relationship short-circuits how we deal with death and loss. Based on extensive interviews, Sally Cline observes that women tend to experience death and loss as interior, relational, and ultimately unresolvable. A woman does not, she says, ever fully "recover" from her great losses but evolves into a new person who carries those losses within her reconstituted self, and continues to "work" them without time limits, quite often for the rest of her life.[4]

Yet women's internalized experience of death, she writes, has been erased into men's experience of death as an external event to be managed, overcome, and put behind them. By this numbing cultural standard, there is something "wrong" with those who don't "get over" their losses and "get back to normal." The consequence of "getting over" death is that we cannot learn, grow, or heal. Our cultural standard for grieving is antithetical to the wisdom attributed to Aeschylus and cited by Bobby Kennedy during his own years of amazing growth: "He who learns must suffer, and even in our sleep, pain that cannot forget falls drop by drop upon the heart. And in our despair, against our will, comes wisdom to us by the awful grace of God."

The Caregiver's Story and the Dance of Death give recognition, structure, and voice to a relational mode of caregiving, and extend relational psychology in a new direction. The Story and the Dance are premised on the caregiver's capacity and willingness to empathically attune herself to the wants and needs of her dying parent, and on their having or trying to have meaningful connection. During their dance, both partners have opportunities to learn and grow in and through relationship, and possibly achieve breakthroughs that previously eluded them. By opening to each other and to the Dance, some of the old and difficult places in their relationship may come unstuck, releasing deeper levels of love, empathy, gratitude, and forgiveness, whose flow is healing and even transformative.

Epigraphs from Published Sources

(sources marked with * are fully referenced in Further Reading)

Introduction

Gerda Lerner, *A Death of One's Own* (Madison: University of Wisconsin Press, 1978/1985), 133. Cited with permission from Prof. Lerner. I found this quote in Sandra Bertman's, *Facing Death, 95.**

Part I: Where are We?

John Briggs and F. David Peat, *Seven Life Lessons of Chaos*. Found in Karen Speerstra's compendium, *Divine Sparks: Collected Wisdom of the Heart* (Sandpoint, ID: Morning Light Press, 2005), 62.

Chapter 2. Hospitalizations

Sharon K. Inouye, "A Practical Program for Preventing Delirium in Hospitalized Elderly Patients," *Cleveland Clinic Journal of Medicine* 71, no.11 (November 2004): 890.

Chapter 7. Building Family of Caregivers

Marie de Hennezel, *Intimate Death*, 95.*

Part III. Rhythms of the Dance

David Hare, screenwriter, from the motion picture, "The Hours," courtesy of Paramount Pictures Corporation.

Chapter 11. Path through the Shadows

Colette, *My Mother's House* (New York: Farrar, Straus & Young, 1953) cited by Hope Edelman at the front of her book, *Motherless Daughters* (New York: Dell Publishing, 1994). Edelman found this quotation in Mary Jane Moffatt, ed., *In the Midst of Winter* (New York: Vintage, 1992 edition), 193.

Edelman, *Motherless Daughters*, xviii, xix.

Adrienne Rich, *Of Woman Born* (New York: Norton, 1986), 237.

Deena Metzger, *Writing for Your Life: a Guide and Companion to the Inner Worlds* (San Francisco: HarperSanFrancisco, 1992), 93.

Peggy Whiting and Elizabeth James, "Bearing Witness to the Story: Responses to Shadow Grief in Diverse Family Contexts," *Journal of Healing Ministry* (Winter 2005), 33. "Shadow grief" italicized in original.

Niels Bohr, in Speerstra, 471.

Whiting and James, "Bearing Witness," 33.

Chapter 12. Retrieving the Understory

Apara Borrowes, "My Ear was Tuned to the Great Below," unpublished poem used with permission from the author.

Chapter 13 Dance of Grace

Kahlil Gibran, *The Prophet* (New York: Alfred A. Knopf, 1923/1952), 81. Used by permission of Alfred A. Knopf, a division of Random House, Inc.

Chapter 14. Unexpected Gifts

Judith Viorst, *Necessary Losses* (New York: Ballantine Books, 1986), found in Speerstra, 343.

Robert A. Neimeyer, "Meaning Reconstruction and the Experience of Chronic Loss," in *Living with Grief When Illness is Prolonged,* 161.★

Chapter 15 Houses Speak

Simone Weil, *The Need for Roots,* found in Speerstra, 342.

Grace Paley, source unknown. Quote is mentioned by Don Murray, "Inside the Writing Process by Don Murray," *Boston Globe* (November 15, 2004).

Chapter 16 Roots and Completion

bell hooks, *Remembered Rapture: The Writer at Work* (New York: Henry Holt & Co., 1999) brought to my attention in a workshop by Maureen Murdock at the June 2006 International Women's Writing Guild conference at Skidmore College, Saratoga Springs, NY.

Hildegard of Bingen, found in Speerstra, 527.

Part V. Giving Form to Dance

Mary Catherine Bateson, *Full Circles, Overlapping Lives,* found in Speerstra, 511.

Chapter 17. Caregiver's Story

Susan Reinhard, Nursing's Role in Family Caregiver Support," in *Caregiving and Loss,* 181.★

Joanne Lynn, "Living Long in Fragile Health," in *Improving End of Life Care,* S14.★

Marie de Hennezel, *Intimate Death,* 25.★

Stephen Connor and Jocelia Adams, "Caregiving at the End of Life," in *Access to Hospice Care,* S8.★

Rosalynn Carter, "Foreword" to *Caregiving and Loss,* iv.★

Connor and Adams, "Caregiving," S8.★

Ira Byock, *Four Things,* 32.★

Andrea Sankar, *Dying at Home,* 7.★

Sandra R. Kaufman, . . . *And a Time to Die,* 28.★

Sankar, *Dying at Home,* 20.★

Bruce Jennings, True Ryndes, Carol D'Onofrio, and Mary Ann Baily, "Access to Hospice Care: Expanding Boundaries, Overcoming Barriers," lead article in *Access to Hospice Care,* S3.★

Chapter 18. Dance of Death

Byock, *Four Things,* 7.★

Sankar, *Dying at Home,* 8.★

de Hennezel, *Intimate Death,* 131, who quotes Michel de M'Uzan, "The Work of Death," in *From Art to Death* (Paris: Gallimard, 1977), 182-199.★

Chapter 19. Dancing

François Mitterand, "Foreword" to *Intimate Death,* ix.★

Byock, *Four Things,* 26.★

Sandra Bertman, *Facing Death,* 81.★

Judith V. Jordan, speaking at a 1999 colloquium, quoted by Christina Robb, *This Changes Everything: The Relational Revolution in Psychology* (New York: Farrar, Straus, and Giroux, 2006), 173.

Notes to Dying into Grace

Introduction
1. Andrea Sankar, *Dying at Home*, xv-xvi.*

Chapter 1. The Call
1. An excellent understanding of Reiki is now available from Pamela Miles, a pioneer in bringing Reiki into conventional medicine, *Reiki: a Comprehensive Guide* (New York: Tarcher/Penguin, 2006). Written with precision and attentiveness to nuance, Miles' book is as subtle as the practice about which she writes. Her website [www.ReikiInMedicine.org] offers excerpts from the book, medical papers about Reiki, and popular articles describing the use of Reiki in medical settings.

Chapter 2. Hospitalizations
1. A clear articulation and development of Toyota thinking can be found in the work of James P. Womack and Daniel T. Jones, *Lean Thinking: Banish Waste and Create Wealth in your Corporation* (New York: Free Press, 1996/2003). The Pittsburgh Regional Healthcare Initiative has pioneered the application of Toyota Production System principles to health care.
2. A panel of physicians working with Public Citizen's Health Research Group in their 2005 edition of *Worst Pills, Best Pills: A Consumer's Guide to Avoiding Drug-Induced Death or Illness* (New York: Simon & Schuster) suggests choosing other, safer antibiotics than the family to which "Q" belongs. Among its "side-effects" is abnormality in heart rhythm that can lead to death.
3. Inouye has summarized her research in "Delirium in Older Persons," *The New England Journal of Medicine* 354, no. 11 (March 16, 2006): 1157-1165.
4. Ibid., 1159.
5. Ibid., 1157.
6. Pointed out by Anne-Marie Audet, MD, in discussing the book, January 29, 2007.
7. Sharon K. Inouye, "A Practical Program for Preventing Delirium in Hospitalized Elderly Patients," *Cleveland Clinic Journal of Medicine* 71, no.11 (November 2004): 893-894; S.K. Inouye, et al., "Nurses' Recognition of Delirium and its Symptoms: Comparison of Nurse and Researcher Ratings," *Archives of Internal Medicine* 161 (2001): 2467-2473.

Chapter 3. Mobilizing
1. My suggestions for pronouncing Welsh names come from Tony Leaver, *Pronouncing Welsh Place Names* (Llanrwst: Gwasg Carreg Gwalch, 1998) with the exception of Gymanfa Ganu which I borrowed from the website of the Welsh National Gymanfa Ganu Association: www.wngga.org
2. The Green House Project exemplifies this approach. Artemis March, "Elder Homes Replace Nursing Homes in Tupelo, Mississippi," *Quality Matters*, 22 (January 2007). www.cmwf.org/publications/publications_show.htm?doc_id=441561#case

Chapter 7. Caregivers
1. Artemis March, "Consistency, Continuity, and Coordination: the 3Cs of Seamless Patient Care," http://www.ArtemisMarch.com; first published in *Quality Matters*, 18 (June 2006). http://www.cmwf.org/publications/publications_show.htm?_id=378546#perspective

Chapter 9. Letting Go
1. Hillary Johnson, *My Mother Dying*, (New York: St. Martin's Press, 1999) 175.
2. Marija Gimbutas, *Civilization of the Goddess* (San Francisco: HarperCollins, 1991); Gimbutas, *The Kurgan Culture and the Indo-Europeanization of Europe*, ed. Miriam Robbins Dexter and

/ 331

Karlene Jones-Bley (Washington, D.C.: Institute for the Study of Man, Journal of Indo-European Studies Monograph no. 18, 1997).
3. Richard Gerber, MD, *Vibrational Medicine* (Santa Fe: Bear & Company, 1988); James L. Oschman, *Energy Medicine: the Scientific Basis* (Edinburgh: Churchill Livingstone, 2000).
4. Brian Greene, *The Elegant Universe: Superstrings, Hidden Dimensions, and the Quest for the Ultimate Theory* (New York: Random House, 1999).

Chapter 11. Shadows

1. Debra Umberson, *Death of a Parent: Transition to a new Adult Identity* (Cambridge, UK: Cambridge University Press, 2003).
2. Peggy P. Whiting, "Walking Through the Shadows—Many Paths, One Journey," presentation at Association for Death Education and Counseling 26th Annual Conference, Pittsburgh, PA, March 2004.
3. The central myth of Sumerian culture tells the story of Inanna, the glorious and beloved Queen of Heaven and Earth (or Queen of the Great Above), who, in her maturity, journeys to her elder "sister", the primordial, enraged, unloved, wounded, fierce Ereshkigal, Queen of the Great Below. Through her descent, initiation, and "death" in the realm of the dark, low, and formless, Innana surrenders her illusions of control and opens to the wisdom of the Great Below, while compassion and witnessing open Ereshkigal to receiving love and healing, allowing the sisters to meet the other side of themselves and become the whole which maintains the balance and cycles of all life. Diane Wolkstein and Samuel Noah Kramer, *Inanna: Queen of Heaven and Earth, Her Stories and Hymns from Sumer*, (New York: Harper & Row, 1983); Sylvia Brinton Perera, *Descent to the Goddess: A Way of Initiation for Women*, New York: Inner City Books, 1981).

Chapter 12. Understory

1. My summary of Welsh culture and history and historical facts in this and the following paragraphs are derived from the classic study by historian R. Merfyn Jones, *The North Wales Quarrymen, 1874-1922* (Cardiff: University of Wales Press, 1982); and Janet Davies, *The Welsh Language* (Cardiff: University of Wales Press and The Western Mail, 1999).

Chapter 13. Dance of Grace

1. Gibran, *Prophet*, 81.

Chapter 15. Houses Speak

1. R. Mervyn Jones, *North Wales Quarrymen*, 25-27.
2. Griff Richard Jones, interview with Artemis March, August 23, 2005.
3. David Gwyn, interview with Artemis March, October 28, 2006.
4. Ibid. See also Gwyn's book: *Gwynedd: Inheriting a Revolution: The Archaeology of Industrialisation in North-west Wales* (Chichester: Phillimore, 2006).
5. In the United Kingdom, registries in each town keep track of births, marriages, and deaths. Records offices or archives are located in larger towns, and hold a much larger collection of documents for their entire shire or county. It is often difficult to find a birth certificate owing to administrative changes, the redrawing of boundaries over time, separate record-keeping by parish and civil authorities, and the tendency of individuals to refer variably to their birth village, county seat, or the shire itself as their place of birth.

Chapter 16. Roots and Completion

1. Merfyn Williams, *The Slate Industry*, (Princes Risborough: Shire Publications, 2002); R. Merfyn Jones, *The North Wales Quarrymen*; Griff Richard Jones, interview, August 23, 2005. Compensation rates varied, but getting paid more than five shillings a day was frequently a bargaining objective that was difficult to achieve.
2. R. Merfyn Jones, *North Wales Quarrymen*.
3. Griff Richard Jones, interview; R. Merfyn Jones, *North Wales Quarrymen*.
4. R. Merfyn Jones, *North Wales Quarrymen*; Williams, *Slate Industry*; Jean Lindsay, *A History of the North Wales Slate Industry* (Newton Abbot: David & Charles, 1973).
5. Gwyn, interview, October 28, 2006.

6. Ibid.
7. Ibid.
8. R. Merfyn Jones, *North Wales Quarrymen;* Alun John Richards, *Fragments of Mine and Mill in Wales* (Llanrwst: Gwasg Carreg Gwalch, 2002). Richards says those who had a bit of land identified themselves as "farmer" to the census takers because its status was higher than quarryman. Jones argues the opposite and marshalls more evidence for his claim.
9. R. Merfyn Jones, *North Wales Quarrymen,* 41-43.
10. Ibid.
11. Barbara Ehrenreich and Deirdre English, *Complaints and Disorders: The Sexual Politics of Sickness* (Old Westbury: Feminist Press, 1973) broke ground on this now well-documented fact.

Chapter 17. The Caregiver's Story

1. Caregiving may be shared or rotated by siblings or another "family" group or network ("family" meaning significant and committed people who may or may not have blood or legal ties), but in Part V, I write about the primary caregiver as being one person who is female. It is the situation I know best. Many of us are in this situation. Even when there are siblings or a family network, one person, usually female, often takes the lead. Surveys suggest women do 75-80% of family caregiving.
   The learning and wisdom I have distilled into articulating the Dance of Death and the Caregiver's Story can be applied to a caregiving relationship with a dying spouse or life partner, or a dying sibling or close friend, or a dying animal companion. My focus, however, is on intergenerational relationships that have the unique emotional power of parent and child, most particularly mother and daughter.
2. Joanne Lynn, "Living Long in Fragile Health," in *Improving End of Life Care* (2005): S16-S17.★
3. Susan Reinhard, "Nursing's Role in Family Caregiver Support," in *Caregiving and Loss,* 181.★ See also Agency for Healthcare Research and Quality, *The Characteristics of Long-Term Care Users* (Silver Spring, MD: AHRQ, 2000).
4. Carol Levine, "Introduction: Nature of Caregiving" in *Caregiving and Loss,* 5-18;★ Peter Arno, Carole Levine, and M.M. Memmott, "The Economic Value of Informal Caregiving," *Health Affairs,* 18, no. 2 (1999): 182-188; Peter Arno, "Economic Value of Informal Caregiving: 2000," presentation to the American Association for Geriatric Psychiatry, Orlando, FLA, 2002. See also an excellent document, "Family Caregiving and Public Policy: Principles for Change," 2003, on the National Alliance of Caregivers' website [http://www.caregiving.org], which organizes salient facts and references under a clear statement of principles developed by a collaborative group of family caregiver advocates.
5. Levine, "Nature of Caregiving." See also the work of Elizabeth Warren at the Harvard Law School on bankruptcies (triggered by medical bills in about 40 percent of cases), and the particular vulnerabilities of single women, divorcing and divorced women, and the elderly.
6. Levine, "Nature of Caregiving," 10-11; R. Schultz and S.R. Beach, "Caregiving as a Risk Factor for Mortality: the Caregiver Health Effects Study," *Journal of the American Medical Association,* 282, no. 23 (1999): 2215-2219; J. Kiecolt-Glaser et al., "Slowing of Wound Healing by Psychological Distress," *The Lancet,* 346 (1995): 1194-1196; Nicholas Christakis, Paul Allison, and Suzanne Salamon, "Mortality after the Hospitalization of a Spouse," *New England Journal of Medicine* 354, no. 7 (February 16, 2006).
7. Christakis, et al., "Mortality." Spouses suffering from dementia, psychiatric disease, hip or other serious fractures, chronic obstructive pulmonary disease, or congestive heart failure increased the risk of death by 12-28%, while other diagnoses had much smaller or no quantifiable effect.
8. Stephen Connor and Jocelia Adams, "Caregiving at the End of Life," in *Access to Hospice Care:* (2003): S8. Connor is research director of the National Hospice and Palliative Care Organization, and Adams is founder/director of the Center for Caregiver Training in San Francisco.
9. Bruce Jennings, True Ryndes, Carol D'Onofrio, and Mary Ann Baily, "Access to Hospice Care: Expanding Boundaries, Overcoming Barriers," lead article in *Access to Hospice Care,* S48.★
10. Jude Rabig, interview with Artemis March, December 22, 2006.
11. Sankar, *Dying at Home,* 5.
12. Surprises noted by Sankar, *Dying at Home,* 5, 128.
13. Sally Cline, *Lifting the Taboo: Women, Death, and Dying* (London: Little, Brown and Company, 1995), 96.

334 / DYING INTO GRACE

14. See, for example, Shirley Ann Smith, *Hospice Concepts*;* Marie de Hennezal, *Intimate Death*;* Ira Byock, *Dying Well*;* Ira Byock, *Four Things*;* Joanne Lynn, Joan Harrold, et al., *Handbook for Mortals*.*
15. Institute of Medicine, *To Err is Human, 1999*.* In mid-2006, the IOM released a new report, *Preventing Medication Errors*, focusing just on medication errors. The study concludes that: hospital patients can expect one medication error each day they are hospitalized, a minimum of 1.5 million of these medication errors harm patients, and that thousands die as a result.
16. Numerous studies showing poor communication with families, less attention to elderly and dying, and poor coordination among physicians can be found or referenced on websites such as those of the Commonwealth Fund [www.cmwf.org], the Robert Wood Johnson Foundation [www.rwjf.org], or the Institute for Healthcare Improvement [www.ihi.org]. See, for example, Dana Beth Weinberg et al., "Beyond Our Walls: Impact of Patient and Provider Coordination Across the Continuum of Outcomes for Surgical Patients," Commonwealth Fund, February 2007; see also my perspective on the "3Cs of Seamless Care," and Sharon R. Kaufman's, *And a Time to Die*.*
17. Kaufman, *And a Time to Die*, explains why. She combines exhaustive knowledge of the literature with in-depth field work to present a searing indictment of how managed care, the DRG structure of Medicare payments, the hospital system and its routines, and providers shape and manage the end of life, and evade the forthright discussion of death.
18. Ibid., 91.
19. Ibid., 29.

Chapter 18. Dance of Death

1. Wider affirmation of our experience and of the Reiki premise that the recipient is in charge of using the energy came out of a conversation with a Reiki master I met recently. From her practice and her students, she has learned that a sick cat will take in Reiki energy for about 45 minutes—just as Pandora did—but a healthy cat will barely sit still for even five minutes.
2. Donald Winnicott, *The Maturational Processes and the Facilitating Environment: Studies in the Theory of Emotional Development* (New York: International Universities Press, 1963), 43-45, 145-146, and passim.

Chapter 19. Dancing

1. Kahlil Gibran, *The Prophet*, 11.
2. Jean Baker Miller, *Toward a New Psychology of Women* (Boston: Beacon Press 1976/1986); Jean Baker Miller and Irene Stiver, *The Healing Connection: How Women form Relationships in Therapy and Life* (Boston: Beacon Press, 1997); Judith V. Jordan et al., *Women's Growth in Connection: Writings from the Stone Center* (New York: Guilford Press. 1991); Judith V. Jordan, Maureen Walker, Linda M. Hartling, *The Complexity of Connection: Writings from the Stone Center's Jean Baker Miller Training Institute* (New York: Guilford Press, 2004); and numerous books, and scores of reports and working papers from the Stone Center at Wellesley College. Carol Gilligan, *In a Different Voice: Psychological Theory and Women's Development* (Cambridge: Harvard University Press, 1982); Mary Field Belenky, Blythe McVicker Clinchy, Nancy Rule Goldberger, Jill Mattuck Tarule, *Women's Ways of Knowing: the Development of Self, Voice, and Mind* (New York: Basic Books, 1986). Christina Robb has told the story of these pioneers and their paradigm-breaking psychology in *This Changes Everything: the Relational Revolution in Psychology* (New York: Farrar, Straus and Giroux, 2006).
3. Robb, 2006, 163.
4. Cline, *Lifting the Taboo: Women, Death, and Dying*, interviewed 150 women and drew extensively on 80 interviews. See especially chapters 1, 3, and 4.

Further Reading and Resources

During my mother's late years, I knew of and had read but one caregiving book, *The 36-Hour Day,* a favorite at the local Office of the Aging. When we were in the thick of things, I had no time to go searching for things to read, and my mind wouldn't have been able to absorb much. The time to read is obviously in advance of late-life hospitalizations and dying. To read at all, we need to be aware of books as well as have access to them, enough money to buy them, or the time to urge our local library to acquire them. Web access through home and libaries is making it easier to find the growing numbers of books on senior issues, caregiving, and death and dying. Still, we need to focus. The readings annotated here and websites of some key organizations can be starting points for your search.

Institutional and Clinical Dying

Sharon R. Kaufman . . . *And a Time to Die: How American Hospitals Shape the End of Life.* Chicago: University of Chicago Press, 2006.
> Based on extensive fieldwork and comprehensive command of literature, a penetrating analysis of how the hospital system, use of rhetoric, and treatment-oriented, reimbursement criteria organize and manipulate the process and timing of dying and frame family decision-making. Extensive notes and bibliography.

David Wendell Moller. *On Death Without Dignity: The Human Impact of Technical Dying. Perspectives on Death and Dying Series,* Richard A. Kalish, series editor. Amityville: Baywood Publishing Company, 1990.
> A thoughtful examination of medical-technological manipulation of the dying process, physician difficulties with death, and social isolation of the dying. Many references.

Sherwin B. Nuland. *How We Die: Reflections on LIfe's Final Chapter.* New York: Alfred A. Knopf, 1994.
> Nuland, a teacher of surgery and the history of medicine at Yale, spells out for the lay person the biological and clinical realities of several terminal illnesses.

Hospice, Palliative Care, and End-of-Life Care

Institute of Medicine. *Approaching Death: Improving Care at the End of Life.* Washington: National Academy Press, 1997.
> Panel of experts tried to distinguish and limit futile treatment, better understand physical and emotional symptoms in life-threatening disease, and design health care (including pain management) to match end-of-life needs.

Bruce Jennings, True Rynes, Carol D'Onofrio, and Mary Ann Baily. *Access to Hospice Care: Expanding Boundaries, Overcoming Barriers.* Hastings Center Report Special Supplement 33, no. 2, pp. S3-S59, 2003.   www.thehastingscenter.org 1-845-424-4040.

Based on multi-disciplinary deliberations among experts in hospice, palliative care, and end-of-life care, a comprehensive framing article is augmented by short essays on increasing access to hospice care and creating new and expanded models of hospice.

Bruce Jennings, Gregory E. Kaebnick, and Thomas H. Murray, editors. *Improving End of Life Care: Why has it been so Difficult?* Hastings Center Report Special Report 35, no. 6, 2005.

Short essays by diverse professionals (bioethicists, geriatricians, legal scholars, etc.) assessing flaws in approaches to end-of-life-care reform since the mid-1970s, gains made, threats to their ongoing viability, and new initiatives.

Marcia Lattanzi-Licht with John J. Mahoney and Galen W. Miller. *The Hospice Choice: in Pursuit of a Peaceful Death.* New York: Simon & Schuster, 1998.

A hospice pioneer and educator worked with leaders of the National Hospice Organization to create a practical, warmly-written resource on the workings of hospice. Intended for families, each chapter uses a story to lead into a set of issues. Notes, Q&A, resources.

Shirley Ann Smith. *Hospice Concepts: a Guide to Palliative Care in Terminal Illness.* Champaign Illinois: Research Press, 2000.

Drawing on her experience as a nurse, hospice director, bereavement counselor, lecturer, and researcher, Smith provides a "succinct, yet comprehensive, overview" of elements of hospice care to orient hospice team members as well as families. Written for ease of reference on specific topics.

See also:
Hospice Foundation of America   www.hospicefoundation.org
National Hospice and Palliative Care Organization   www.nhpco.org

Psycho-Spiritual Possibilities and Relationship Completion through Dying

Sandra L. Bertman. *Facing Death: Images, Insights, and Intervention.* New York and London: Brunner-Routledge, 1991.

A highly honored innovator and pioneer in bringing the arts and humanities into death education has created a book filled with images—and diverse audiences' and students' reactions to them—from her double-slide presentations to assist death educators, frontline professionals, the dying, and their families.

Ira Byock. *Dying Well: the Prospect for Growth at the End of Life.* New York: Riverhead Books, 1997.

Loosely woven around Dr. Byock's gradually deepening understanding about how to create openings through well-timed questions with dying patients whose resistance to dealing with unfinished business was hindering their completing important relationships.

Ira Byock. *The Four Things that Matter Most: a Book about Living.* New York: Free Press, 2004.

Byock, an activist physician-champion for palliative care (see www.dyingwell.com), has distilled his experience into eleven words.

Maggie Callanan and Patricia Kelley. *Final Gifts: Understanding the Special Awareness, Needs, and Communications of the Dying.* New York: Bantam Books, 1992/1997.
Two experienced and gifted nurses explore "nearing death awareness" through warmly told stories which decipher dying patients' symbolic language about what they are experiencing or needing for completion—language often missed or ignored by family and providers. Invitingly and accessibly written. Annotated reading suggestions.

Marie de Hennezal, *Intimate Death: How the Dying Teach Us How to Live.* Translated by Carol Brown Janeway. New York: Alfred A. Knopf, 1997.
Beautifully written, translated, and produced book by a psychologist in a French palliative care unit who brings compassionate presence and witnessing to dying patients whose stories thread through the book. Foreward by François Mitterand is stunningly poetic.

Joanne Lynn and Joan Harrold, et al. *Handbook for Mortals: Guidance for People Facing Serious Illness.* New York: Oxford University Press, 1999.
Synthesizes the experience, knowledge, and collaboration of a numerous professionals into a single, graceful voice. Practical advice on making decisions, controlling pain, foregoing treatment, getting what is needed from doctors, and facilitating meaningful and honest conversations between the dying and loved ones. Topic-related resources.

Family Caregiving

Claire Berman. *Caring for Yourself While Caring for Your Aging Parents: How to Help, How to Survive.* New York: Henry Holt and Company, 1996.
Emapthically explores the emotions of caregivers, a range of issues (siblings, long distance, being the only child) and the line between dedication and martyrdom.

Kenneth J. Doka and Joyce D. Davidson, editors. *Caregiving and Loss: Family Needs, Professional Responsibilities.* Washington, DC: Hospice Foundation of America, 2001.
Designed for professionals who support and advocate for family caregivers, this book is also a fine and accessible introduction to the issues for anyone by several luminaries in the field.

Kenneth J. Doka, editor, with Joyce Davidson. *Living with Grief When Illness is Prolonged.* Washington, DC: Hospice Foundation of America, 1997.
Another book from HFA's annual bereavement teleconference to educate hospice workers, volunteers, and others through accessible articles by leading professionals.

Nancy L. Mace and Peter V. Rabins. *The 36-Hour Day: A Family Guide to Caring for Persons with Alzheimer Disease, Related Dementing Illnesses, and Memory Loss in Later Life.* Johns Hopkins Press, 1981/1999.
A classic which warmly and empathically affirms the frustrations of caregivers while providing an excellent compendium of advice on a full spectrum of medical, practical, behavioral, and self-care issues while demystifying "dementia."

Virginia Morris. *How to Care for Aging Parents.* New York: Workman Publishing, 1996/2004.
Comprehensive, easy-to-read and easy-to-use caregiver's bible for the full spectrum of medical, financial, housing, legal, familial, and other practical issues, with an extensive yellow pages of resources. Thoroughly researched by a healthcare journalist whose style is compassionate, forthright, and wise.

Andrea Sankar, *Dying at Home: A Family Guide to Caregiving.* Baltimore and London: Johns Hopkins University Press, 1991/1999.

An empathic ethnographic account of the challenges, stresses, and issues experienced by caregivers of people who are actively dying. Practical advice on how to manage hospitals, support services, strangers in the house, intra-family conflict, informal support networks. Excellent appendices on the medical and physical tasks and problems of caring for people in the last months, weeks, and days of their life.

See also:
Family Caregiver Alliance   www.caregiver.org
National Alliance for Caregivig   www.caregiving.org
National Family Caregivers Association   www.nfcacares.org
Rosalynn Carter Institute   www.rosalynncarter.org
American Association of Retired Persons   www.aarp.org

Healthcare System Safety, Quality, and Redesign

Institute of Medicine. *To Err is Human: Building a Safer Health System.* Linda T. Kohn, Janet M. Corrigan, and Molly S. Donaldson, ed. Washington: National Academy Press, 1999. www.nap.edu, 1-800-624-6242.

This study's revelations about the magnitude of often deadly, preventable hospital errors and infections rocked the medical world and raised the profile on safety.

Institute of Medicine. *Crossing the Quality Chasm: a New Health System for the 21st Century.* Linda T. Kohn, Janet M. Corrigan, and Molla S. Davidson, editors. Washington: National Academy Press, 2001.

This second and final report by the Committee on the Quality of Health Care in America offers principles and guidance for redesigning the healthcare system around six aims: patient-centeredness, safety, effectiveness, timeliness, efficiency, and equitability.

See also:
Pittsburgh Regional Healthcare Initiative   www.prhi.org
Institute for Healthcare Improvement   www.ihi.org
Robert Wood Johnson Foundation   www.rwjf.org
Picker Institute   www.pickerinstitute.org
Commonwealth Fund   www.cmwf.org

Acknowledgments

During the months after my mother died, I knew the telling of this story would begin with The Call. The day after Christmas, I was suddenly able—and needed—to start writing. When I had drafted a few chapters and introductory material, I wondered if anyone was going to want to read this account of a dying woman and her daughter. My first inkling that yes, I should continue writing, came from an unusually late evening phone call from Linda Clarke. Riding in a car and reading chapters by streetlight and flashlight because she could not put them down, she had had to let me know immediately that she was mesmerized by Olwen, our story, and my writing.

Several early readers—Sue, Mary Jane, and Mary Wirth—affirmed my reconstruction of the story and its emotional and relational veracity based on their deep and/or long knowledge of Olwen and our relationship. They wanted to get to Olwen's story sooner, however; the preface and introduction were in their way. I began pulling material from the front to the back, eventually developing part V from those embryonic and initially mislocated ideas. A new introduction later emerged in tandem with my increasing clarity about why I was writing this book, for whom, how to position it, and how I wanted to guide reader expectations.

Later on, I asked my cousin Michael to read and vet the manuscript, giving particular attention to the years before and after I was born—years during which he, considerably older than I, was part of my natal household. To my surprised delight, he, a discerning and critical reader, found my writing "superb." Our conversations reaffirmed dynamics and patterns from those times, resurfaced moments we hadn't recalled in years, and triggered his remembering other incidents. He wondered, however, as a couple of others had, if I were not idealizing Olwen? No, the difficulties—hers, mine, ours—are right there. What has intervened is our transformative journey which catapulted me into the After, from which I cannot get myself back to the ever-ambivalent Before. In the

Before, "I spake as a child," but now I see Olwen "through a glass," *clearly*, and "face to face" (1 Cor. 13:11-12).

When I had drafted chapters 1-14, and part V was still enfolded into a dense, single chapter, I asked several people who are psycho-spiritually gifted and have rich language for interior life to read the book critically: Lynn Roberson, Eurydice Hirsey, Lindsa Vallee, and Sharon Bauer. I asked them to evaluate things like: Is this scene, passage, or incident essential to the story? Why? How do I round off this too-sharp edge? Where do you get bogged down? What feels redundant? What does the reader need to know about the daughter that supports rather than intrudes into the story?

We interrogated these and other issues in depth, to the great benefit of this book. Our conversations were nourishing on many levels. For example, as we were exploring what the introduction should be, Lynn suggested thinking about it as an antechamber where one prepares before entering ritual space and welcomes the reader into an intimate journey. These women began to give me language for talking *about* the book and articulating its value because they saw into it so deeply, yet through eyes other than my own.

During this time, I was also grappling with how to end the book and bring the reader to closure. Clearly, the author must take the reader forward from the deathbed, but how far? The answer seemed inseparable from knowing *whose* story must be concluded. Olwen's certainly—in which case, the first two pages of chapter 14, then called epilogue, could suffice. We need a bit more, however, if I pull the story forward into new reflections about Olwen and our relationship emerging after her death. But if the book is also about the daughter's reconstitution of meaning and identity—a process which some grief educators as well as myself believe is the core of our inner work following the death(s) of our parent(s)—then it should complete that part of my story as well. All four of these women noted above, along with Sidney Abbott and a panel of women who had written about illness and death, said the same thing: The book has to be about *your* story, too. Readers want to know how you come out of your passage and are changed by it.

Reconstituting one's identity and place becomes even more salient when we have lost both parents (especially when those losses occur close together), are only children, and/or do not have children ourselves—all of which apply in my case. It is not surprising that I found myself overwhelmingly pulled to return to the "old country" and reconstruct whatever I could of my ancestral history. Never envisioned at the outset, chapters 15 and 16 emerged from sorting out my ancestral research and finding an unexpectedly deep connection with my roots and my lineage. The question of how to complete *my* story thereby emerged organically.

My cousins Robin, Emrys, Gwen, Gwenan, and Eric provided stories, photographs, documents, press clippings, and other bits. Robin generously compiled, copied, and organized written materials about my grandfather, transported me (I was on foot during the second trip) from the airport to a remote village, and made it possible to visit again with Emrys, his dear father. Emrys and Olwen had corresponded for years, and, at 92, while caregiving his failing wife during my first trip, he had gone out and copied a photograph of my grandfather's mother—my only photograph of her. On my grandmother's side, Gwen is the primary inheritor of family stories which she has shared with our cousin Eric and myself, and the three of us have had conversations with one another about our speculations, our questions, and what we think we know. Despite their greater proximity, they, too, feel they know little about our family, and my research findings were as new for them as they were for me. Gwenan drove me around the Welsh countryside, drawing on a faint memory to locate the grave of our great-great-grandfather in a tiny village cemetery as well as the farm location where his two sons, including my mother's grandfather, Robert, grew up.

Clerks in several North Wales records offices and registries were patient, and several went out of their way to be helpful. Farmers and local history enthusiasts helped to fill in the context of my great-grandparents' lives. Falcon Hildred was generous with his hospitality, transportation assistance, and my nascent explorations of industrial archaeology. Slate historian Griff Richard Jones made visually and physically vivid the process of quarrying slate in underground chambers. Industrial archaeologist-historian David Gwyn brought his extensive knowledge to bear on my specific questions, such as when certain towns became connected by railway links. Historian R. Merfyn Jones, now a university vice-chancellor, suggested I contact David. Nesta became my primary informant in Pen-y-Dyffryn. She clarified puzzles about family houses, and took me to visit Mrs. Parry, possibly the last person alive who can clearly remember Olwen's grandmother, Anne.

Because it is extra work for readers to track names of people who make only a brief or occasional appearance, I have not named people who do not figure repeatedly in the story. It is more useful for you to know the *roles* of peripheral people (night nurses, on-call nurse, hospital social worker) than have another name to absorb. Similarly, I have pulled back the scattered references to friends who provided critical support at key moments but are not characters in Olwen's drama. A dozen or so friends were "regulars" in this process, and form a Greek chorus surrounding and supporting our story.

Editing my own work seemed to have reached its limit after I had pared about 25 percent of the book. I consulted with Kathleen Spivack, a highly-regarded writing coach, about how I might further compress or revise the book, especially certain challenging passages. To my surprise, she did not say "cut," but, in her perusal, spotted places where she wanted to see a little more. We explored tenses and what Kathleen calls "pentimento layers" of the past, and she observed that books written in the present tense and/or with a first-person narrator tend to be flat. Through our conversation, I began to form a conscious, editorial rationale for what I had done intuitively: as the main storyline moved inexorably toward death, it needed the counterpoint movement into progressively deeper backstory to impart the magnitude of their ultimate convergence. Kathleen was certain I could tackle the main problem—overwriting—myself, and, as a by-product, achieve my goal of cutting another 12,000 words. She was right.

Still, I sought and found editorial input. I knew that part V, which is written in a more didactic voice, could use a little polishing, and Terry Hiller helped me on that account. Through Melissa Rosati who coached me on the labyrinth of distribution issues, I found Anya Achtenberg who lived up to her website endorsements: seeing to the heart of complex issues, saying more with less, and knowing how to give feedback in ways an author can hear. I gave Anya only the most challenging material—problematic passages out of context, and key backstory chapters. Her keen eye for issues of voice and our rich conversations gave me a new though hardly perfect alertness to word choices that "pull you out of the story," and to paragraphs that go past themselves and fall apart.

Through Melissa, I also found my literary attorney, Sheila Levine, who read the entire manuscript from the perspective of legal vetting, and has been most generous with her time and commitment to me and this book. I found Melissa, in turn, through Hannelore Hahn, who founded the International Women's Writing Guild thirty years ago. Although my work has demanded for decades that I write, my understanding of the art of writing escalated to a new level through my exposure to outstanding faculty and students attending the Guild's 2006 conference at Skidmore College. I was encouraged when a workshop leader and attendees became so absorbed in my reading that they forgot to call the time limit.

Pre-production had its crises when the cover designer could not execute my cover concept, let alone take it to another level, while the interior designer backed away from a collaborative mode of working; I lost several weeks, and the clock was ticking. Five people—Gail Bryan, Annette Robichaud, Lynn Roberson, Lindsa Vallee, and Sharon Bauer—made time to meet with me within a twenty-four hour period. We explored and critiqued design possibilities and the ever-morphing title and subtitle. Only two things were still certain: the front cover would use a photograph Mary Wirth took of my mother's and my hands a few days before Olwen died, and the back cover would use a photograph of us from long ago. Everyone who had viewed my collage of Olwen's life had immediately gravitated to this picture of us.

Gail called a colleague, Maureen Roche, whom she knew had the artistic imagination and skills to make the cover soar—*if* she was willing to take on this project. Maureen's ability to capture the complex soul of the book in visual form was breathtaking. A conventional route might have been hushed tones and pastels—as if the spiritual dimensions of dying were antiseptic, ethereal vapors. Maureen did the unexpected—which is, of course, what I had hoped for. Her complex visual metaphor binds the spiritual journey to the physical, the raw, the intimate—the essence of my story. Death rips through all the layers, separating the living from the dying, the quick from the dead. Yet by ripping away the illusions, the veils, the layers, it can bind the living and the dying on a primal level which can never be torn asunder.

Maureen also attuned immediately to the ancestral backstory, and wanted to work with the original prints. Her scanning and digitally retouching so many fading photographic treasures was a great gift, and working together on the collages was a delight.

My first conversation with Alvart Badalian, president of Arrow Graphics, told me I had found the right graphics firm to translate my manuscript into a book. Her knowledge of the business and commitment to excellence shown through everything she said. Given the precision of Alvart's questions and the thoroughness of our handoff discussion, it was no surprise when her partner's design and layout conveyed the elegant simplicity and gracefulness I sought, and the proofs came back in such good shape even though we were working on an expedited path. Alvart graciously but firmly kept us on track, listened and translated exceedingly well, and Aramais tailored his design of epigraphs and elements for their size and sensibility while designing the book as a seamless whole.

In the chaos of having had no designers, my nagging dissatisfaction with two years of title and subtitle variants had imploded. Eight years after the concept of the "dance of death" first came to me during another dying process, I gave up my attachment to it as the title of the book. Here I was, about to go press, and I had no title! Knowing the answer I was seeking lay within the story, I skimmed chapters while scribbling words in a stream of consciousness, went to bed at a weird hour, and woke up with the title that, finally, simply, and elegantly captured the outcome of our dance.

Now, the subtitle had to change, and include "mother" and "dance." My roving "focus group" members all seemed to be coming up with "mother and daughter" as part of the subtitle, as was I. Lindsa suggested ellipses between its two parts, which was perfect. On the way back from meeting with Maureen, Gail popped out with, "a healing dance." Lynn e-mailed back: "'a dance of healing' keeps the feeling of flow and grace." Yes! Finally, the title and subtitle *are* the story we lived and that I am telling.

So, with the help of my village, my journey with Olwen and the ancestors enters the wider world.

About the Author

Artemis March, PhD, MBA, has been evolving her own brand of narrative non-fiction for the past twenty years without realizing it was preparing her to write this book. A sociologist by training, she first got into the storytelling business at the Harvard Business School where she designed case studies for students and executives. Her research consulting practice has migrated toward fostering fundamental change in healthcare safety and quality from the standpoint of the patient. A signature uniting her work is the discernment of structural simplicity and story underlying complexity and chaos. (www.artemismarch.com)

Reader Commentary about *Dying into Grace*

"An extraordinarily valuable book. I wish I had had it. I wish [my mother's caregiver] had had it. I wish the nurses at the hospital had had it."

—**Gail Bryan,** artist and writer

"I have never read a book that was so poignant, deep, nuanced, and able to hold so many dimensions: the historical and the present, the individual and the system, the practical and the spiritual, the tough and the tender, the ordinary and the extraordinary. The story is deceptively simple yet so powerful—it took my breath away ... *Dying into Grace* invites us into a profound journey that gives us a relational model for dying well."

—**Lynn Roberson,** psychotherapist and Reiki practitioner

"Artemis March is inviting us into a new paradigm—death as a dance with our dying parent in which we must follow, yet anticipate how she will lead. We must listen with our whole body, beyond and through the words, and be willing to move with whatever is happening ... She shows us how to notice and capture and string on a necklace many tiny treasures that may otherwise seem small and mundane and not part of the sacred, but it is all those little contributions from many people that allows dying to become a dance, and freed Olwen to open spiritually. I would love for this book to be read by my family and loved ones, with the hope that someday, when my time comes, they might 'dance' with me."

—**Lindsa Vallee,** psychotherapist

"I couldn't put this book down. It is so primal and personal. If I had had it before my mother died, it would have helped me. It captures everything I went through and couldn't articulate because it was below the surface. What a great gift to our generation! Artemis March is exploring death at so many levels. She is showing us how the dying person can be an active participant in their own process, and helping us find ways to engage more spiritually with our dying parents so that we can help them to die well."

—**Dr. Eurydice Hirsey,** chiropractor and cranial-sacral therapist

"This book is riveting. I could not put it down. It renders with such care and compassion the author's dying mother. Artemis March has managed to recede her own brilliance so as not to outshine the fading light of her mother. Hardly anyone pays close attention to such a small light, but the reader gradually discovers the essence of an elegant and earnest soul trying to master the terrifying and bewildering process of dying. Olwen carries into her dying her great sense of responsibility, of following through, of doing things the right way so that she can leave her body with the dignity that befits her inner being."

—**Dr. Linda J. Clarke,** author of *On a Planet Sailing West*

"*Dying into Grace* is extremely rich. I have taken away many insights as I engage with my own mother's long descent into death. This is a book not only for daughters but also for aging mothers and the conversations they might have. When Olwen says something important, no matter in what form or syntax, her daughter does not dismiss her, but is really paying attention. Like a gifted psychologist who listens for underlying coherence and meaning, Artemis is teaching us to 'listen through' unconventional speech, apparent randomness, and surface confusion ... This is quite a miraculous and hopeful story. It tells about the last months as having the potential to heal the deepest wounds of a lifetime. As we gradually learn what underlies the life Olwen created for herself while also forming the patterns of self-denial that now threaten to sabotage the best efforts and best hopes of mother and daughter, we see a depth of change and opening that was not previously possible, and are all the more able to appreciate the enormous breakthroughs and transformation during Olwen's final days of dying."

—**Sharon Bauer,** psychotherapist

"Through the immediacy of a riveting story and models she draws from it, Artemis March has captured the complex essence of family caregiving. A wealth of clinical and psychological insight arises seamlessly from a story that reads like a novel, yet challenges professionals and families to bring thmselves fully to the moment, and with greater awearenes of how they contribute to situations they see as independent of themselves. Profound yet practical, this book is essential for anyone involved with end-of-life care."

—**Sandra Bertman,** PhD, Director, Medical Humanities and the Arts Program, Boston College; pioneer in death education for healthcare professionals

"Artemis March asks and answers an essential question: how can we enhance the possibilities for mutual growth and healing as a parent moves closer to death? Her book shows us that the mother-daughter relationship can be transformed even at the very end of life, affirming the possibility for transformational movement throughout the lifespan. This book will help to empower caregivers in a culture that too often denies and avoids the process of dying. And it will be useful to therapists who are working with clients who are engaged in this process."

—**Judith V. Jordan,** PhD, Director, Jean Baker Miller Training Institute, Wellesley College; co-creator/developer of Relational Psychology

"Artemis March has a special gift. She is able to tell a very personal and intimate story, that of a daughter accompanying a parent during the last phases of life into death, in a way that is like being engaged in a conversation with a sage. She is a source of incredible understanding for a phase of life we all experience. Dr. March invites us to a table where we can have a real conversation about death and dying. She gives us the words and a framework to navigate a territory from which we have been isolated and about which we have been silenced, yet yearn to speak . . . This book is simply extraordinary. If healthcare professionals understood and applied her insights and wisdom, it would be a huge step towards achieving a healthcare system that is truly patient-centered."

—**Anne-Marie Audet,** MD, MSc, Fellow, American College of Physicians; Fellow, New York Academy of Medicine; policy change agent for healthcare quality improvement and patient-centered care